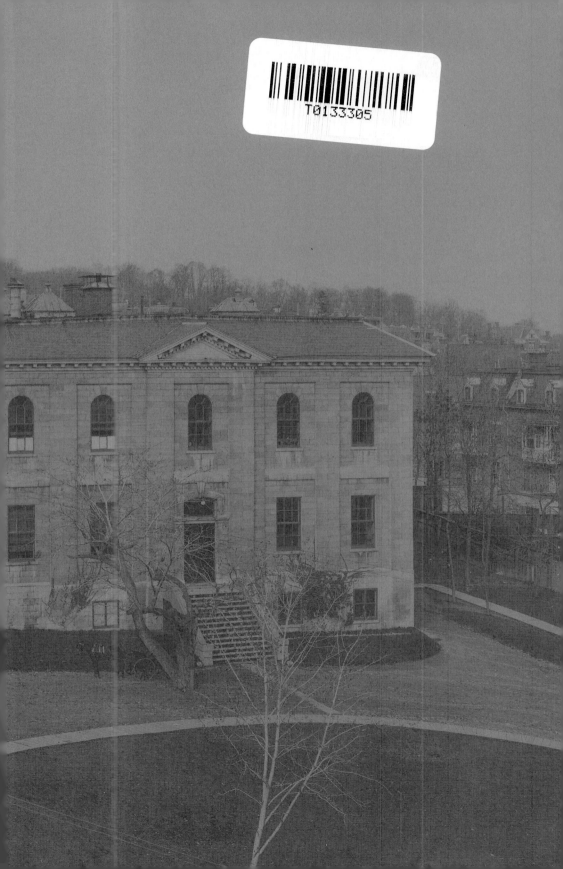

McGill Medicine
Volume 2
1885–1936

McGill Medicine

Volume 2
1885–1936

JOSEPH HANAWAY

RICHARD CRUESS

JAMES DARRAGH

McGill-Queen's University Press
Montreal & Kingston · London · Ithaca

© McGill-Queen's University Press 2006
ISBN 0-7735-2958-6

Legal deposit first quarter 2006
Bibliothèque nationale du Québec

Printed in Canada on acid-free paper that is 100% ancient forest
free (100% post-consumer recycled), processed chlorine free

This book has been published with the help grants from
Associated Medical Services Inc. and the Office of the Dean,
Faculty of Medicine, McGill University.

McGill-Queen's University Press acknowledges the support of the
Canada Council for the Arts for our publishing program. We also
acknowledge the financial support of the Government of Canada
through the Book Publishing Industry Development Program
(BPIDP) for our publishing activities.

Library and Archives Canada Cataloguing in Publication

Hanaway, Joseph, 1933–
McGill medicine / Joseph Hanaway, Richard Cruess.

Vol. 2 by Joseph Hanaway, Richard Cruess, James Darragh.
Includes bibliographical references and index.
Contents: v. 1. The first half-century, 1829–1885. – v. 2.
1885–1936.
ISBN 0-7735-1324-8 (v. 1).– ISBN 0-7735-2958-6 (v. 2)

1. McGill University. Faculty of Medicine–History.
I. Cruess, Richard L. II. Darragh, James, 1924– III. Title.

R749.M34H35 1996   610'.71'171428   C95-920944-1

End papers: Front, Medical Building, 1894
Back, Medical Building, 1911

This book was designed and typeset by studio oneonone
in Sabon 10/12.5

Contents

Illustrations

Abbreviations

AMA American Medical Association
CAMC Canadian Army Medical Corps
Can Med Surg Canada Medical and Surgical Journal
Canad J Surg Canadian Journal of Surgery
CB Companion of the Order of the Bath
CM Member of the Order of Canada
CMA Canadian Medical Association
CMAJ Canadian Medical Association Journal
CMG Companion of the Order of St Michael and St George
CMH Children's Memorial Hospital (later Montreal
   Children's Hospital)
COTC Canadian Officers' Training Corps
*Dtsch Med Wochenschr Deutsche Medizinische
   Wochenschrift*
FRCP Fellow of the Royal College of Physicians
FRCS Fellow of the Royal College of Surgeons
J Hist Med Journal of the History of Medicine
JAMA *Journal of the American Medical Association*
LMCC Licentiate of the Medical Council of Canada
LRCP Licentiate of the Royal College of Physicians
M B Gov Minutes, Board of Governors of McGill University
M Fac Med Minutes, Faculty of Medicine (McGill)
MCH Montreal Children's Hospital
McM McCord Museum

Med-Chi Montreal Medico-Chirurgical Society
MGH   Montreal General Hospital
MNI   Montreal Neurological Institute
MQUP   McGill-Queen's University Press
MUA   McGill University Archives
MUL   McGill University Library
NA   Notman Photographic Archives, McCord Museum
   of Canadian History
OBE   Officer of the Order of the British Empire
OL   Osler Library
RCPSC   Royal College of Physicians and Surgeons
   of Canada
RF   Rockefeller Foundation
RVH   Royal Victoria Hospital
SMB   Strathcona Medical Building

Acknowledgments

We would like to praise and thank the staff of the McGill University Archives – Joanne Pelletier, Gordon Burr, and previous staff Jane Kingslin, Rob Michal, and Phebe Chartrand – for help in completing the first century of the history of the McGill Faculty of Medicine. The staff of the Osler Library, the present Osler librarian, Pam Miller, former director June Schachter, and former assistant director Wayne LeBel have continued to help, along with the able assistance of Lily Szczygiel and Mary Simon.

Our history could not have been completed without the help of the staff of the Notman Photographic Archives in the McCord Museum. Special thanks to our friends Tom Humphry (retired photographer), Nora Hague, and Heather McNab, who over the years have helped in many ways. Brenda Klinkow (retired) and Susanne Morin made valiant attempts to find special pictures. Special thanks to an old friend, Roy McGregor, retired professor of geology, St Andrew's University, Scotland, who found and explained Lainchoil, the name of the gift of $50,000 that Donald Smith gave to the Faculty of Medicine in 1883.

Special thanks are due to Richard Bachand from McGill's Department of Geology for a splendid rendition of the map of Roddick's movements during the 1885 Riel Rebellion. Others to whom we owe special thanks are: Frances Groen, director of the McGill University Libraries, for her support; Kendall Wallis, for his unfailing enthusiasm and expertise as a reference librarian; and Martin Entin, author of a biography of Edward W. Archibald, for supplying valuable information about Archibald and the C.F. Martin years. Dean Abraham Fuks has been an enthusiastic supporter of this project and has an abiding interest in the history of medicine. William Feindel, honorary Osler librarian, has asked probing questions that have helped. We are grateful to Sean Murphy, retired chairman of ophthalmology at McGill and Frank Buller's grandson, who allowed us to use a portion of his unpublished history of ophthalmology at McGill. We thank James Baxter who let us use his *History of Otolaryngology in Canada* as a reference for the section on his specialty. He was chairman of his department. Robert Fortuine and Donald MacIntosh, both knowledgeable scholars and McGill graduates, read the manuscript and provided detailed reviews and invaluable editing services for the authors.

Hyman Casselman, M.D., C.M. 1927, one of McGill's oldest medical graduates, was helpful in answering questions about his experiences at McGill. He died at ninety-eight in 1998.

Faye Mills typed early sections of the manuscript. Marcia Sweet helped with chapter 1 of volume 2. Special thanks go to Paul and Carol Mills, whose computer expertise was invaluable for the early manuscript; to Phil Cercone, director of the McGill-Queen's University Press, who supported our project from the beginning; to Joan McGilvray, our favourite editor, who can laugh while reading and editing this kind of work; to Alan and Alice Ryan, who provided relaxed hospitality in Bridgehampton, New York, in the fall of 1997 when the introductory chapters were written; and to Barbara Darragh, who put Joe Hanaway up in her home in Ottawa on numerous occasions while he worked on this project.

Special thanks go also to generous publication grants from the Associated Medical Services of Toronto and Abraham Fuks, dean of the Faculty of Medicine, McGill University.

Introduction

Volume 1 of *McGill Medicine, The First Half Century, 1829–1885*, described the evolution of medical teaching at McGill University. Volume 2 continues the narrative for the second half century ending in 1936, which coincides with the retirement of Charles Ferdinand Martin, the Faculty of Medicine's first full-time dean.

Medical teaching at McGill began on 29 June 1829, but its origins can be traced back to 1801 when the Royal Institution for the Advancement of Learning was established to promote Protestant education in Lower Canada. The Royal Institution languished for ten years until James McGill, who had made a fortune in the fur trade, bequeathed £10,000 and his country estate, Burnside, to found a college bearing his name. His wife's family did not agree with this decision, so when he died in 1813, his bequest was contested by her son, Francis Desrivières, who wanted the money and the estate. This delayed the implementation of James McGill's plans for sixteen years.

While a prolonged battle over the McGill bequest moved through the British law courts at a slug's pace, the War of 1812 with the United States ended in 1815. After the war a flood of immigrants, mainly from the United Kingdom, arrived in Canada. Most of them landed in Quebec or Montreal, often in the late fall. Had they arrived earlier, many would have gone to the countryside to seek work. The severe winter weather, an agricultural slowdown caused by drought, and the predominance of French language in the countryside resulted in many of those unfortunate people remaining in the cities. Their economic situation was precarious, and their plight did not go unnoticed. In 1815 some Montreal citizens began to provide food, shelter, and education for the poor, and later that year the Female Benevolent Society began to coordinate and manage the charitable work. In 1816 and 1817 several doctors joined the cause and offered to treat the sick poor, providing there was an institution in which to do it. The Benevolent Society responded by renting a four-room house in 1818. Thirty-seven people were admitted as patients over a period of months. The success of this endeavour led to leasing a bigger house in 1819, ambitiously called the Montreal General Hospital. Rules and regulations were published dealing with the activities of the hospital.

At the same time a group of civic-minded men made a formal proposal to the Government of Lower Canada for money to build a permanent public hospital in Montreal. Unfortunately religious zeal interfered with this proposal, resulting in a strong and vitriolic objection by a Catholic member of parliament who felt that an expansion of the francophone hospital L'Hotel Dieu would be more appropriate. A challenge resulted in a duel between the parliamentarian O'Sullivan and Dr William Caldwell in which both were wounded, thus ending the debate. Money was raised from private donations, and the cornerstone of the permanent Montreal General Hospital (MGH) was laid with ceremony on 6 June 1821, the hospital's official founding date.

Four doctors who had helped to found the MGH – Caldwell, William Robertson, John Stephenson, and Andrew Holmes – decided to start a medical school associated with the hospital, and thus the Montreal Medical Institution (MMI) opened for teaching on 10 November 1823. Henry Loedel, one of the original founders of the MGH and the MMI, resigned before the MMI opened.

Meanwhile the legal problems of the paper university progressed. The Royal Institution was incorporated in 1819 and on 31 March 1821 obtained a charter for McGill College from King George IV. Thus the college was nominally established but it had no statutes, students, or staff. James McGill's will stipulated that a college had to be started within ten years of incorporation – that is, by 1829. By 1824 time was running out, and the governors appointed a faculty of prominent educators to make the college look official.

In 1828 the Privy Council of England found in favour of the McGill bequest, and the Burnside property was claimed by the board of governors of McGill College. Moving as fast as possible to meet the deadline, the governors called a meeting on 24 June 1829 at the Burnside cottage and asked the four teachers of the Montreal Medical Institution if they would accept the offer to be the first teaching faculty of McGill College, which they did. In 1833 William Logie became McGill's first medical graduate and also the first medical graduate in Canada.[1]

Initially the new medical school utilized buildings in the city; it moved to the McGill grounds in 1845 and back to the city in 1851. It was not until 1872 when the Faculty of Medicine moved to a new building on the McGill grounds (the present James Building site) that proper facilities for teaching were available. In 1872 William Osler graduated in medicine from McGill and after two years of study in Europe returned to Montreal full of modern teaching experience. He convinced the faculty that the use of student laboratories where "learning-while-doing" took place was a better way of teaching pre-clinical science than the lecture room. In the 1880s McGill Medical School had student laboratories for anatomy, histology, chemistry, and physiology. However, in spite of the facilities at the Montreal General, clinical education was neglected.

Volume 1 of this history includes lists of the staff of the medical faculty from 1829 to 1885, the graduates in medicine, and the prize winners and medallists, as well as the examinations for M.D., C.M for 1854–55 and biographical sketches of thirty-one professors.

For the second volume a wealth of information is available, including material about the Montreal General and Royal Victoria hospitals, the development of the specialties, the full-time system for pre-clinical and clinical faculty, and research programs. By the turn of the century the classes had enlarged to over one hundred per year so that the names of the graduates are not included in this volume. The Gold Medal winners, the examination papers for the 1900–1901 session, the officers of the faculty, the teaching hospitals and university, and biographical sketches of the thirty-one prominent members of the medical faculty are included. Twenty-six of the professors whose biographical sketches are included in volume 1 continued to play a prominent role after 1885; they are cross-referenced in the present volume.

In the mid and late nineteenth century, few questioned the prevailing belief that exposure of medical students to scientific thought in student laboratories would result in more scientifically oriented medical practitioners. That belief was the result of the exciting discoveries in chemistry, physiology, pharmacology, and bacteriology in Europe, where medical education was state supported and professors could work full time at teaching and research.

When students who had taken postgraduate training in Europe returned to Canada and the United States, they expounded the view that medical education should have a strong scientific orientation. Some

dissenters in the United States felt that training students in sophisticated laboratories did not contribute to their clinical practice of medicine;
however, the former attitude prevailed. Sir William Osler was a good
example of a convert who returned from Europe having had experience
in basic histology and with knowledge that was lacking at McGill.[2]
Abraham Flexner also believed that strong basic science teaching and
laboratory facilities made the best medical schools, and he virtually
neglected details on the integrity of clinical training in any of the medical schools he evaluated.[3] It became apparent after World War I that
clinical excellence did not necessarily result from basic pre-clinical subject knowledge alone but from an equal emphasis on clinical training
of senior medical students. Also, there needed to be a shift in research
emphasis from the medical school to the hospital, from pre-clinical to
clinical science.

No one thought that this was important because there was very little
research on patients in hospitals before World War I – that is, research
in laboratories with facilities close to hospital beds, or with hospital
beds included in the research units. Flexner's glowing report on McGill's
medical facilities and policies in 1910 stressed the quality and quantity
of the laboratories, the extensive medical library, the number of professors, and the faculty's finances. His report neglected to mention anything
about how clinical medicine was taught, whether students were satisfied
with their clinical training, and whether they thought they were prepared to practise medicine on graduation.

The gradual change in pedagogical emphasis to clinical medicine
after the turn of the century paralleled the gradual rise in academic professionalism and the prestige of academic medicine. For several years
McGill professors with private medical practices such as F.J. Shepherd
and A.D. Blackader dominated the faculty with their influence and
income status. But with the arrival of J.C. Meakins at McGill in 1924 as
the first full-time professor of medicine and with his dominant position
in the Faculty of Medicine, the standard of academic professionalism in
clinical subjects was set. In Europe full-time clinical professors were paid
by the government to teach and do research without the need for income
from a private practice. In Canada and the United States the full-time
concept developed because foundation money was available to support
the salary requirements of those members of medical faculties who were
willing to accept full-time positions. This was not accomplished without
disappointment and opposition. At Johns Hopkins, where three of the
four founding professors were in private medical practice, the full-time

program sputtered, and Osler vigorously opposed the idea after he left Hopkins in 1904.[4]

The idea of full-time clinical staff did not surface at McGill until C.F. Martin initiated it at a meeting in 1918 when he was chairman of the Faculty Education Committee. It took six years for the faculty to implement the concept that, just as the basic subjects needed full-time teachers to keep up, so the clinical subjects also needed full-time teachers and researchers to keep abreast of progress. Research as well needed to be clinically oriented and to move into the hospital setting adjacent to the patients on the wards. This was accomplished with a funded unit for research where patients with many different diseases were studied – the McGill-Royal Victoria Hospital University Clinic. This gradual recognition of the need for better clinical education and the need to give equal emphasis to clinical subjects improved with the rise of academic professionalism in medicine to the point where the full-time research-oriented professors eventually gained greater prestige than the once dominant private-practitioner teachers of the past.

McGill Medicine
Volume 2
1885–1936

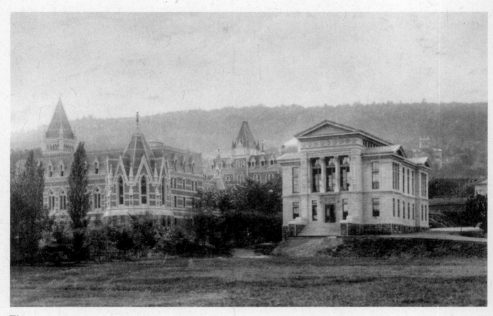

Figure 1
Redpath Museum, 1884. Photo by William Notman, 1884

1 Period of Expansion, 1885–1901

We can only instil principles, put the student on the right path,
give him methods, teach him how to study and only discern
between essentials and non-essentials.
WILLIAM OSLER[1]

THE UNIVERSITY

In 1885 McGill University was on the verge of a period of unprecedented growth in its scientific facilities that would continue until after
1910. By the turn of the century the university had added four science
buildings, a library, an agricultural college, and a women's college; the
Medical Building had been enlarged twice.[2] As the teaching facilities expanded, more students could be accommodated, and the enrolment in
the medical school increased. In 1872 there were 154 students in the
Faculty of Medicine, 232 in 1884, and over 400 by 1900.

The construction and development of scientific facilities on the McGill
grounds began seriously in 1882 when the Redpath Museum (fig. 1)
was completed. Considered a landmark scientific building in a Canadian university,[3] it was prized greatly by Principal Sir William Dawson.[4]
Additional science buildings were built on the east side of the campus
– the Macdonald Physics (1890), Engineering (1893), and Chemistry
(1898) buildings. They were balanced on the west side of the campus
by the Redpath Library (1893). The benefactors who provided funds
for this development were Peter Redpath, who gave the money to construct the museum and the library named for him, John H.R. Molson,
Sir William Macdonald (fig. 2), and Sir Donald Smith (fig. 3). The extraordinary insight and wealth of these men supported the programs
that Principal Dawson suggested to expand the university.[5] In 1883 Sir
Donald Smith gave the medical faculty its first major gift in the name

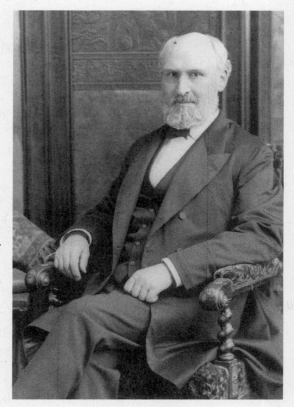

Figure 2
Sir William Christopher
Macdonald, 1831–1917.
Photo by William
Notman, 1890

of the Lainchoil Endowment,[6] stipulating a matching amount from
the public, which was collected in one year under the name of the
George Campbell Fund. This provided the faculty with a little more
than $100,000 for its first endowment fund.

THE FACULTY OF MEDICINE

In response to growing student enrolment and the need for more laboratory space, between 1885 and 1888 the faculty added a wing to
the north of the 1872 Medical Building. Funding for the new addition
came from the recently established endowment fund, because the university did not have money to lend to the faculty for construction. The
plan was to renovate the Medical Building to accommodate an enlarged library, a medical museum, and student laboratories for histology, pharmacology, and gross anatomy, and to construct an addition
with two large lecture theatres and two large, fully equipped labora-

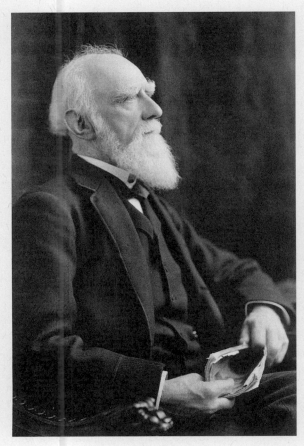

Figure 3
Sir Donald
Alexander Smith
(later Lord
Strathcona and
Mount Royal),
1820–1914.
Photo by William
Notman, 1895

tories for physiology and chemistry.[7] The much-needed addition cost $25,403 and almost doubled the size of the Medical Building. Although the building plan did not seriously challenge the didactic tradition, it did provide greatly enlarged laboratories for students in the pre-clinical subjects.[8] The new laboratories would provide the first exposure to scientific apparatus and experimentation for most medical students. No one questioned the need to introduce them to scientific concepts in the basic disciplines and to provide hands-on exposure. It was thought that gaining some sense of the scientific method in solving simple laboratory problems early in the medical course would introduce future practitioners to solving clinical problems. No one dared challenge this apparently progressive concept until C.F. Martin in 1918 made the first move to upgrade the clinical services to equal the quality of the pre-clinical subjects.

THE CURRICULUM

The curriculum of 1885–86 had changed little in a decade. Most pre-clinical subjects were still repeated in the first and second years of the four-year course. The lectures in chemistry and botany were given at high-school level to bring students up to a uniform standard. By 1890 some of the courses had basic and advanced levels to accommodate the expanding volume of information. The basic course was taught in the first year and the advanced course in the second year.

When Osler departed from McGill in 1884 for Philadelphia, the course that he taught (the institutes of medicine) was abandoned and replaced by separate courses in each of its three components – histology, physiology, and pathology. George Wilkins (fig. 4) taught histology, although he had had no special training in the subject. He gave a lecture/laboratory course two days a week. More important, Wilkins continued Osler's course in practical histology and microscopy along with Wyatt Johnston.[9] In this course students were taught to fix, mount, section, and stain tissues and to examine body fluids, including blood. These techniques and procedures could be of inestimable value for practitioners who would have a microscope in their office but no available clinical laboratories.

T. Wesley Mills[10] taught a lecture and demonstration course in physiology and conducted a two-hour laboratory session on Saturday morning. A McGill graduate and a trained physiologist, he could have requested more time for the physiology course, but the new laboratory wasn't equipped for extensive student use, and by nature he preferred to develop his own career. Mills was a maverick who had scientific skills, but his personality separated him from the students and the rest of the teaching staff.[11]

Wyatt Johnston taught pathology, the third part of the institutes of medicine, to the third-year students. Instruction on materia medica was moved to the second year, but also remained mostly a lecture course. Chemistry was the exception, with a major student laboratory requirement taught at basic and advanced levels. The reason for the emphasis on laboratory work in chemistry and its lack in physiology and materia medica can be ascribed to the professors directing the courses, not to the faculty. Gilbert Girdwood was a sophisticated chemist and scientist. He was a full-time member of faculty and devoted to developing chemistry at McGill and to his own research.[12] In contrast, James Stewart (fig. 5), who taught materia medica, was a practising physician assigned to the job with no particular training in the subject. He went on

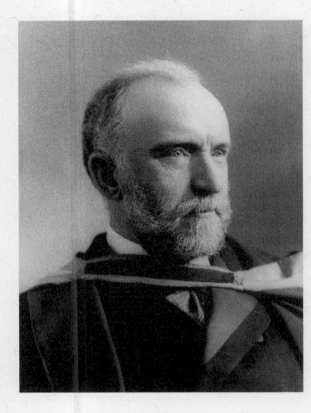

Figure 4
George Wilkins,
1842–1916.
Photo by William
Notman, 1897

to be professor of medicine at McGill and physician-in-chief at the Royal Victoria Hospital after George Ross died in 1892.[13]

By 1885 the optional summer course for the medical students was in its tenth year.[14] It had become a major commitment to supplement and extend the teaching in the regular October to March academic sessions. The students paid a fee of $20 for the course, which consisted of bedside instruction in medicine and surgery and weekly clinics in medicine, surgery, venereal disease, ophthalmology, laryngology, and gynecology and diseases of children, the skin, and the nervous system. Most of the teaching staff participated in the lectures and demonstrations. Stewart, the first person at McGill to develop a special interest in neurological disease,[15] gave the clinics on the nervous system.

In 1894 the academic term was extended from six to nine months, and the elective summer course was discontinued. The faculty made its first commitment to teaching about mental diseases with the appointment in 1895 of T.J.W. Burgess as a lecturer in the subject. He demonstrated patients at the Verdun Asylum.[16] Before this McGill

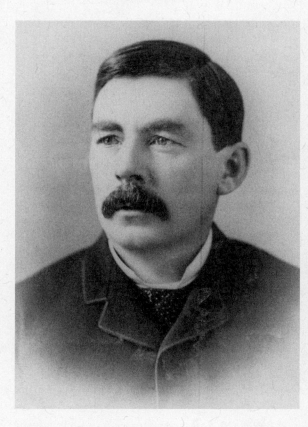

Figure 5
James Stewart,
1846–1906.
Photo by William
Notman, 1885

had not seen the need for the specialties of neurology and mental diseases, which had been established in the United States and Europe. Mental patients were kept in a custodial fashion, with little therapy provided except sedation.

Diseases of infants and children were traditionally part of the obstetrics course. Gynecology was separated from obstetrics in 1883 with the appointment of William Gardner as professor of gynecology.[17] Alexander Blackader, who was a trained pediatrition, held clinics for children's diseases at the general hospital. His interest in pediatrics was in competition with the obstetricians who strongly objected to a separate specialty for children, so he was wise enough not to challenge the system for a department at that time. Despite his position as professor of pharmacology and therapeutics in 1891, and the Faculty of Medicine's reticence to establish a department of pediatrics, Blackader was McGill's first and leading advocate for a separate specialty for children's diseases.

By 1897 Blackader's interest had prevailed. He and James Cameron began a course of student lectures on diseases of infants and children. Both were professors in other subjects.[18] The professors of obstetrics, who had substantial pediatric practices, did not want to give up or lose patients, so they opposed the formation of a McGill department of pediatrics. So influential were these men that a department of diseases of infants and children was not established until 1937 when Harold Cushing, who had practised pediatrics for more than two decades, was appointed McGill professor and chairman of pediatrics.[19]

To graduate M.D., C.M in 1900 required considerable effort. A candidate had to attend four nine-month sessions at the McGill medical faculty. Transfer students from other medical schools had to spend at least one academic year (usually more) at McGill and pass the final examinations in order to get a McGill medical degree. For McGill students, there had been little change in the requirements over the previous twenty years – two years of anatomy, physiology, chemistry, and pharmacology; the courses on the theory of medicine, surgery, obstetrics, and gynecology; and instruction in clinical medicine and surgery on the hospital wards. One year only was required for medical jurisprudence, histology, pathology, practical chemistry, public health, bacteriology, mental disease, ophthalmology and otolaryngology, biology, pathologic anatomy, pediatrics, and medical and surgical anatomy. In addition to cards verifying completion of those courses, students had to have cards signed for twenty-four months of hospital attendance, divided between medicine, surgery, and obstetrics and gynecology. They had to work up and record ten medical and six obstetrical cases, dispense medicine for three months in the hospital pharmacy, give twenty vaccinations, and attend six post-mortems. In addition, as had been the tradition for many years, graduating students had to submit notarized statements that they were over twenty-one years of age and swear an oath of morality in Latin, the *sponsio academica*.[20]

THE DOUBLE COURSE

On 1 February 1902 the faculty executive appointed a committee to confer with the Faculty of Arts and the Faculty of Applied Science regarding a proposal to establish a six-year double course for the B.A. or B.S.C. and the M.D., C.M. degrees. The Faculty of Medicine approved such a course on 22 March 1902. Students would enter McGill having completed the senior matriculation examinations and register in the Faculty of Arts or the Faculty of Applied Science. After two years they

would automatically enter the medical faculty and be awarded B.A. or
B.S.C. after the second year and M.D., C.M. after completing the four-
year course. Only a few students with outstanding ability, however, registered for the double course.[21]

THE POSTGRADUATE COURSES

The demise of the undergraduate summer course in 1894 coincided
with a new interest in advanced education for medical graduates. Practitioners who wanted to keep up with advances in medicine welcomed
this new initiative. In 1896 the faculty sponsored the first postgraduate courses at the Montreal General and the Royal Victoria hospitals.[22]
At the RVH there were short practical clinical sessions for physicians
in general practice consisting of advances in medicine, surgery, and pathology. The sessions at the MGH were devoted to clinical experience in
the specialties of ophthalmology, gynecology, and laryngology. In addition, a diploma course in public health was instituted in 1899. The
candidates had to be medical graduates and had to have spent a year
in the field, on the hospital wards, and in the laboratory to qualify for
the diploma.[23]

PATHOLOGY AND THE MEDICAL MUSEUM

Another serious need in the 1890s was for a faculty chair in pathology.
The faculty had insufficient funds, so Sir Donald Smith was approached
for support. In 1893 he donated $100,000 to endow chairs in patholo-
gy and hygiene.[24] The Strathcona Chair of Pathology was filled the
same year by thirty-year-old John George Adami (fig. 6) from Cambridge. Adami was trained in research but did not have extensive experience in pathology. With his energy and enthusiasm he soon became
a university pathologist. He developed a department for teaching and
research and wrote a two-volume textbook of general pathology published in 1908 and 1909 (fig. 7).[25] This was the second medical textbook
to originate from McGill.[26] The pathology department in 1893–94
was in the north-east end of the Medical Building where Adami had a
small office and laboratory. Autopsies were performed in the hospitals
– the Montreal General and the Royal Victoria (after 1894) – where
gross material was prepared for tissue presentations and for the weekly
clinico-pathology conferences on Saturday mornings. Adami, as McGill's
professor of pathology, taught the student course. He was pathologist to
the Royal Victoria, but there was a controversy at the Montreal General,

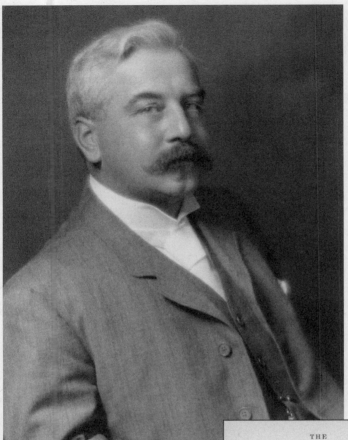

Figure 6
John George Adami, 1862–1926.
Photo by William Notman, 1908

Figure 7
Title page of *Principles of
Pathology*, volume 1, by John
George Adami, 1908. Volume 2
was published in 1909. Copy
in the Osler Library

THE

PRINCIPLES OF PATHOLOGY

BY

J. GEORGE ADAMI, M.A., M.D., LL.D., F.R.S.
PROFESSOR OF PATHOLOGY IN McGILL UNIVERSITY, AND PATHOLOGIST TO THE ROYAL VICTORIA HOSPITAL,
MONTREAL; LATE FELLOW OF JESUS COLLEGE, CAMBRIDGE, ENGLAND

VOLUME I
GENERAL PATHOLOGY

WITH 322 ENGRAVINGS AND 15 PLATES

PHILADELPHIA AND NEW YORK
LEA & FEBIGER

which insisted on appointing its own pathologist and giving Adami the title of advisory pathologist.[27]

The Medical Museum was an adjunct to the teaching facilities in pathology unique to the times (fig. 8). The concept of the museum originated in Europe when there were few illustrated texts to depict the interesting anatomical and pathological specimens found in dissections and post-mortems. A medical museum was considered an important feature in all well-developed medical schools in Europe and North America. Although a room was devoted to the McGill Medical Museum from the beginning of the faculty, it was limited to a professors' collection of interesting specimens over the years without a definite purpose. Physicians in Canada had little experience in assessing internal disease on examination prior to the 1850s.[28] Andrew Fernando Holmes reported his use of the stethoscope at McGill in 1850.[29] Despite Laënnec's great work of 1819,[30] anglophone Canadian physicians seldom went to France and were slow to accept the use of the stethoscope, and so they could make little clinico-pathological correlation with the physical findings in chest and abdominal diseases and autopsy findings.

More important, no one at the Montreal General had had serious training in pathology prior to the appointment of William Osler to the medical faculty in 1874. Prior to the promotion of antisepsis by Roddick between 1877 and 1880, surgery was superficial. The head, chest, abdomen, and pelvis were not accessible because of the threat of sepsis, and hence the surgical services contributed only a negligible number of specimens to the museum.

After 1875 F.J. Shepherd contributed many specimens from the dissection room to the museum's anatomy section. Models in wax, papier-mâché, and plaster, loose bones, and comparative skeletons were added. The pathological collection by the time of Osler's departure from Montreal in 1884 had changed its focus. Osler had contributed about five hundred specimens supplied from post-mortems at the Montreal General and the Montreal Veterinary College.[31] Aneurysms, endocarditis, and cancer of the stomach were Osler's major interests, as well as an array of other organ pathologies.

Wyatt Johnston followed Osler as pathologist at Montreal General. He made many contributions to the museum collection up to the mid-1890s. When the MGH Pathology Building was constructed in 1895, he resigned as pathologist in order to devote his time to bacteriology and forensic medicine. He perfected and published new techniques dealing with the handling of infected materials.

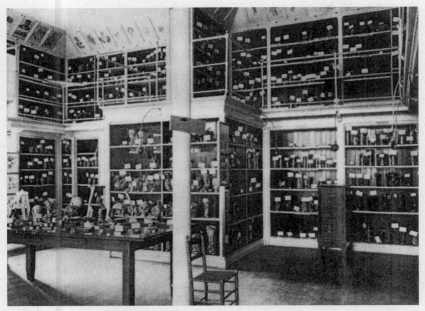

Figure 8
McGill Medical Museum, 1905. Photographer unknown

Despite the rapidly growing collection of specimens, the job of the curator of the Medical Museum was given to a junior member of the faculty. It was a purely custodial job, to ensure that specimens looked presentable and did not dry out and that there were enough jars for new specimens. By 1894 the museum occupied two rooms in the Medical Building and had a set of obstetrical models of deformed pelves, wax models illustrating the normal stages of the pregnant uterus, new skeletons, and a set of brain sections purchased in Germany. All this was under-utilized, poorly catalogued, and occupied valuable space. Although interested in the museum, Professor Adami gave it a low priority except to appoint M. Ballie, an osteologist and articulator, to put the bone collection in order. The museum remained dormant until one day in 1898 when Charles F. Martin, assistant physician at the Royal Victoria, met Maude Abbott (fig. 9) walking through the McGill campus. He invited her to come to the hospital to work with him on a research project. He also introduced her to George Adami. She so impressed Adami that he asked her to be assistant curator of the museum and to catalogue the collection.

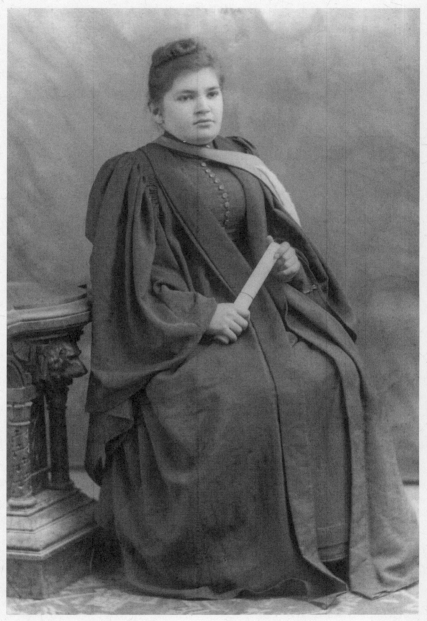

Figure 9
Maude Elizabeth Seymour Abbott, 1869–1940. Graduation photograph,
McGill University Bachelor of Arts, by William Notman, 1890

Martin had heard of Maude Abbott's interest in pigment cirrhosis and gave her a project. Adami gave her another – to work up a case involving hemochromotosis of the liver. Both projects were published – Martin's in 1899 and Adami's in 1900. Abbott's work secured for her the first female membership in the Montreal Medico-Chirugical Society in 1899 and the honour of the first paper prepared by a woman to be read before the Pathological Society of London in January 1900.

In 1899 Maude Abbott was promoted to curator of the Medical Museum, and a corner of the museum was screened off as her space. She had prodigious energy and an extraordinary ability for organizing and cataloguing the numerous specimens to make them more useful and accessible for teaching. Eventually she became restless in her role of cataloguer, surrounded by hundreds of specimens that were not used for student teaching. Her knowledge of the collection led her to hold optional demonstrations of specimens to groups of fourth-year medical students. These became so popular that the class had to be divided into sections so that all could come to the early-morning sessions. By 1904 student acclaim was so great that her museum demonstrations were made a compulsory part of the pathology course.[32]

HYGIENE AND PUBLIC HEALTH

The specialty of hygiene and public health was of equal importance to pathology and to the community but never captured the interest of the students. This field dealt with water and air purity, tracking of infectious diseases, compiling statistics on common diseases that affected the community, supervising laboratories for testing for venereal disease, and establishing legislation to support public health issues. To give the course a boost, Dean Robert Craik was appointed professor of hygiene in 1889; he was Strathcona Professor of Hygiene from 1893 to 1901.

At the turn of the century there were many public health problems in Montreal – epidemics of infectious diseases, poor housing, and issues of air quality, water supplies, and sanitation. The expertise in the McGill Department of Hygiene contributed to amelioration of some of those problems.

STUDENT LIFE

Medical students in the 1890s lived mostly in boarding houses or apartments east of the McGill campus, paying approximately $14 to $18 a month for a double room and board.[33] Most of the city streets were packed earth, only a few streets having been paved with macadam or crushed rock with help from private funds. This was practical in the severe winters, but the streets were muddy in the spring and fall and dusty in the summer. Streetcars in the late 1880s ran on St Catherine Street as far west as Greene Avenue and east to St Lawrence Boulevard via Windsor and St James Streets. By 1895 streetcars travelled from Place d'Armes two and a half miles west and three and a half miles east. Since the Montreal General was so far downtown and not accessible by streetcar, most students walked there from the McGill campus. The enormous snow accumulation of the Montreal winter posed considerable obstacles to this trek. It was not unusual for snowbanks to rise six to eight feet with sidewalks partially cleared behind them. The difficult footing slowed walking considerably. However, most of the students came from central Canada, and the difficult conditions did not deter them but were accepted as part of living in Montreal.

MONTREAL GENERAL HOSPITAL

Despite the major effort in updating and maintaining the facilities for pre-clinical training in the medical school, the environment for clinical training at the Montreal General deteriorated progressively. The physical condition of the hospital in the 1880s and the early 1890s was deplorable and demanded serious attention in order to maintain the quality of medical care and student teaching. This was documented in a record book[34] containing handwritten comments by the members of the hospital board of management, who would make annual visits and describe (at times in detail) the disrepair and rundown state of the facility.

Many years later C.F. Martin (fig. 10) described his personal experience with the deteriorating conditions at the hospital in this period from the point of view of one student giving another student a tour of the hospital.[35] In this amusing reminiscence, he described dark and dingy walls, ceilings in need of paint, and corridors dimly lit by gaslight. The floors in many rooms were worn through. At least one bathroom had a hole through the floor. The toilet and bathroom facilities were inadequate – there was only one on each of the male wards and the plumbing was frequently in disrepair. The wards were poorly ventilated, poorly illuminated, and crowded – the men's wards so overcrowded at times that some of the patients had to sleep on mattresses on the floor. In warm weather a tent was pitched on the hospital grounds to accommodate the overflow. Under such conditions, separating patients with infectious

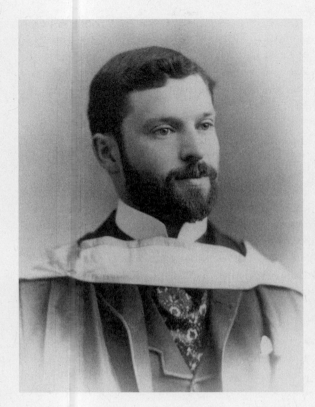

Figure 10
Charles Ferdinand
Martin, 1868–1953.
Photo by William
Notman, 1896, four
years after Martin's
medical graduation
in 1892

diseases such as typhoid, tuberculosis, and diphtheria was impossible.
Frequently patients with these diagnoses were the majority on the
wards, intermixed with general medical and surgical patients. The situation was partially alleviated in 1882 when separate medical and surgical wards were established in the old Montreal General buildings
following the efforts of Ross, Roddick, and Shepherd.

The laundry was located under the first floor wards on one side of
the hospital, with noxious vapours ascending to the patients above –
their lives were dismal enough without such added distress. Temperature control was irregular, in the winter sometimes too cold and at
other times too hot. The walls were infested with roaches, which flourished in warm weather. It is no wonder that the hospital had difficulty
attracting young women to work as nurses under these circumstances,
despite the construction in 1889 and 1890 of accommodation for them
on the top floor.

The autopsy room in the basement was small and dark, equipped
with a long table, a shelf for books and instruments, and a few chairs

and pails. Osler performed 780 post-mortems in that room between 1874 and 1884.[36] Later Johnston performed post-mortems in the same room, and reported many of his interesting cases. Unfortunately in the late 1880s the autopsy room was adjacent to the kitchen. The staff and governors agreed that for hygenic reasons it should be moved out of the hospital to a separate building, and this was done in 1895.

Patients with mental disease who were noisy presented a problem on the open wards and had to be confined in a few isolation rooms in the basement. There was no instruction or special interest in that area of medicine until T.J.W. Burgess was appointed in 1895.[37]

The original operating room, designed forty years before antisepsis came to Montreal, was an open theatre where students stood in tiers to observe surgical procedures. The table, floor, and walls were wooden, making them impossible to clean; assistants and staff wore street clothes, and medical staff curious about the surgery being performed would wander in and out, oblivious of the risk to the patient. By the early 1880s this practice was less frequent, since the air in the room would have been saturated with carbolic acid steam. Antiseptic technique had by then developed to the point where the surgeons who were believers would scrub their hands with soap and water and then rinse in chloride of mercury before going into surgery. By this time many surgeons wore rubber aprons over their street clothes, with sleeves rolled up. Surgical gloves[38] had been tried in different places; the early use of surgical gloves in the United States, however, was usually because of allergy to soap or iodoform, not because of better technique. Antisepsis was fairly well established at McGill by the 1890s, but there were still a number of sceptical surgeons who had tried adaptations of Joseph Lister's technique without good results. Despite this, there was a steady development in antisepsis after Roddick introduced carbolic spray in 1877. This evolved to the use of dry sterile dressings and clean techniques by 1890, which continued to control the infection rate.

The board of management was cognizant of poor conditions at the hospital and the urgent need for new beds, renovations, construction, and funds to improve patient care and teaching facilities. The hospital received an unexpected bequest of $40,000 in 1884 on the death of David Greenshields. Sir George Stephen,[39] a long-term friend of the hospital and member of the board of governors, contributed another $50,000 in the same year to establish an endowment and building fund. Unfortunately, the mid-1880s was a time of recession in Quebec, and public support for additional funding was limited. New construction and renovation were postponed until after 1887. Then plans were developed for new and separate surgical wings to the south of the existing buildings and a complete renovation of the old buildings along Dorchester Street as medical wings (fig. 11). The Greenshields and the Campbell wings were built in a U shape (fig. 12), with the open end facing south towards Lagauchitière Street. These surgical wards (fig. 13) were completed in 1892, adding 120 beds and completely separating the surgical department from the old medical wings along Dorchester Street.

The cost was more than expected and more than the available funds; there was no money for a new operating room and the accompanying preparation rooms that were the heart of the surgical department. Another public appeal was considered to complete the job. Then, quite unexpectedly, the MGH received a remarkable windfall – a young man named George Hamilton, the son of the Honorable John Hamilton from Montreal, died of tuberculosis in Colorado and bequeathed $100,000 to the hospital. This legacy provided funds for modern operating and ancillary rooms to complete the surgical wings. Additional money was available to renovate the original central building and the Richardson and Morland wings in 1896 for the department of medicine. Each open ward could accommodate about thirty patients. Separate rooms were added at the end of each ward to segregate patients requiring special attention.

To complete this phase of construction and renovation, a two-storey pathology building was built on the east side of the Richardson wing facing Dorchester Street, containing a post-mortem room, a laboratory where Wyatt Johnston did his bacteriology work,[40] and a chapel. The money was provided by a gift from Mrs Charles Phillips who donated $10,000 for the project.

THE ROYAL VICTORIA HOSPITAL

By 1887 Queen Victoria had occupied the British throne for fifty years, and there were golden jubilee celebrations throughout the empire. Sir George Stephen (fig. 14) and his cousin Sir Donald Smith (fig. 3) decided to commemorate the great occasion by pledging money for the construction of a new hospital for Montreal and McGill on the south side of Mount Royal, north of the McTavish Street reservoir. The donors wanted a charter dated in 1887, the Jubilee Year, and the name to be the Royal Victoria Hospital. Queen Victoria granted her permission without delay. This was a momentous event for the McGill medical faculty – an opportunity to gain a new clinical facility of modern design to be staffed by faculty members. It must have pleased the faculty

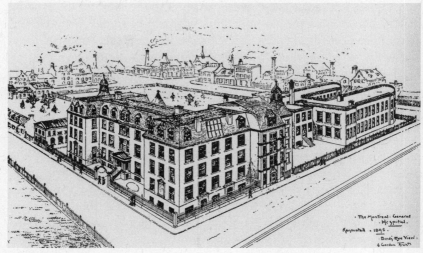

Figure 11
Building plan of the MGH after new wings and renovations, 1895. E.H.
Bensley, R.R. Forsey, and J.C. Grout, *The Montreal General Hospital Since
1821*, Montreal, 1971

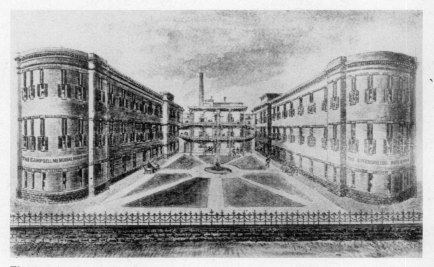

Figure 12
MGH Greenshields and Campbell surgical wings, completed in 1892, looking
north from Lagauchitière Street. Illustrator unknown

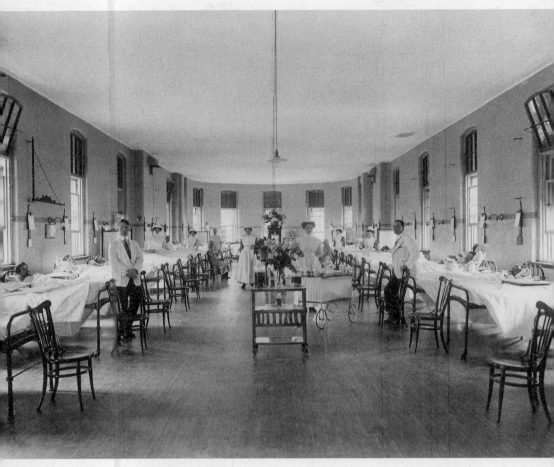

Figure 13
MGH Surgical Ward M, opened in 1892. Note the charts on the wall and the electric lighting. Photo by William Notman, 1910

immensely to know that Stephen and Smith wanted a first-class institution and were prepared to pay to make it that way.

Agreement on plans for the Royal Victoria met with obstacles when the board of management of the Montreal General objected to not being consulted. In 1889 the General's board proposed an amalgamation of the new hospital with the old and construction of new buildings on the Montreal General's Dorchester Street property. Representatives from the two hospitals started negotiations. Since neither side would concede to the other, both dropped plans for amalgamation in the same year.[41] Other obstacles arose in the potential pollution of the McTavish Street reservoir and cost overruns. Both problems were resolved, so that construction was delayed for only a short time.

The Royal Victoria's proponents and donors decided to proceed with plans prepared by a British architectural firm,[42] and construction began on 20 June 1891. The plans called for a central administration and teaching building flanked by east and west wings that faced north and south. Bridges (fig. 15) connected the three units. Construction was completed in 1893 at a cost of $650,000. The remaining $350,000 of the original $1,000,000 donation was left for endowment. The new hospital was a formidable baronial structure with stone turrets and large windows. It contained 265 beds, electrical lighting with gaslight backup, and central heating. Figure 16 depicts one of the thirty-bed wards.

The opening of the Royal Victoria required the appointment of new staff for the departments of medicine and surgery. It was necessary to establish a balanced political arrangement with the Montreal General, from which most of the staff would come. This posed a delicate situation because the General had been unchallenged as McGill's teaching hospital since the 1820s. But to everyone's general satisfaction a healthy competitive environment eventually arose. Thomas Roddick was appointed chief surgeon at the Royal Victoria. This appointment was balanced by Francis Shepherd remaining at the General as senior attending surgeon, an arrangement satisfactory to both hospitals. By 1893 Roddick had almost given up operative surgery because of an allergy to iodoform and increasing interests in medical politics.[43] James Bell (fig. 17), the 1872 Holmes Medallist,[44] was appointed assistant surgeon at the Royal Victoria. He had worked with Roddick at the General and during the Riel Rebellion in 1885. After one year Bell was promoted to chief surgeon at the Royal Victoria when Roddick resigned.

In 1893 James Stewart (fig. 5), the taciturn Scot who was known for his pauciloquent manner, was appointed physician-in-chief. George Ross would have been the first physician-in-chief at the Royal Victoria but

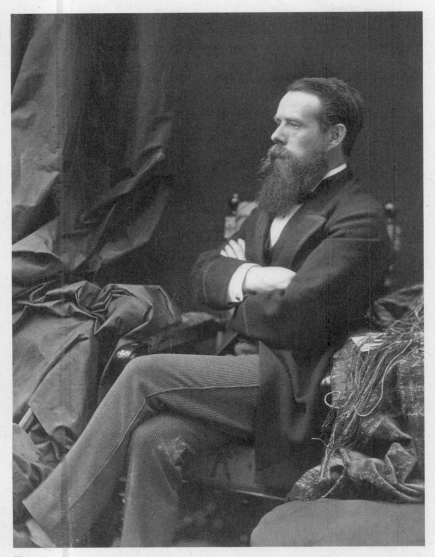

Figure 14
Sir George Stephen (later Lord Mount Stephen), 1829–1921.
Photo by William Notman, 1871

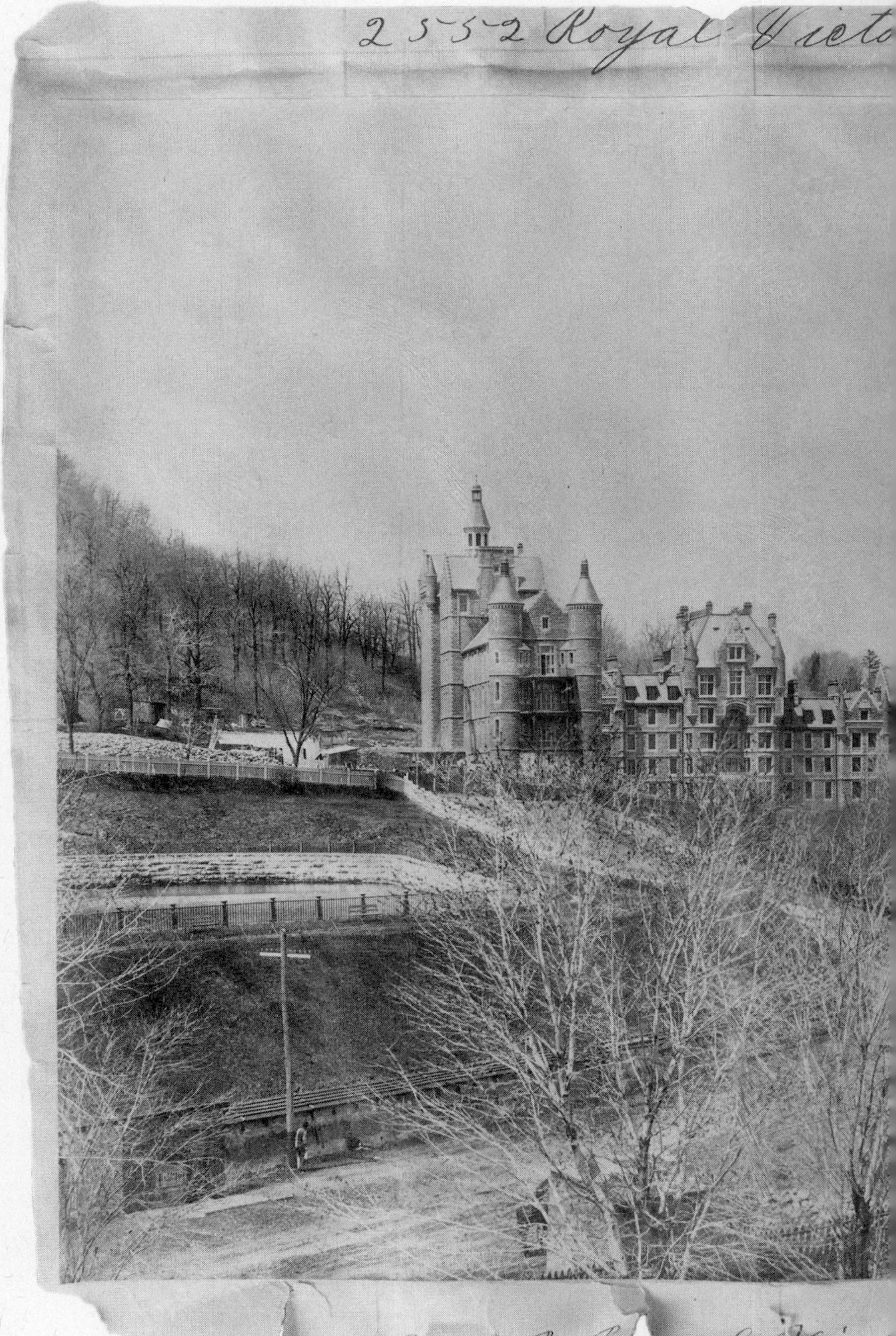
2552 Royal Victo

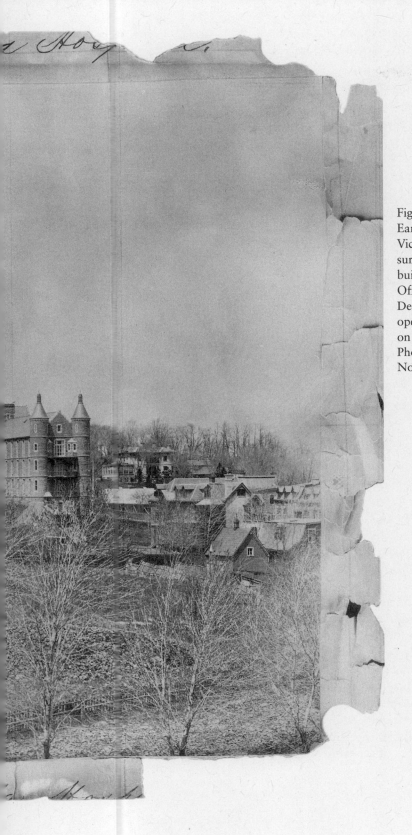

Figure 15
Early photo of Royal
Victoria Hospital
surrounded by
builders' refuse.
Official opening
December 1893;
opened for patients
on January 1894.
Photo by William
Notman, 1893

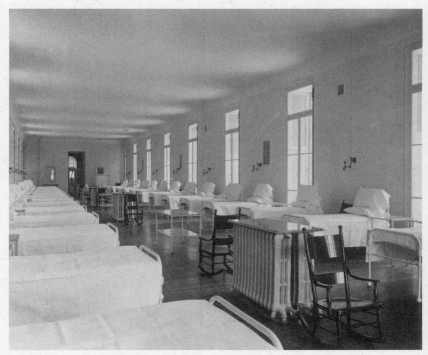

Figure 16
Typical Royal Victoria Hospital medical ward (before occupancy). Note the
double windows and inside shutters. Photo by William Notman, 1894

unfortunately died in 1892. To fill in the other departments at the new
hospital, Frank Buller was appointed chief of ophthalmology and otology, and William Gardner head of gynecology. The assistants in medicine were W.F. Hamilton, who had been an excellent student, and C.F.
Martin (fig. 10), who went on to be physician-in-chief, professor of
medicine, and an influential dean from 1923 to 1936. Bell's assistant in
surgery was A.E. Garrow, the 1889 Holmes Medallist. William Gardner's assistant in gynecology was A.W. Gardner, who resigned in 1896
to be replaced by J. Clarence Webster, a gold medallist from Edinburgh
University in 1890. The last brilliant addition to the clinical staff was
Herbert Stanley Birkett (fig. 18), the 1886 Holmes Medallist, who had
been trained in eye, ear, and throat disease. He came to the Royal Victoria as a laryngologist in 1898, concentrating on nose and throat disease, while Buller specialized in eye and ear diseases. The two specialists
shared private offices in Montreal for years.

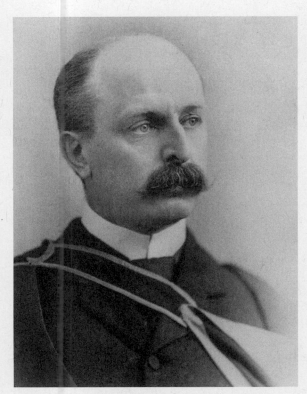

Figure 17
James Bell,
1852–1911. Photo
by William Notman,
1895

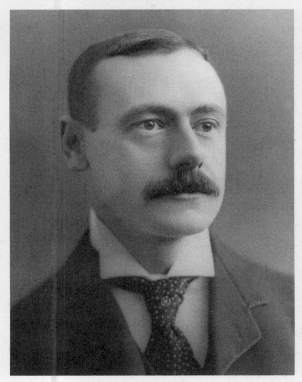

Figure 18
Herbert Stanley
Birkett, 1864–1942.
Photo by William
Notman, 1898

HOUSE SURGEONS

The house surgeons were appointed from the leading students in the graduating class and were assigned to different members of the medical and surgical attending staff on rotation. They were "handmaidens" of the attendings. This apprenticeship system worked only because there were few house surgeons. They learned quickly, faster than the average student, and as their numbers were kept low, each learned a great deal of medicine in four to six years. The house surgeons did not receive a salary or honorarium but were provided with uniforms, meals, and a place to sleep in the hospital. Any income they had came from relatives or from money made in private practice. After four years a house surgeon would be sent a few patients for his own and would gradually develop a practice at the hospital. Members of the attending staff when on vacations and holidays would have the house surgeons take care of their patients and would send their carriages around to the hospital for the house surgeon to use for home visits. This was done until a house surgeon had enough patients and a reputation that would allow him to afford a place to live and a carriage so that he could leave the hospital environment.

As could be expected, the new Royal Victoria and its brilliant staff attracted a brilliant group of house surgeons. N.D. Gunn, W.A. Brown, and W.E. Deeks – all Holmes Medallists[45] – were the first three to be appointed. The most noticeable was Neil Gunn, who went to Johns Hopkins for a doctorate in anatomy and histology, then returned to Montreal to teach histology at McGill for fifteen years. When A.A. Robertson, 1894 Holmes Medallist, was appointed an RVH house surgeon, the Montreal General became concerned that it was no longer attracting the most qualified medical graduates. In addition to being an older facility and only partially renovated, the General had a tradition that all prospective house surgeons, even Holmes Medallists, had to solicit individual approval of the numerous life governors of the hospital.[46] This archaic imposition was more than most prospective house surgeons were willing to accept. The new institution and a brilliant medical staff made the Royal Victoria more desirable and accessible. The Montreal General realized its disadvantage and rectified the situation in 1895 by rescinding the required approval of house surgeons by the life governors and getting on with its construction and renovation projects.

In 1891 there were five house surgeons at Montreal General and in 1895, seven. In 1895 the Royal Victoria had eight house surgeons –

four in surgery, three in medicine, and one in obstetrics and gynecology. At the MGH the house surgeons took care of about 250 patients. They worked with individual members of the medical and surgical staff, admitting and examining all patients on their particular service and recording the history, examination, diagnosis, treatment, and ultimate disposition in the medical and surgical casebooks.[47] They did this as well as assisting in the operating room and clinics and were on call for their individual attending staff man day and night. They also performed rudimentary laboratory tests such as urinalysis and hemoglobin, in an eight-by-twelve foot converted storeroom that was the hospital laboratory at that time.

The Royal Victoria in its first decade was expanding and had its own ambulance service.[48] When an emergency call was made to the hospital, a gong would ring and house surgeons would sprint to the front door. The winner would take the doctor's bag and run to meet the horse-drawn ambulance, which was kept at the stables down University Street. The house surgeon rode with the driver. Frequently patients called more than one hospital, so that if two ambulances appeared on the scene at the same time, there would be a contest for the patient. Ambulances had regular wheels in warm weather and runners in the winter. Sometimes it took hours to draw an ambulance through the snow. Even after the first motor ambulance was presented to the RVH in 1909,[49] the horse-drawn vehicles were still used because they were more reliable, and the horses frequently had more power to get either the wagons or the sleighs up Pine Avenue or University Street to the hospital.

MEDICAL STUDENTS

Clinical training for medical students in the hospitals still seriously lagged behind the teaching level found in the pre-clinical courses. House surgeons were essentially apprentices in a hospital setting, admitting and examining patients and helping, but with little responsibility for patient care. The situation of the medical students was even more difficult. There was no universal internship as we now know it. Upon graduation most would go directly into practice. Only a very few could receive further training as house officers. There was no concept of a team, and within the hospital students were usually only tolerated. Although they examined patients and reported to the clinical professors of medicine and surgery three times a week, the emphasis was on physical findings, and treatment did not involve student input. It is a paradox that so much effort was put into developing student participation in pre-clinical laboratory courses where students were given good opportunities to learn scientific methods in a hands-on way; yet in their third year, ready to tackle clinical problems in a scientific way, they were thwarted because they were only allowed to examine patients on the wards. They listened to lectures on patient management but could not participate in decisions for treatment and disposition for which they would be responsible after graduation.

One of the basic political facts that led to this state was a lack of control over hospital policy by the medical faculty. The same doctors staffed the hospitals and the medical school, but each institution had its own governing board. The policies in the hospitals regarding teaching on patients by students and house officers were made by the hospital governors, who acted independently of the medical school and made decisions for the benefit of the hospitals, not the school. Another part of the problem was that members of the hospital staff still believed in the old concept of watching the masters perform – at surgery in the operating rooms or on the wards – and that this was sufficient to provide the students with the skills to practise. This attitude persisted up to mid twentieth century in the surgical specialties, gradually changing as the older members of the medical staff retired.

This problem with the teaching hospitals affiliated with a major medical school was not unique to McGill.[50] It persisted for many years at McGill until the hospital governing boards finally acknowledged that a full union[51] with the medical school, such as existed at Johns Hopkins and Washington University,[52] was to the advantage of both institutions. Staff appointments were made independently at the Montreal General and the Royal Victoria, although almost invariably doctors were appointed to the Faculty of Medicine as well as to the hospital by mutual agreement. There would be at least one case in the future, however, when the Royal Victoria made a major appointment and the medical school refused to accept the candidate.[53]

MEDICINE AND SURGERY IN THE 1890S

The medical and surgical casebooks that appeared in 1863 on the hospitals wards provide a glimpse of the types of patients admitted during this period. These extraordinary volumes of folio size were kept in the medical and surgical offices. When a patient was admitted, a history was recorded by the house surgeon. The majority of medical patients had an infectious disease. Typhoid, tuberculosis, dysentery, bronchitis, erysipelas, unclassified pneumonias, heart and kidney disease, infected glands, syphilis, fever of undetermined origin, debility, dyspepsia, and rheumatism were the most common diagnoses. Some patients had suffered strokes or heart attacks. Temperature charts clipped to the ends of the beds or on the wall at the heads of the beds were kept on each patient (figs. 19A and B); and on the same sheets the urine output, pulse, and respirations were noted. Many of these sheets have been preserved in the casebooks. The house surgeon assigned to Drs Stewart or Blackader, for example, would admit all the patients for these doctors while on their services, write the histories, perform physical examinations, and write any follow-up notes weekly in the casebook until the patient was either discharged or died.

The most interesting part of those histories was the physical examination, particularly of the chest, which reached a sophisticated level in the late 1800s. Details of the appearance, expansion, percussion, and auscultation of the chest with comments about vocal fremitus, thrills and bruits, murmurs, and rubs were recorded. Dullness was often percussed precisely on one side of the chest to a single rib level. Ophthalmoscopy[54] was performed along with a reasonably precise neurological exam. Babinski's sign was described by 1896.[55] Strength, sensation, and reflexes were recorded, including clonus and hyperreflexia in cases of cord and brain involvement. The medical histories were brief, and follow-up notes were sporadic – weekly or less frequent – and undoubtedly dictated by the attending staff. There was no attempt to record daily progress notes because the patients' conditions changed slowly, although the attending doctors undoubtedly saw their patients daily. The house surgeons had no independent responsibility to write notes unless dictated by the attending staff.

The surgical admissions were managed similarly, for example, for Roddick's and Shepherd's patients. Their house surgeons would admit, examine, diagnose, and record the findings in the surgical casebooks. Surgical therapy had also undergone a remarkable change in scope since the 1840s, mainly because of anesthesia, first used in Montreal in 1847,[56] and, later, antisepsis, first used in 1868[57] but really introduced to the community by Craik in 1869 and Roddick in the 1870s. As the surgical staff accepted antisepsis more and more, the number and type of surgical procedures and the diagnoses increased with less worry about infection.

Another extraordinary record – the Operation Book – exists from the Montreal General, covering procedures from 1881 to 1890.[58] It records all the operations, surgeons, and dates, in addition to the names, ages, and diagnoses of the patients. Scanning this volume, one notices that in

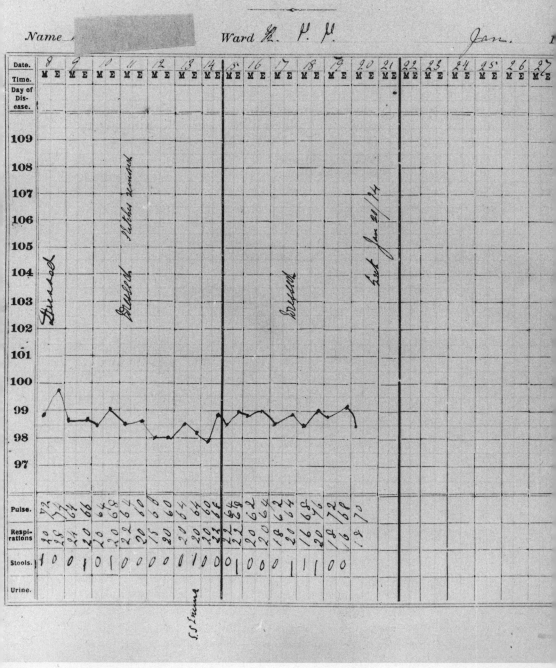

Figure 19A and B
Temperature charts from MGH medical casebooks. These pages are from a chart of a patient with typhoid fever, December 1893 to 20 January 1894. Note pulse and respirations but no blood pressure recordings.

Name _____ Ward 12 _____ Dec & Jan _____ 187

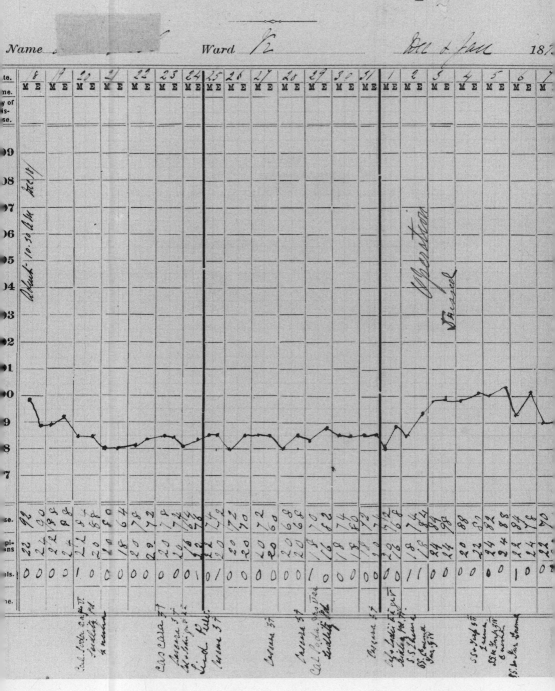

the month of May 1882, nine surgical procedures were performed. In May 1890, twenty-seven procedures were performed, consisting mostly of lancing abscesses and buboes, casting fractures and sprains, amputations, removing tumours, hemorrhoid tissue, and cataracts, with occasional cancer and eye muscle surgery. Laparotomies were done occasionally for suspected intestinal obstruction. Appendectomy[59] was reported occasionally. Trephining the head after a trauma of the skull to look for a skull fracture was reported. By 1890 the Operation Book recorded hemorrhoidectomy, amputations, casting of fractures, mastectomy, appendectomies, laparotomy, and nephrectomy as having been done and the patients leaving the hospital having survived the procedures. Although x-ray had been developed and was available by the late 1890s at McGill, it was still only useful for bones and chest. Contrast material (barium) was used for the radiological gastrointestinal tract starting around 1910;[60] otherwise it was difficult to determine the nature of internal diseases except by inference.

By the 1890s medical therapy had changed drastically from what it had been in the 1840s when medical treatment was limited to bleeding, purgatives, laxatives, mercury and chalk, and blistering, which were used for many conditions.[61] There was no science behind those forms of treatment – only dogma that had been passed on from previous generations. Fifty years later, medical therapy in the hospital and in practice was based on scientific observations that, given a certain clinical presentation, an appropriate drug could alter the findings.[62] It was observed, for example, that digitalis could strengthen the heartbeat and could reverse heart failure and edema.[63] In contrast, to purge the unfortunate victim in heart failure would hardly do him any good and might further aggravate the condition because of electrolyte problems.

Pharmacological research had progressed to such a degree in the 1890s that many specific medicines were available to the knowledgeable physician. However, most therapy remained symptomatic. Opiates (opium and morphine) were available, mainly as tinctures, and were used to control pain, cough, and intestinal disturbances (colitis); they were also found to be useful for persistent hiccups that were common in typhoid fever. The hypodermic syringe was available at this time,[64] but morphine was more conveniently administered as a tincture in water. Quinine was used for malaria, which was well known in Upper Canada[65] in Osler's childhood but less common in Montreal. It was also useful for sundry fevers. Bismuth, mercurials, iodides, and bromides were used as powders for a multitude of illnesses including syphilis and seizures. Chloral hydrate in small doses was used as a tranquillizer and for sleep. Sodium salicylate was prescribed for arthritis and fevers. Belladonna compounds quieted upper gastro-intestinal symptoms, and apo-morphine was used as an emetic for toxic ingestion. Iron compounds were used for anemia; syrup of rhubarb, bismuth, and potash with bismuth were given to quiet dyspepsia. Colchicum (colchicine) compounds or mixtures were used to treat gout. Cod liver oil, iron compounds, and compounds of strychnine and arsenic were used as tonics. Alcohol in the form of whiskey, brandy, rum, or gin was used liberally in the hospital and at home as a stimulant to give patients a feeling of well being. Diphtheria antitoxin (horse serum) was available in the 1890s,[66] and smallpox vaccine had been available for decades.[67] Osler's textbook, first published in 1892,[68] described these various forms of treatment, which were still mainly symptomatic.

RODDICK AND THE RIEL REBELLION

Thomas Roddick, who had a reputation for expediency, was always looking for new challenges. In 1885 he found an unusual opportunity. At the outset of the Riel Rebellion in western Canada on 22 March 1885,[69] the Canadian government sent more than five thousand troops under General F.D. Middleton to the Northwest to quell the uprising, which lasted until 2 July 1885. It was apparent that the army did not have a medical service to handle casualties in the field and particularly when the troops were embarked on an arduous trip to Manitoba and Saskatchewan from Central Canada. Darby Bergin, an 1847 McGill medical graduate from Cornwall, Ontario, had been appointed surgeon general.[70] In Bergin's opinion, Roddick was the only man medically trained and physically fit to tackle the front-line job of establishing a medical care system in the field and nearby cities, and an evacuation plan for the wounded.

On 3 April 1885 Bergin appointed Roddick chief of the medical staff in the field. Roddick chose James Bell from Montreal as his assistant. Bergin and Roddick had the enormous task of organizing a group of doctors and nurses, planning base and field hospitals, acquiring supplies, and planning transportation for wounded patients as well as the medical personnel.[71] One merely has to look at a map of southern Manitoba and Saskatchewan (fig. 20) and note the distances from Winnipeg to Regina and Saskatoon to see the wide territory Roddick had to cover in his effort to establish proper medical care for the Canadian troops. Bergin and Roddick also had to arrange for beds and referral hospitals in Winnipeg and Saskatoon with the help of personnel from

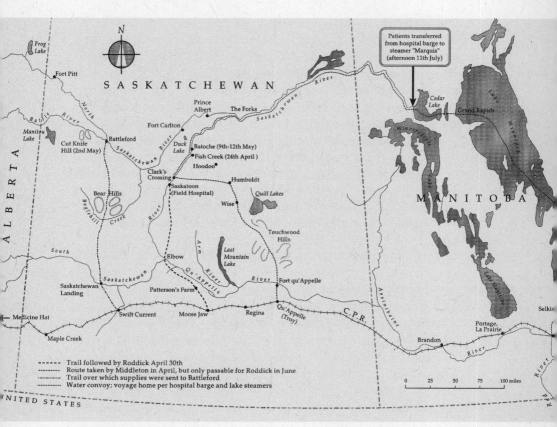

Figure 20
Map of territory covered by the Canadian Army Medical Services during
the Riel Rebellion 1885. Drawn by Richard Bachand, McGill University, after
map in H.E. MacDermot's *Sir Thomas Roddick* (Toronto: Macmillan, 1938)

McGill and University of Toronto. They then had to get the medical
staff to the field where the fighting was by train, boat, and wagon in
order to treat and evacuate the wounded. Moving from Saskatchewan
to Moose Jaw and Winnipeg, Roddick eventually evacuated the wounded after the various battles with remarkably good results despite the
lengthy journeys. He attributed the good results to the lack of germs in
the open air. In his opinion germs saturated the Montreal General and
caused frequent infections.

At the conclusion of the rebellion, Roddick had accomplished a difficult mission under unpredictable circumstances and demonstrated his
single-minded genius and capacity for organization.

STAFF DEATHS

Untimely staff deaths robbed McGill of a few of its outstanding teachers during this period of expansion and improving standards of education. Dean Palmer Howard died in 1889, ending one of the most influential careers in medicine of the first seventy years of McGill's existence. Craik and Ross prepared a resolution for the faculty minutes:[72] "This Faculty desires to record its profound grief at the unexpected death of its Dean and Professor of Medicine, Dr. Robert Palmer Howard. One of its own graduates, he had risen from the lowest office to the very highest position which it is in the power of the University to bestow. To his students he was the master respected and revered, but at the same time thoroughly appreciated and loved. To his colleagues he was the trusted friend and adviser. To his University he was a tower of strength. This Faculty deplore the loss of a remarkable able and successful teacher and one who had for a number of years filled with great credit to himself and much usefulness to the University the responsible and honourable position of Dean."

Howard's last effort as dean was to encourage the faculty to establish chairs in pathology and hygiene, funded by Lord Strathcona in 1893.

Richard MacDonnell, who had a promising career in medicine, died in 1891 at age thirty-eight. George Ross, the brilliant clinician and professor of medicine, died in 1892 at age forty-seven. Howard, Ross, and Mac-Donnell had formed the backbone of the medical department at McGill.

ADDITIONS AND RENOVATIONS, 1892–95

From 1889 to 1893 the student enrolment had increased by sixty-four students. The faculty was again faced with the need to expand the facilities to accommodate the increased numbers. To do so, it was going to have to borrow money from the university for the land and use the remaining funds in the endowment for the construction. The cost of the land was estimated at $25,000, the costs for building renovation and new construction at about $30,000. When the faculty presented its plans to the McGill board of governors, to everyone's surprise, J.H.R. Molson, one of the governors, offered to purchase the land and pay for the building, giving the faculty $60,000 for the project.

The result of this gift was a new wing of the Medical Building (fig. 21) to the north, which expanded student laboratory facilities and lecture theatre capacity to accommodate almost double the enrolment. An adjacent building was attached to the side of the new wing and reno-

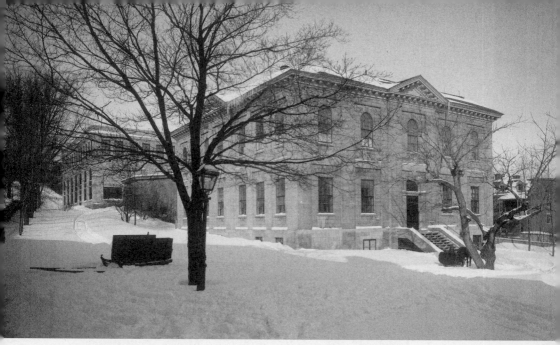

Figure 21
Medical Building in midwinter. Starting from the right, buildings built in 1872, 1885, and 1894. Photo by William Notman, 1894 or 1895

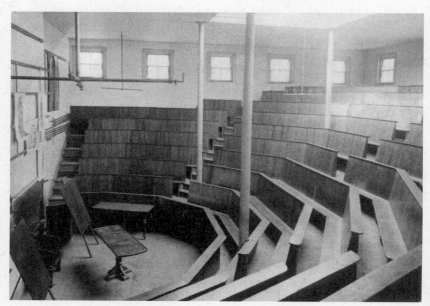

Figure 22
McGill Faculty of Medicine, anatomy lecture room, constructed 1885.
Photo by William Notman, 1894

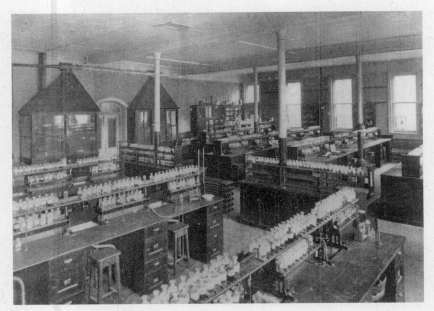

Figure 23
McGill Faculty of Medicine, main chemistry laboratory.
Photo by William Notman, 1894

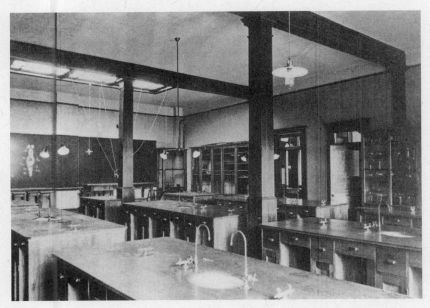

Figure 24
McGill Faculty of Medicine, physiology laboratory.
Photo by William Notman, 1894

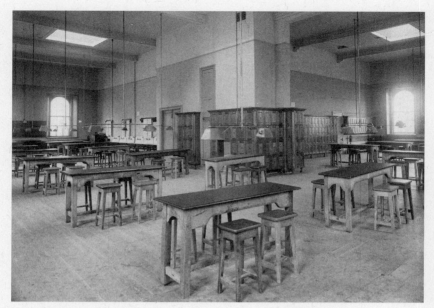

Figure 25
McGill Faculty of Medicine, anatomy dissecting room.
Photo by William Notman, 1894

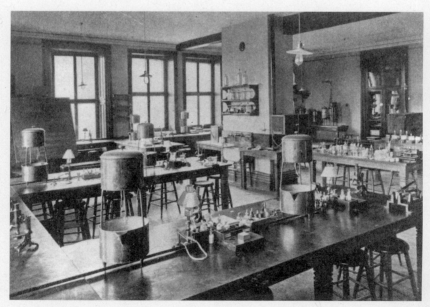

Figure 26
McGill Faculty of Medicine, bacteriology laboratory.
Photo by William Notman, 1894

vated for an academic pathology department to accommodate the recently appointed professor of pathology, John George Adami.

On 3 January 1895 a grand opening was held to celebrate the completion of the construction. The governor general of Canada, the Earl of Aberdeen, attended and addressed the audience. Dean Craik reviewed the history of the medical faculty from 1829 to date.[73] Acting Principal Johnson and Emeritus Principal Sir William Dawson also spoke.[74] The ceremony closed with three cheers for the queen and the university, led by the governor general, followed by an open house and tour of the lecture rooms (fig. 22) and modern laboratories – chemistry (fig. 23), pharmacology and physiology (fig. 24), anatomy (fig. 25), and bacteriology (fig. 26).

DEANSHIP OF ROBERT CRAIK

Robert Craik (fig. 27) succeeded Howard as dean of the faculty in 1889. At the time he was professor of hygiene and the senior member of faculty, having served continuously in various appointments since 1856.[75] For the twelve years of his deanship he gave the annual address at the medical convocation. The carefully edited manuscripts for those addresses, together with some of his other addresses and lectures, were published, providing one of the most valuable sources of information about the first seventy-five years of the medical faculty.[76] His valedictory address on 5 May 1863 included the following remarks on the "doctor's life":

But, gentlemen, supposing that you surmounted all the difficulties incident to the earlier part of your career, and have established yourself in ample practice, your troubles are by no means at an end. The public can have no conception, and you yourselves but a faint one, of all the stern realities of a doctor's life. How few will give him credit for his quiet endurance, his anxious watchings, his baffled hopes, and his untiring self-sacrifice? See him in the full tide of his professional career; what a life of anxious troubled unrest, what exorbitant expectations are made upon his resources, what unthinking demands upon his time and vital energies? By day and by night, sunshine and storm, on work day and the day of rest, for rich or for poor, with or without recompense, he must ever obey the call of suffering humanity.[77]

In 135 years there has been little change in the reality of medical practice. In his opening address for the 1890–91 session, Craik addressed the issue of the cost of educating doctors:

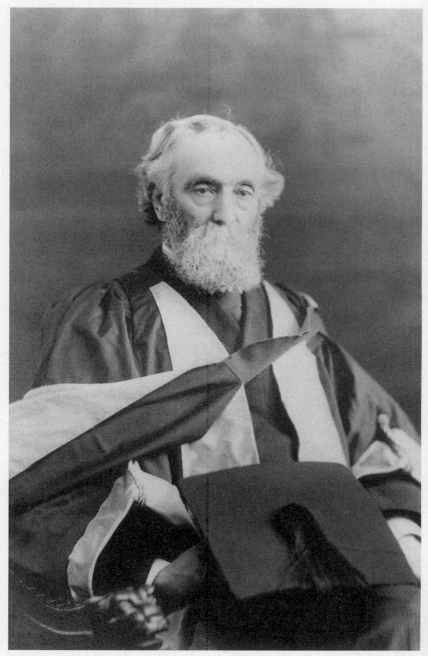

Figure 27
Robert Craik, 1829–1906. Photo by William Notman, 1901

But, it may be asked, are not the fees from the students intended to meet [the expenses of medical school], and has not the cost of medical education been increased to the student in proportion to the cost of providing it? The answer is, that medical teaching, properly so called has never been self-supporting and is now less so than before. It is true that the aggregate amount of a student's fees is now greater by some 20 to 30 percent than it was 5 and 20 years ago; but in the same period, not only has the aggregate of school expenditure been more than doubled, but in some departments it has been trebled and quadrupled, and all this while practising the most rigid economy in every particular. Nor does there seem at present to be any remedy for the disparity for the price paid for medical education and the cost of providing it.[78]

With a few changes in the numbers, this speech could be repeated to explain the cost of medical education today.

Fortunately, there was always Lord Strathcona to turn to when school expenditures had to be defrayed. In 1898 in the names of Lady Strathcona and their daughter, the Honorable Mrs Jarred Howard,[79] Strathcona came to the aid of the faculty once again and gave $100,000 towards future extensions and renovations of the Medical Building. Instead of investing the money to pay faculty salaries and laboratory costs and developing long-term plans, the faculty decided on another Medical Building expansion. This ambitious addition, constructed in 1901, consisted of three wings, one down each side and one in the middle of the complex (fig. 28). A laboratory wing in the north corner where the Molson Pathology Building stood was connected down the east side of the building to the original 1872 structure. A second part connected the Molson Wing to the 1872 building on the west side. A third part was the replacement of the 1885 wing with towers added to the east and west sides. These additions and the renovations provided 1,50,000 cubic feet of space, sufficient for twice the student enrolment of 1900.[80] There were four lecture theatres – three for 250 students and one for 400 to 450. The library stacks had room for 40,000 volumes.

Overleaf: Figure 28
Medical Building with additions and cupolas, 1901. Note the original Royal Victoria Hospital buildings, 1893, in the background and the portico over the front steps of the Medical Building. Photo by William Notman, c. 1901

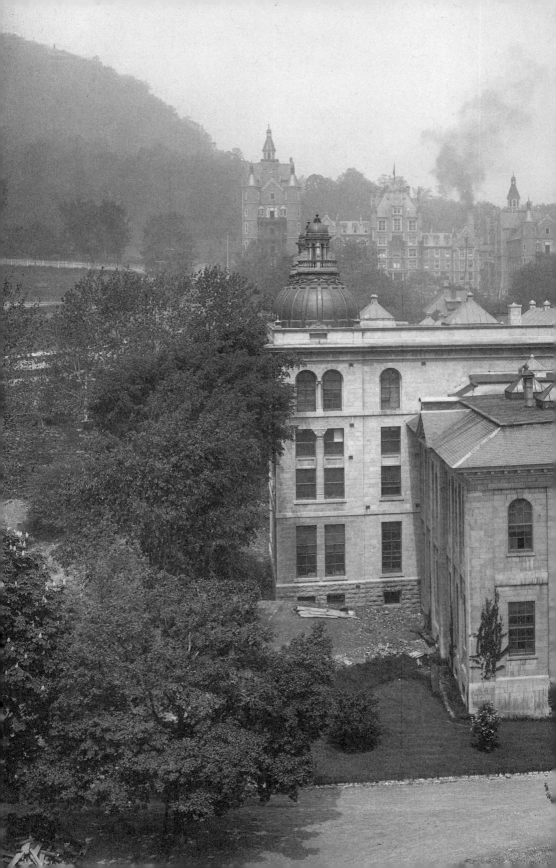

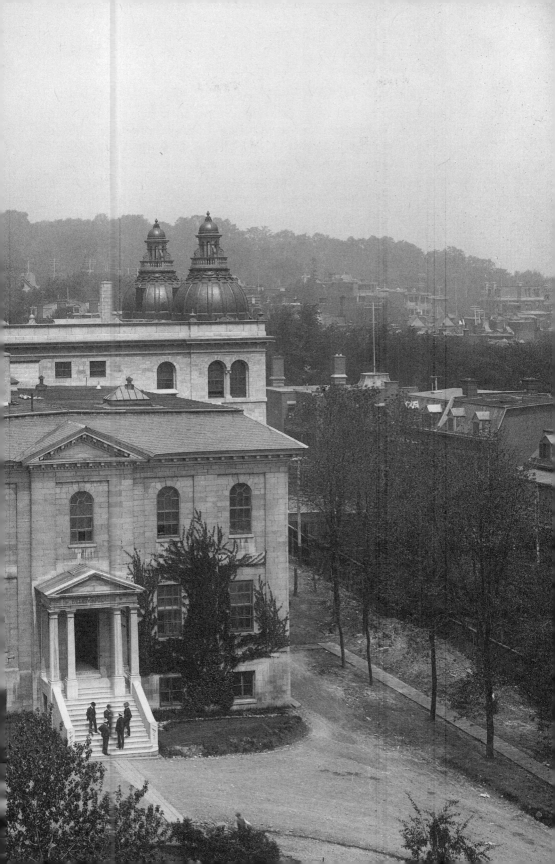

The official opening in September 1901 was a grand occasion. Lord Strathcona, then Canadian high commissioner in London as well as chancellor of McGill, returned to Montreal for the occasion. He entertained the Duke and Duchess of Cornwall and York (the future King George V and Queen Mary), Governor General Minto, Prime Minister Wilfred Laurier, and other dignitaries at his home on Dorchester Street. The royal guests received honorary doctorates at Royal Victoria College before going on to open the Medical Building at the university and visit the Royal Victoria Hospital. When the royal guests left Montreal the following day, they might have been forgiven for wondering if there was any part of Montreal for which Lord Strathcona had not been responsible.[81]

THE MEDICAL SCHOOL AT THE TURN OF THE CENTURY

In his address at the medical convocation on 14 June 1901, Dean Craik reported on the origin of the students in the Faculty of Medicine:

Of the 490 [students] in attendance during the present session, 467 have been undergraduates, proceeding to the [M.D., C.M.] degree; while the remaining 23 were graduates and partial students pursing special courses of study. The area from which the students have been drawn has also increased, more particularly of late years, almost in proportion to their numbers. For many years the provinces of Ontario and Quebec, or Upper and Lower Canada, as they were formerly called, furnished all but a very small minority of our students, and these provinces together still furnish a majority of the whole; but the homes of the others are every year becoming more and more widely distributed, over an area covering the whole dominion, and stretching out over the whole of this continent, through the United States, Newfoundland and the West Indies, as well as across the Atlantic to Great Britain and Ireland; and this session even across the Pacific Ocean, to China and Japan. The number from different provinces and countries are as follows: Ontario, 156, or nearly 32 percent; Quebec, 142, or almost 29 percent; New Brunswick, 52, or 10½ percent; the United States, 47, or 9½ percent; Nova Scotia, 29, or nearly 6 percent; Prince Edward Island, 27 or 5½ percent; British Columbia, 13, or 2½ percent; Newfoundland, 9, or nearly 2 percent; Manitoba and Northwest Territories, 4; the West Indies, 4; Great Britain and Ireland, 4; China, 2; and Japan, 1; all of the last 5, less than 1 percent ... Indeed, it seems not too much to claim that the Medical Faculty of McGill University is being recognized as one of the representative medical schools of Anglo-Saxondom.

In spite of this apparent successful and prestigious position, the faculty had some major problems at the turn of the century.

First was the proprietary mentality of the medical faculty that it could still continue to manage its own financial affairs. By 1900 the income from student tuition fees was $57,125 a year; however, this amount was not enough to run the faculty's increasingly expensive scientific laboratories for students, and there were annual deficits in the operating accounts. Since 1885 the faculty had received gifts and some funds for professorships. Instead of establishing an endowment fund and using the income to offset the deficits, it used the gifts for capital expansion. As a result it had to go annually to the university or outside sources to make up the deficits in the operating accounts. The long-term effect of this was that the faculty had no money to develop new programs or establish needed professorships.

From 1829 to 1890 the medical students paid separate fees for classes directly to the individual professors. This system worked when there was one professor per class but became increasingly complicated and unsatisfactory after 1885 when junior instructors were appointed for some of the practical classes. Starting with the 1890–91 session, students were charged a fixed sum of $100 for each of the four years. In addition they paid a graduation fee and hospital fees.[82] After 1901 the fees were increased, and 457 students paid $125 each per year. The revenue was used to pay debts, laboratory expenses, building maintenance, and the salaries of the fifty-seven faculty members. A full professor's salary ranged from $2,400 to $3,600 per year; lecturers received about $400 to $600 a year, depending on the number of lectures they gave. Despite a lack of endowment funds, construction of new facilities continued in a cavalier way with little consideration for how to pay for the increased operating expenses.

Secondly, the persistence of didactic teaching in all four years – too many lectures and not enough practical experience – continued to be a problem. This was cited by sources both outside and inside McGill for all of the basic sciences except for anatomy, which had only one-third of its total hours spent in the lecture room. Osler and Shepherd proved without a doubt that practical exposure in visual subjects such as anatomy and histology was the best way for students to learn those disciplines. Lectures had a role, but a balance was necessary. The same principle applied to chemistry, physiology, pharmacology, and pathology. Although chemistry did have a practical emphasis under Gilbert Girdwood before the turn of the century, other subjects were still lecture courses with token laboratory time. It took new personnel, money, and many years to correct this. McGill had made a major effort to improve its teaching programs and had accomplished much in the area of laboratory experience in the pre-clinical subjects. The teaching in the clinical subjects in the hospitals, however, lagged behind and did so for many years.

Thirdly, interest, space, and funding for research were sadly lacking, mainly because McGill had emphasized the development of teaching and student facilities almost exclusively. Wyatt Johnston, Wesley Mills, and Girdwood, nonetheless, carried on personal research, published regularly, and had scholarly reputations. These exceptions did not influence the policy of the medical school.

A further problem was the failure to develop a true clinical clerkship in the hospitals, in spite of its great success at the Johns Hopkins Medical School under Osler, who still had a significant influence at McGill. The broader problem essentially was that the practical training to which students had been introduced in the first and second year of the medical course was not continued to the same degree in the hospitals in the third and fourth years. The fault lay with hospital boards and with the clinical professors who had no experience in training students and house staff properly. Most of the staff were self-trained or had only passive exposure to bedside medicine while walking the wards in Europe. By the turn of the century neither Stewart, who gave the lectures in medicine, nor Roddick, who gave the lectures in surgery, were up to date in their subjects. The same cycle had occurred in 1872 when the older staff members were teaching what they had learned thirty years before. This continued until World War I when many of the older men went overseas and younger teachers replaced them in the lecture rooms.

Another area of difficulty was the entrenched opposition to admitting women to medical school because of persistent Victorian beliefs of the role of women as ladies. Women had been admitted in the McGill undergraduate college in 1884 under an endowment from Sir Donald Smith, and had been admitted to Bishop's University Medical School as early as 1890.[83] Despite the performance of outstanding undergraduate scholars at McGill such as Maude Abbott and Octavia Ritchie, however, chauvinism, prudishness, stubbornness, and tradition contributed to keeping women out of medical school. In his address to the Medical Convocation of 1 April 1890, Dean Craik had reported: "Urgent and repeated applications have been made to us to admit female students to our classes; and influential deputations, composed of persons of both sexes, have waited upon us, and urged their views in support of both sides of the question. The Faculty, while far from denying the desirability, under suitable conditions, of admitting women to the practice of medicine, could not see its way to the admission of female students to its classes, hitherto designed exclusively for men; and was, therefore, reluctantly compelled to withhold its consent."[84] Even the male students were openly opposed to admitting women, feeling that they were not mature enough or as prepared for the stress as were men.

Paradoxically, for men, entrance (matriculation) requirements by 1900 were relatively low. A senior high-school certificate was not required, because a student could leave high school with a junior matriculation certificate, take the McGill Matriculation Examination, and be admitted to the Faculty of Medicine as long as he was over seventeen years of age. The matriculation examination was a test for median, not extraordinary, ability. Knowledge of Latin (or Greek), high-school level mathematics, English grammar, composition, literature, and history were required. French and German language examinations were optional. McGill did not hesitate to increase the difficulty of its courses but was not going to make it too difficult for an applicant to be admitted to the medical faculty. The faculty also admitted applicants who had passed provincial or state high-school leaving examinations. A college degree was acceptable for entrance, but only a minority of applicants had that qualification.

THE SCHOOLS FOR NURSES

Although not directly related to the medical school, important developments in the related profession of nursing in the last half of the nineteenth century greatly improved medical care. These developments included the staffing of hospitals by trained nurses and the establishment of training schools for nurses. Faculty members participated in the instruction of the student nurses. At the teaching hospitals, medical students and house officers benefited from practical instruction by senior nurses.

Florence Nightingale had started one of the first training schools for nurses at St Thomas's Hospital in London, England, in June 1860.[85] The movement spread to North America where the first training school was started in Roxbury, Massachusetts, in 1873. In 1874 Dr Theophilus Mack started the first training school for nurses in Canada in St Catharines, Ontario. By 1900 there were schools for nurses in most large Canadian hospitals,[86] at the same time as it became socially acceptable for women to work outside the family or marital home. Teaching and stenography were already established careers for women, and gradually nursing too became increasingly popular. The applications for admission to schools for nurses exceeded their capacity for enrolment.[87]

In February 1890 the board of management at Montreal General appointed Nora Livingston as lady superintendent. A graduate of the New York Hospital's Training School of Nurses, she was the third person with special training in nursing to hold that position. The first was Maria Machin from 1875 to 1877, the second Anne Maxwell from 1880 to 1881. Miss Livingston started the Montreal General's School for Nurses in April 1890. In the ensuing years she introduced several innovations: a three-year course, lectures by the medical and surgical attending staff and senior nurses, practical instruction on the wards, distinctive uniforms while on duty to distinguish nurses from other female hospital employees, a residence for the student nurses near the parent hospital, and, after 1906, a three-month probationary period of instruction with no assigned duties. Many of the schools for nurses followed Livingston's model. She directed the School for Nurses from 1890 to 1919. During her term of office 649 students completed the three-year course. Many graduate nurses went on to occupy important positions in the nursing profession in Canada and other countries.[88]

The Royal Victoria's School for Nurses was equally popular and successful. Prior to the official opening of the hospital, in June 1893 Edith Draper was appointed lady superintendent. A Canadian by birth, she was a graduate of the Bellevue Hospital in New York. At the time of her appointment she was in charge of the Illinois Training School for Nurses.

When the first patients were admitted to the Royal Victoria in January 1894, trained nurses staffed the hospital. The first probationary student was admitted to the RVH School for Nurses on 10 January 1894. Initially the course spanned two years. The first class of twenty-six nurses graduated 28 April 1896. Later the course was extended to three years. By the turn of the century the RVH School for Nurses received more than five hundred applications each year. Only a fraction of the applicants could be admitted as probationers or students due to limited accommodation. Miss Draper resigned in 1897 and was succeeded by Annie Murray until 1901, and then Florence Henderson until 1908. In 1908 Mabel F. Hersey was appointed lady superintendent and director of the RVH School for Nurses. She held those positions with distinction until 1938. By the fiftieth anniversary of the school in 1943, nearly two thousand nurses had trained at the Royal Victoria and were practising their profession in all the corners of the earth.[89] When the McGill School for Graduate Nurses started in 1920, many graduates from the MGH and the RVH schools enrolled to gain a higher degree.[90]

2 Planting the Seeds for Change, 1901–14

To have lived through a revolution, to have seen a new birth of science, a new dispensation for health, reorganized medical schools, remodelled hospitals, a new outlet for humanity, is not given to every generation.
WILLIAM OSLER[1]

DEANSHIP OF THOMAS GEORGE RODDICK, 1901–08

Roddick attended his first faculty meeting as dean in January 1902.[2] He was professor of surgery, chairman of the Royal Victoria's medical board, and a member of the Canadian Parliament for the St Antoine District of Montreal. He had given up operative surgery in 1893, partly because he had dermatitis from antiseptic solutions, but also because he was busy in Ottawa promoting his "Roddick Bill." It's aim was to establish a dominion registry for Canadian doctors so that they could move between provinces without taking additional qualifying examinations.

THE DENTAL DEPARTMENT

The first major development that required the new dean's attention concerned a dental department at McGill.

Dentists appeared in Quebec in the 1850s; however, they had been trained elsewhere, because there was no dental school in the province. The Dental College of the Province of Quebec was founded in Montreal in 1892. Seeking a university affiliation, the dental college suggested to the McGill board of governors that McGill establish a degree course in dentistry. After discussing the proposal, the governors decided that the Faculty of Medicine would run the dental department. The medical faculty, however, wanted to award a diploma of "Graduate in Dentistry" and not a doctorate. This meant that dental graduates would have a qualification inferior to that of the veterinarian students who received the degree of Doctor of Veterinary Medicine (D.V.M.) on graduation.[3]

Finding the McGill proposal unacceptable, in 1896 the dental college, decided to found an independent school of dentistry affiliated with Bishop's University in Lennoxville, Quebec,[4] thereby providing a university association so that the degree of doctor of dental surgery (D.D.S.) could be conferred. Bishop's Dental School required three years of training, extended to four in 1901, and had facilities on St Catherine and St Lawrence Streets in Montreal. It remained open from 1896 to 1904 and graduated eighty-six dentists.[5]

In 1903 discussions regarding the establishment of a dental school associated with McGill were resumed because Bishop's medical school was near closing. The dental college communicated with McGill and the Faculty of Medicine, stating that it would be interested in forming a dental school at McGill which, according to the McGill board of governors, would have to be a department of the medical faculty. The faculty, not wanting a new expenditure, insisted that the dental school would be an independent department and responsible for its own finances. The professors of the new school would run it, teach and examine students, and make policies. Recalling the stumbling block of 1896, the medical faculty proposed a four-year course leading to a degree of Master of Dental Science (M.D.S.) and a doctorate degree (D.D.S.) after one to three years of extra work on a thesis or on advanced dentistry. After further discussion, some felt that the D.D.S. degree should be awarded after four years of dental school, as was the case in medicine. No further decision was made on this issue.[6]

A list of nine items was sent to the McGill Corporation,[7] the body which regulated the academic affairs of the university; it agreed with the general principles proposed. Soon afterward in 1904, coincident with the closing of Bishop's medical faculty in 1905, the Bishop's University dental faculty requested that its teaching staff[8] be considered for the staff of the Dental Department of McGill, and that presently enrolled students continue at McGill and be eligible for a degree in the usual manner.

McGill's Faculty of Medicine later agreed to accept part of the Bishop's proposal – the Bishop's dental faculty would be the professional staff of the Dental Department of the McGill medical faculty. According to the agreement, the Dental Department had to run economically, and the staff would be responsible for the department's financial affairs

– an unusual commitment for a purely part-time staff. As regards the transfer of enrolled Bishop's dental students, McGill refused to accept them unless they started in first year in 1904. One student did, and others continued at McGill and were granted Bishop's degrees in 1905–06.

In 1892 a dental clinic had been established at the Montreal General under the direction of R.H. Berwick, and in 1921 the space for the clinic was enlarged, doubling its capacity. This is where dental students gained practical experience in their third and fourth years and provided service to the community.[9]

In May 1911 and again in February 1912, the head of the Dental Department requested a full-time assistant professor for the department. The Faculty of Medicine did not grant this request until December 1912 when the first full-time instructor, A.W. Thornton, was appointed to the department as professor, director of the Dental Clinic, and head of the Dental Department. In 1920 the Dental Department was established as the Dental Faculty, and Thornton was named as its first dean in 1920. A.L. Walsh succeeded him as dean in 1927 and continued in the position until 1948. The first McGill degrees in 1908 were the controversial Master of Dental Science, awarded to three graduates. This was changed to Doctor of Dental Surgery (D.D.S.) in 1917. The unfortunate consequences of the McGill takeover were the refusal to teach in French and to accept women applicants – both had been features of the Bishop's Dental Faculty.[10] McGill refused to accept women applicants for the dental school, an injustice that remained a faculty policy until 1926.

FULL AMALGAMATION OF THE FACULTY OF MEDICINE WITH McGILL UNIVERSITY

In 1904 the medical faculty had to face the problem of poor financial management. The newly enlarged Medical Building with its advanced facilities gave no hint of the serious financial state of the faculty. In 1902 the faculty finance committee submitted a detailed report of the assets and liabilities of the medical school. It stated that unexpected costs from the new construction of 1901 had exceeded Lord Strathcona's $100,000 gift, and the faculty was in dire need of $25,000 for operating expenses. There wasn't enough money for faculty development, and even a $400 telephone system couldn't be afforded, so the faculty borrowed $25,000 from McGill University. This typified the faculty's ineptness in financial planning – running a deficit because of its ambitious capital building program. Despite bequests and income from the students' tuition fees, the faculty had insufficient income to pay salaries and the annual expenditures for the upkeep and maintenance of the Medical Building, thereby incurring a deficit in the thousands of dollars. Yet, nowhere in the faculty minutes was there a word questioning the progressive indebtedness, which suggests that no one was worried as long as Lord Strathcona was alive to rescue the school from debt.

In 1903 the McGill governors had urged the medical faculty, through Secretary Vaughn and Dean Roddick, to develop a schedule to repay its indebtedness to the university. The university also wanted the faculty to make an annual contribution to the university's general operating funds to which the other three faculties contributed.[11] The medical faculty reluctantly agreed to give all graduation fees to the university – a rather meaningless gesture since in January 1902 the faculty had borrowed $25,000 from the university to pay its debts.

In 1904 the faculty's finance committee reported a deficit of $7,509 for the year and a total indebtedness to the university of $37,000. It was decided to ask Lord Strathcona for the money, so Dean Roddick and Professor Adami visited him in England, where he was Canadian high commissioner from 1896 to 1914. After they outlined the problem, he gave the faculty $50,000 to pay off the debt of $37,000, leaving $13,000 to be held by the university board of governors for future requirements. Strathcona then questioned the faculty's poor financial management and recommended to Roddick and Adami that the faculty should work toward better financial arrangements with the university. He implied that he thought the faculty should get out of the business of running its own school and that he wasn't going to live forever.

Roddick and Adami took his advice seriously and produced an amalgamation plan. As regards the arrangements between the university and the medical faculty, the faculty wanted to retain control of its appointments and a guarantee that it could retain its bequests and some of its other income. The university governors, however, could make no such guarantees. By McGill's charter, the governors controlled appointments to the university and furthermore could not guarantee that all the money that came to the faculty could be used exclusively for its purposes while other faculties might be in deficit. The governors were not going to let the Faculty of Medicine dictate the policies and terms for this full amalgamation. They wanted the faculty to carry on its own affairs as before and did not want major changes in the relationship except for better financial management. The faculty had little choice and at a meeting on 26 November 1904 agreed that "in the opinion of the

Medical Faculty, its welfare and the interests of medical education in Montreal would best be served by the faculty seeking full union with the university, and to this end a committee be appointed to convey the above resolution to the Governors of the University to discuss with them the conditions under which full union could best be accomplished, and to report to the faculty the results of the conference."

Dean Roddick and Professors Shepherd and Adami represented the faculty in the discussions with the university governors. They reported at the monthly faculty meetings, and in May 1905 it was further resolved that the faculty recognized "that the time has arrived when it is to its own best interests and those of the university that there should be full amalgamation of its affairs in the hands of the university."

The university governors received this resolution and responded with one of its own: "The Governors desired to place on record in the minutes the expression of the great gratification with which it received intimation that the Medical Faculty has resolved to place the management of its affair in the hands of the university, thereby securing complete union with that body, and with the said resolution the Board of Governors heartily and unanimously concurred."

This agreement ended seventy-six years of the Faculty of Medicine's proprietary existence and its tenuous dependence on the aging Lord Strathcona in later years.[12] Lord Strathcona died in 1914 at age ninety-four while living in the U.K.

ROBERT TAIT McKENZIE

An important personality – whose influence is still felt – arose from the medical faculty during the 1890s and the first years of the new century. Robert Tait McKenzie (fig. 29) was one of the first persons at McGill to recognize the importance of physical fitness in human health.[13] In 1898 he was appointed medical director of physical training at McGill, one of the first such positions held at a Canadian university (fig. 30).[14] He introduced compulsory physical examinations for all students entering university to determine suitable sports and exercise programs for them.

McKenzie conceived the idea of developing a department and school of physical education, but McGill did not have funds or adequate athletic facilities to support such programs. On the other hand, the University of Pennsylvania in Philadelphia, which had offered him a position, had a gymnasium, a football stadium with a running track, and other recently constructed athletic facilities. In 1904 McKenzie accepted

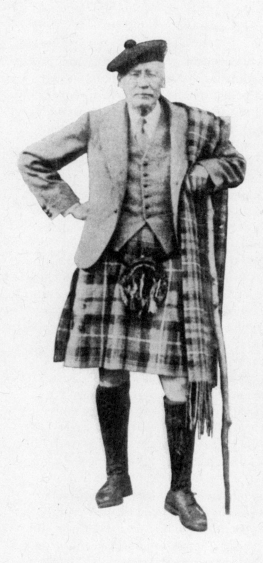

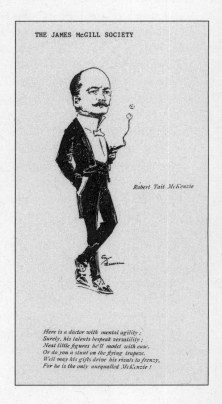

Robert Tait McKenzie

Here is a doctor with mental agility ;
Surely, his talents bespeak versatility ;
Neat little figures he'll model with ease.
Or do you a stunt on the flying trapeze.
Well may his gifts drive his rivals to frenzy,
For he is the only unequalled McKenzie !

Left: Figure 29
Robert Tait McKenzie, 1867–1938. Photographer and date unknown

Right: Figure 30
Cartoon of Robert Tait McKenzie. From F.M. Johnston's *People We Meet:
McGill Outlook* (Montreal, 1903). Collection of cartoons of McGill faculty

a position as director of the physical education department at the University of Pennsylvania where he would have greater opportunities to put his theories to work. Committed to athletics and to athletic training, he had an abiding interest in getting people to participate in athletics rather than watching, and so imposed compulsory physical education for all students at the University of Pennsylvania.

In addition to his pioneering careers in physical education and later in rehabilitation medicine,[15] McKenzie became equally renowned for his artistic ability, which he incorporated into his overall interests in medicine and athletics. He began to sketch at an early age and was quite accomplished by the time he entered medical school. He became interested in sculpture as a way of showing the faces and muscles of athletes. His first untrained effort was to sculpt four heads or masks called *The Progress in Fatigue*, with faces of athletes showing Violent Effort, Breathlessness, Fatigue, and Exhaustion (fig. 31),[16] completed after years of studying photographs of runners. As a demonstrator of anatomy (1894) he also conceived the idea of an anatomical model of a sprinter in the starting position in order to demonstrate the surface anatomy of muscles. He proposed the idea to several sculptors, but they were not interested. Undaunted, he decided to sculpt the figure himself. He measured the limbs and torsos of many athletes and obtained the services of McGill medical students who were willing to model for the figure. After many sessions he completed *The Sprinter* in 1902, revealing his remarkable untrained ability. *The Sprinter* was the second in the extraordinary series of over two hundred athletic and military figures, busts, masks, friezes, and medallions which he created, now displayed in Canada, the United States, and England. His statues stand in the Parliament Buildings in Ottawa, at McGill University, at the University of Pennsylvania, in the British House of Commons, at Cambridge University, Greenwich Park, England, Princess Street Gardens in Edinburgh, and in the Queen's Collection at Balmoral. More recently, Canada Post issued two commemorative stamps of *The Sprinter* and *The Plunger* for the 1976 Olympic Games in Montreal.

The Falcon is considered one of the best of his sculptures and the last great piece he created before his death in 1938 (fig. 32). The origin of the idea was the death in 1931 of John Webser, son of Dr Webster of Shediac, New Brunswick, in an accident during a flying race. The parents asked McKenzie to create a memorial, which turned out to be an aviation trophy for which he created a miniature figure of a man about to fly. After completing the trophy in 1934, McKenzie began to work on a sculpture depicting man's conquest of the air. He created a plaster

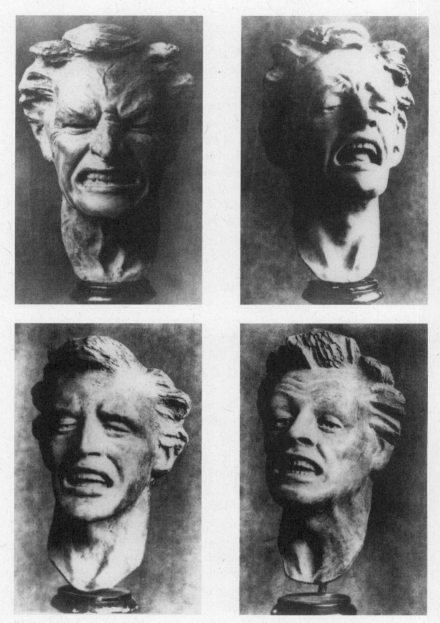

Figure 31
Masks of Facial Expressions by Robert Tait McKenzie. Four masks express-
ing "Violent Effort," "Breathlessness," "Fatigue," and "Exhaustion," 1899.
These copies of the original masks are in the MGH Library. Photo by Tom
Humphry, 1994

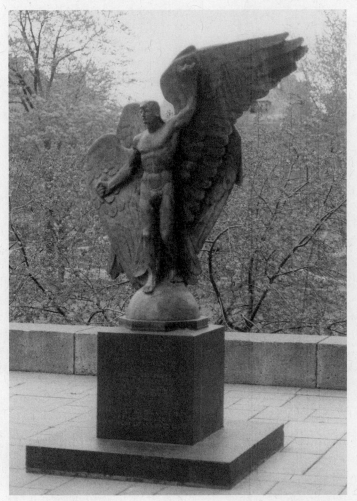

Figure 32
The Falcon by Robert Tait McKenzie 1931. One of McKenzie's finest statues donated to McGill and unveiled 1951. Photo by Tom Humphry, 1994

figure of a man with huge wings that he wanted to be erected at McGill as a record of his affection for his alma mater. The original sculpture was created in his Philadelphia studio. After his death in 1938, McKenzie's widow tried for years to have the sculpture cast in bronze. Finally in 1951 an anonymous donor gave $9,500 to have the statue cast and installed at McGill. The formal unveiling was held on the plaza outside the McLennan Library building in the summer of 1951 in the presence of F. Cyril James, principal and vice-chancellor of McGill.[17]

Although McKenzie's time at McGill was brief and few now know his name, his recognition of physical training as an important element in health education pioneered the emphasis on fitness in Canada and is an important chapter in McGill's history.

AMALGAMATION WITH BISHOP'S
MEDICAL FACULTY

As if a major enlargement of the Medical Building, the founding of a dental department, and full amalgamation with McGill University were not enough changes for the first five years of the twentieth century, Dean Roddick received a letter on 7 January 1905 that was to top all of these and change medical education in the Province of Quebec. The letter from Dean F.W. Campbell of Bishop's University Medical Faculty referred obliquely to an interest in amalgamating with McGill.

A group of Montreal doctors had founded the Medical Faculty of Bishop's University in 1871. A.H. David was dean from 1871 to 1880, and then F.W. Campbell, one of the founders and a professor at the school, succeeded him.[18] Bishop's Medical Faculty had fifty students enrolled and 246 graduates, but lacked adequate laboratory, museum, and library facilities to carry on efficient medical education. The school ran on a limited budget with volunteer clinical staff and had no debt. Among its graduates were Casey A. Wood, William Henry Drummond, Octavia Grace Ritchie, and Maude Elizabeth Seymour Abbott.[19]

The McGill Faculty of Medicine found Dean Campbell's letter of 7 January so vague that no decision could be made until Bishop's stated what it wanted. Committees from both faculties met, but Dean Campbell broke off negotiations in a letter to Roddick on 8 February 1905. Concerned with personal and family problems, he resigned as dean in April 1905 and died the following month.[20]

On 18 February 1905, Dean Roddick had received a letter from the Vice-Dean J.B. McConnell of Bishop's Medical Faculty indicating a continued interest in amalgamation. The letter clearly stated that once its medical faculty was dissolved, Bishop's had no desire to renew medical teaching. A second appeal was being made for resumption of committee meetings between the two faculties:

Dear Sir:
Being concerned that we had arrived at a wrong interpretation of the true attitude of your faculty in regard to the proposed fusion of the two faculties and feeling assured that if the statements made to us were placed before our members

that they would view the matter in a more favourable light, I have at the earliest opportunity conferred with them. They now state that we are prepared to reopen negotiations, if we hear from you that it is the desire of your faculty to have the discussion continued. It is, however, necessary to point out that action on your part cannot be greatly delayed if anything definite is to be accomplished.

[signed: J. B. McConnell]

Meetings were held in February, March, and April 1905 in the McGill faculty board room, attended by William Gardner (acting dean in Dean Roddick's absence), Principal William Peterson, and Robert Ruttan from McGill, and Vice-Dean McConnell, W.H. Drummond, and F. England from Bishop's. The following points were discussed on 29 February 1905:

1 The right of the University of Bishop's College to carry on instruction of medicine in Montreal: to be surrendered for a few years or permanently.
2 The status of students already enrolled in Bishop's (fifty in all). Initially it was thought that Bishop's students would be accepted at McGill on an equal basis, but consideration by the latter required transferring students to start in the first year if they wanted a McGill degree or continue at McGill and be given a Bishop's degree on graduation.
3 The appointment of Dean F.W. Campbell as a McGill professor emeritus.
4 Bishop's students at McGill to be listed as Bishop's students in the McGill calendar.
5 Bishop's faculty members to be given an *ad eundem* M.D., C.M. degree from McGill.
6 The future management of the $2,000 endowment of the Wood and Nelson medals.
7 The movable property of Bishop's Medical Faculty: all to go to McGill.
8 The lease on the F.W. Campbell Building in downtown Montreal: Bishop's requested that McGill assume the remainder of the lease.
9 The status of the Women's Hospital (Bishop's obstetrical facility, which was not in debt): to be determined.
10 Appointments to the Western General Hospital (fig. 33)[21]: Bishop's requested that McGill not interfere with the Bishop's staff at the Western General Hospital (Bishop's teaching hospital) and that

Western General Hospital continue to make its appointments independent of McGill.

11 English representatives to the Quebec College of Physicians and Surgeons: an application would be made to the Quebec Medical Board to maintain the English representation.

12 Appointment of members of Bishop's Medical Faculty to that of McGill: such appointments would be made on a need basis at McGill.

14 Financial status of Bishop's Medical Faculty: it was noted that Bishop's had no debt and a surplus of $1,200–1,300 for the year.

In the summer of 1905 the two universities signed an agreement of amalgamation, and the Bishop's Medical Faculty ceased to exist.[22] On 21 August 1905 Vice-Dean J.B. McConnell sent a letter to Bishop's medical graduates:

[Dean F.W. Campbell's] resignation, a few months before his death, precipitated the necessity for a reorganization of the Faculty, and with this end in view it had under consideration the strengthening of the teaching staff, a new college building, enlarged hospital facilities, &c. To have realized the ideals proposed for the prosecution of the Faculty's work on adequate lines, would have meant the raising of a considerable amount of money and the existence of a much larger degree of enthusiasm and unity of purpose than was then apparent.

Notwithstanding the difficulties in the way, a determination to make the attempt was being seriously entertained. About this time the question of amalgamation with the Medical Faculty of McGill University was suggested as a solution of our Faculty's future. After many conferences, an agreement was finally adopted by the Faculties and Corporations of each University.

By this agreement the University of Bishop's College will not teach medicine, nor confer degrees in medicine in this Province, for at least 15 years. All students are taken over *ad eundem statum*. The *ad eundem* degree has been conferred upon those members of the staff who had only Bishop's College degrees. The application of any graduate of our College for the *ad eundem* degree will be considered. A list of our graduates will appear in the McGill College Calendar, a copy of which will be sent to you annually.

As regards the McGill degree, the arrangement was made that any Bishop's medical graduate could apply to the McGill Faculty of Medicine for a McGill M.D., C.M. *ad eundem*. On review of the application by the McGill faculty, this would be considered but by no means guaranteed. This was particularly attractive since after 1908 there was reciprocity between the Medical Board of the College of Physicians and

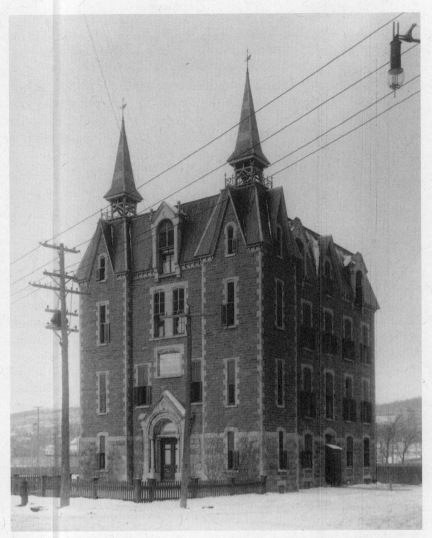

Figure 33
Original Western General Hospital near St Catherine Street and Atwater
Avenue. Later it became the Western Division of the MGH, then a part of the
Montreal Children's Hospital. Photo by William Notman, 1902

Surgeons of Quebec and the General Medical Council of Britain.[23] Initially most of the Bishop's medical graduates who applied resided in the Montreal area and were known to the faculty so there was little difficulty in making positive recommendations to the McGill Corporation. However, the faculty continued to receive applications for the McGill degree from Bishop's graduates through 1914.[24] Applications from doctors living at a distance from Montreal who were not known to the faculty were approved only after appropriate investigation of the professional standing of each applicant. Bishop's medical graduates had to attend a regular McGill convocation to receive the McGill M.D., C.M. degree.

THE FIRE IN THE MEDICAL BUILDING

In the spring of 1907 it appeared that Roddick's trials and pressures were about to end, and he intended to resign as dean in June. However, on the night of 15 April 1907 Professor John Cox was walking up University Street north of Milton at 1:00 A.M. when he noticed flames coming from upper windows on the east side of the Medical Building. (These were later tentatively identified as the windows of the Faculty Conference Room where a meeting had terminated at 10:00 P.M., although students who were in the building when the fire started reported smoke in the upper floors but saw no fire coming from the Conference Room.) Cox and other observers notified the fire brigade. They arrived in minutes, but to their consternation found low water pressure, so at first the blaze was not fought. This was corrected shortly, according to eyewitnesses.[26]

The fire started in the central part of the Medical Building (fig. 34),[27] which had been renovated in 1901. The construction was mainly of wood. Despite the efforts of the fire brigade, the major conflagration in the central portion of the building[28] was soon out of control. Ablaze with flames leaping high into the night, the roof and cupolas of the central wing eventually collapsed. The fire brigade then concentrated its efforts on preventing spread to the north and south wings and brought the fire under control by 3:00 A.M.

Miraculously, the library on the south end of the Medical Building was saved, but two-thirds of the 23,000 volumes in the library suffered water damage and had to be dried and repaired. The anatomy and pathology museums were not as fortunate, with part of the collections accumulated since the opening of the Montreal Medical Institution destroyed. This included many of the specimens collected by

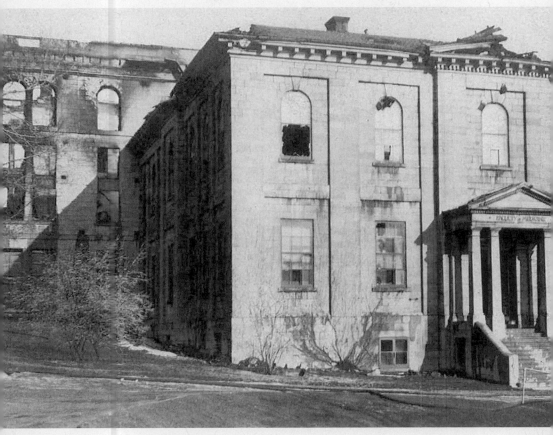

Figure 34
Ruins of the McGill Medical Building the morning after the fire on 17 April
1907. *Old McGill*, 1909

Osler and Shepherd. Many other pathology specimens, including original ones in jars, survived with the help of Maude Abbott and medical
students who carried them out or dropped them from the windows.
The northernmost portion of the building with the pathology and hygiene laboratories was also saved. Tragically, the notes, photographs,
and unpublished manuscript of Adami's *Textbook of Pathology* burned
in his office. Adami was disappointed, but he reassembled the manuscript and submitted it for publication the following year.

On-site descriptions of the fire by reporters are remarkably vague as
to what was actually destroyed. The best estimate is that approximately one-third of the Medical Building was unusable or destroyed by the

fire. The following noon the faculty executive met in an emergency session in the Arts Building to discuss the disaster, assess the damage, and make plans for the short and long term.[29] The first priority was to make arrangements to continue teaching for the balance of the academic year. The medical school lectures resumed in the Arts, Physics, and Chemistry buildings and the intact parts of the Medical Building. The second priority was to arrange short-term repairs to the burned building. The building committee met that night and decided to repair the roof of the laboratory wing (north side) and renovate the usable laboratories so that the spring session of 1907 could finish with the least inconvenience. Roddick revised his plan to retire in June 1907, agreeing to continue as dean until June 1908.

When questioned about the origin of the fire, Dean Roddick felt that there was evidence of arson because of a statement by a young Bank of Montreal employee who happened to be walking through the McGill grounds and noticed suspicious characters in the bushes outside the main entrance to the Medical Building at about 12:30 A.M. Even more important was the unexplained fire in the Engineering Building a week or so before the fire in the Medical Building. The suspicion that students had caused the fire was discounted when no record of disgruntled students could be found. Roddick felt strongly that someone had set both fires, perhaps a discharged employee who thought he had a grievance. Another possible explanation was faulty electrical wiring. The Fire Commission of Montreal held hearings, reviewed all available information, and decided that the fire was accidental because there was no firm evidence to the contrary.[30]

Money for repairs had to come from outside donors because there was insufficient insurance on the building. Many institutions and individuals sympathetic to McGill's plight contributed funds for reconstruction. The fire evoked sympathy from McGill graduates, the governor general of Canada, the deans of Queen's and Laval universities, the Quebec government, the City of Montreal and Quebec City, and many individuals such as William Osler, Charles Moyse, Stephen Leacock, and Lord Strathcona. Many of them contributed money for the reconstruction; even the Montreal General Hospital contributed $500.

The third priority was to develop plans for a completely new fireproof building. On 20 April 1907, five days after the fire, the faculty engaged Percy Nobbs, McGill's professor of architecture,[31] to make preliminary plans to accommodate the needs of the medical school. He suggested a competition for the design of a new medical building. The approximately $360,000 paid out from the fire insurance was far short of what was needed for both the repair of the old building and construction of a new one. Once again Lord Strathcona came to the rescue. He purchased the property at the southwest corner of Pine Avenue and University Street (opposite the Royal Victoria) and presented it along with $450,000 to the medical faculty. Strathcona's generous gift together with the insurance provided enough money for both projects. The former Medical Building was repaired and renovated. The east wing of the new building was completed in 1910. A formal opening was planned in that year but then postponed until June 1911 because of the death of King Edward VII and the coronation of King George V.

THE FIVE-YEAR COURSE

In 1894 Professor Adami had proposed that the medical course be extended by adding a fifth year to provide more clinical experience for students before they started to practise. However, money was not available for the expense of an additional year, so no action was taken.[32] The plan for a five-year program was discussed again in 1907 and was finalized as the fire disaster was being settled. Specific schedules for the fourth and fifth years were presented at faculty meetings. The extra expenditures required for the fifth year were made possible in 1907 when Lord Strathcona donated $50,000 to fund the program for the next five years.

The fifth-year curriculum was planned for senior students to gain further practical experience in the medical and surgical clinics and on the hospital wards. Student hospital training was still seriously lacking because of the unwillingness of the hospital authorities to allow students to be involved in the treatment of patients. Hospital authorities were so strict about this that it was clearly stated on the back of student perpetual cards[33] that a student was forbidden to discuss a patient's illness without the permission of attending staff. Resident training remained the same at this time, although there was an increase in the number of house officers at the Montreal General and the Royal Victoria.[34] Ward training at the bedside for house officers and medical students still lacked any sense of teamwork.

The problems of practical training were recognized, but resistance from the hospital boards of governors persisted for decades. Buller as well as others had been aware of this many years before. In a frank statement to medical students, he debunked the tradition of passively walking the wards in Europe as a useful alternative experience to a proper student clerkship or housemanship. He criticized the bogus belief of students who claimed this experience qualified them for practice.[35] It would appear that he was striking directly at McGill's policy of passive clinical training on the wards.

In 1919 the medical course was extended to six years to enhance the medical students' clinical experience. Most of them started medical practice immediately after graduation. There was a feeling that clinical training had not been extensive enough because residency training was available to so few. Students who had been in the Canadian Army Medical Corps (CAMC) during World War I, or who had entered the medical faculty before 1919, were exempted from the sixth year.

FURTHER CHANGES IN THE CURRICULUM

By 1910 the medical school curriculum had changed in only one major way – it took five years to graduate instead of four. The five-year course started with the 1908–09 session. The first-year class of 1908 started their fourth year in September 1911, their fifth year in September 1912; they graduated in May 1913.

The curriculum for the first three years was unaltered. The major courses taught for two years were anatomy, physiology, chemistry, and pharmacology and therapeutics. The theory and practice of medicine, surgery, obstetrics, diseases of infants, gynecology, and clinical medicine and surgery were taught in the senior years. All other courses were taught for one year (nine months) or one semester for minor subjects. Chemistry, physics, and biology (botany and zoology) remained in the medical school curriculum because the majority of medical students were high school graduates with minimal or no training in science subjects.

The education committee was charged with the responsibility of determining the curriculum for the fourth and fifth years. After numerous discussions and several reports, in May 1911 the faculty executive approved the curriculum for the additional years.[36] Regular clinics in mental diseases were established in the fifth year.[37] Otherwise students spent most of the time in the clinics, seeing and examining patients. The new curriculum also included a course on clinical microscopy. Starting in 1910 medical students had the use of microscopes in the hospitals for doing simple laboratory tests such as blood smears and urinalysis. Fourth and fifth year students were required to purchase a hemoglobinometer and to learn to use it. Examinations were conducted annually, and failure in one or two subjects meant a supplementary examination in the autumn. If a student failed in more than two subjects, or in anatomy or physiology, he had to repeat the year.

The fire that destroyed the central portion of the Medical Building in 1907, although a tragic loss for the faculty and a tremendous inconvenience, was an impetus to make changes in the organization of the teaching facilities and the future location of laboratories for courses such as chemistry, physics, and biology that were also being taught in the Faculty of Arts and Applied Science. The development of sophisticated undergraduate science departments as well as influence from Europe had already convinced many university medical schools to utilize other faculties for teaching science courses rather than duplicating them in the medical school. The fire disaster created an opportunity to reorganize the medical curriculum so that some of the primary subjects were eventually taught in undergraduate faculties.

The faculty executive referred this matter to the education committee. After several reports the faculty executive decided that medical chemistry, anatomy, histology, embryology, pathology, and physiology would be taught in the new Strathcona Medical Building (SMB). Biology and organic chemistry, still taught in first-year medicine, would be taught in other buildings. The old Medical Building was renovated for biology and organic chemistry. When the Biology Building was opened in 1922, it housed biology (botany and zoology), biochemistry, physiology, and experimental medicine. In 1924 pathology and bacteriology moved into the new Pathological Institute on Upper University Street opposite the Royal Victoria Hospital.

Science courses and the construction of laboratory facilities were not the only interest of the faculty. A small group interested in the history of medicine wanted to introduce to the curriculum an element of humanity that was missing on the hospital wards. As a result, in 1907 Andrew Macphail was appointed professor of history of medicine at McGill. This was an interesting appointment because at that time McGill had a limited library collection in the history of medicine, and no one heretofore had considered it an important subject. Macphail gave an annual series of lectures in the history of medicine in the late afternoon or evening. This was an optional course open to all medical undergraduates, with no examination.

After the onset of the war Macphail went overseas with No. 6 Field Ambulance CAMC. When he returned to McGill after the war, he continued as professor of history of medicine and wrote the history of the Canadian medical services during the war.[38] William W. Francis, Osler's nephew[39] started at McGill as demonstrator of pathology before the war. He went overseas with No. 3 Canadian General Hospital. In 1919 he went to Oxford to work on Osler's bibliography. In 1929 when Osler's library came to McGill, Francis became the Osler Librarian, and when Macphail retired in 1937, McGill's second professor of medical history.

RODDICK AND THE MEDICAL COUNCIL OF CANADA

Between 1885 and 1893 Roddick was at the peak of his teaching and surgical activities. He had developed and promoted Listerian antisepsis and improved operating room procedures.[40] In 1885 he did a masterful job as deputy surgeon general and chief of the medical staff in the field during the Riel Rebellion. When he stopped operative surgery in 1893, by nature he needed another cause. He found one at the Canadian Medical Association meeting in St John's, Newfoundland, in 1894. The members discussed the issue of uniform standards of medical education and registration in all Canadian provinces. Palmer Howard had advocated this for years. Roddick realized the importance of this issue and accepted the chairmanship of a CMA committee to further this end.

Initially he had to convince the association members of the need for general guidelines in establishing a qualification for dominion registration. Such a qualification would allow physicians to move amongst the provinces without having to take additional provincial qualifying examinations. The main obstacle was the lack of cooperation between the provincial medical boards. They did not want to compromise their authority in educational affairs or their control over the standards of medical training and the issuing of licences to practise medicine. There was a misunderstanding because Roddick's idea was for central registration, not for control of premedical or medical education or the discipline of doctors. He provided convincing arguments in favour of a dominion medical board. With his remarkable persuasive powers and tempered approach, he finally prevailed upon the medical representatives on his CMA committee to draw up a bill to be read to parliament in March 1901.

The second obstacle was to convince members of parliament and the Liberal prime minister, Sir Wilfred Laurier,[41] that the bill would not infringe on the provincial authority to control medical policy. Initially Sir Wilfred did not clearly understand all the ramifications of the bill, but he agreed to send it to committee for further study. With extraordinary statesmanship Roddick (fig. 35) – a Conservative member of parliament – lobbied for the bill, by now known as the "Roddick Bill" (fig. 36),[42] stressing that although a central medical board would be in the best interests of the medical profession of Canada, it would not require any provincial medical board to join. Once Laurier realized that the

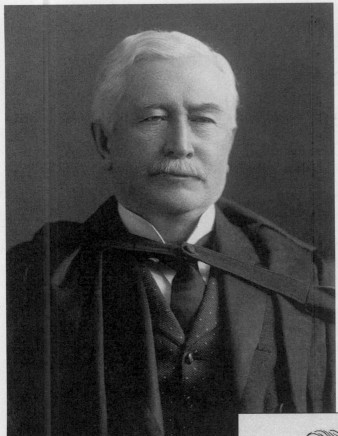

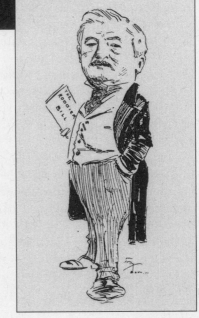

Figure 35
Sir Thomas George Roddick,
1846–1923. Photo by William Notman

Figure 36
Cartoon of Roddick carrying the
"Roddick Bill." From F.M. Johnson's
People We Meet: McGill Outlook
(Montreal, 1903)

bill would actually improve reciprocal relations with the provinces, he gave his support. The Canadian Medical Act passed the third reading in 1902 and provided for the establishment of the Dominion Medical Council.[43]

Having already spent eight years promoting this important issue, Roddick had a greater struggle to convince all of the provinces to agree to a Dominion Medical Council. The provincial medical boards were to remain intact, since the new council had no intention of assuming a disciplinary role. Once the provinces consented to the Canada Medical Act establishing the Medical Council of Canada, an amended bill was passed by parliament in 1911 ending an eighteen-year effort by Roddick to establish a central medical council whose diploma would enable the holder to practise throughout the Dominion of Canada, be qualified for military service, and be admitted to the British Registry with reciprocity. In 1912 Roddick was unanimously elected the first president of the Medical Council of Canada and later was elected "Honorary CMA President for Life" in recognition of his remarkable accomplishments. Dean Shepherd represented McGill at the council's first meeting in 1912. The first examinations for the Licentiate of the Medical Council of Canada (LMCC) were held in Montreal in October 1913, conducted in both English and French.[44]

In 1907 Roddick resigned as professor of surgery and was succeeded by James Bell, previously professor of clinical surgery. George Armstrong, attending surgeon at the Montreal General, was appointed professor of clinical surgery.[45] Roddick attended his last faculty meeting in June 1908, receiving a tribute:[46]

The members of the Medical Faculty desire at this meeting to place on record their high appreciation of the services of Dr. Roddick to the faculty and to the university during the 36 years in which he has been connected with the teaching staff, and especially during the past six years when he has so ably filled the post of dean.

During his tenure of the deanship, among other advances, the Bishop's Medical Faculty has been absorbed by this university, the [McGill] Medical Faculty has assumed a closer relationship with the university at large, the dental department has been instituted, and the medical course has been lengthened from four to five years. In all of these Dr. Roddick has taken a very active part. During the whole period of his connection with the teaching staff, the Faculty desires at this time to recognize the great earnestness, capacity and tact which Dr. Roddick has invariably shown in forwarding the best interests of the Faculty and the University.

DEANSHIP OF FRANCIS JOHN SHEPHERD,
1908–14

In 1908 the university governors appointed Francis Shepherd (fig. 37)[47] to succeed Roddick. He was well qualified to serve as dean of the medical faculty. He had been a member of the teaching staff for thirty-three years and had served the faculty in many capacities: professor of anatomy since 1883, librarian, member at one time or another of all five of the faculty's standing committees, and the faculty's elected representative to the McGill Corporation. When Shepherd accepted the post of dean on a part-time basis, he already had many commitments. For the next six years he devoted a great deal of time to the affairs of the faculty while gradually reducing his other activities and responsibilities.

In 1893, when Roddick moved from the Montreal General to assume the post of chief surgeon at the Royal Victoria, Shepherd had become senior attending surgeon at the General.[48] Shepherd stopped operating in 1911 because of developing cataracts. He retired as attending surgeon in 1913 and was appointed to the MGH consulting staff.[49]

In addition Shepherd held several administrative appointments. He was chairman of the MGH medical board from 1904 to 1914, and a member of the committee of management from 1906 to 1918. A connoisseur of art, he was president of the Art Association of Montreal from 1906 to 1910 and again from 1918 to 1929. From 1910 he was a member of the Advisory Arts Council of the National Gallery of Canada. He attended numerous medical association meetings in Montreal and other cities, such as the American Dermatology Association and American Surgical Association meetings in 1912 in Washington, D.C.

In his personal life, Shepherd, a widower since 1892, continued to live in his residence at 152 Mansfield Avenue at the corner of Burnside.[50] Whenever possible, he went to his country home, "Kanastake," in Como.[51] His son Ernest was married in 1908. In 1909 his older daughter, Cecelia, married Percy Nobbs, McGill's professor of architecture. His younger daughter, Dorothy, acted as his hostess and travelled with him frequently.[52] While he was dean, Shepherd went to Europe three times in 1909, 1912, and 1913[53] during the summer months. Nearly every May or June, and especially during the years when he did not travel to Europe, he went salmon fishing on the Pabos River in the Gaspé Peninsula.[54]

The faculty had made four important decisions during Roddick's deanship. During Shepherd's deanship, there remained a great deal of work to be done to implement those decisions. When the faculty executive held the

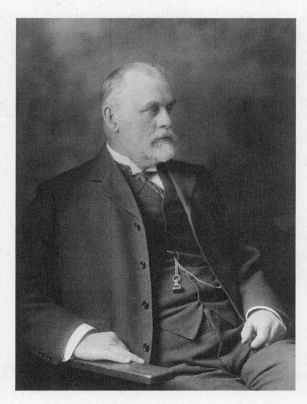

Figure 37
Francis John
Shepherd, 1851–1929.
Photo by William
Notman, 1914

first meeting for the 1908–09 session in September 1908, an urgent agen-
da item was the completion of the plans for the new Medical Building. By
1908 the east wing (University Street) had been designed to house anatomy, pathology, bacteriology, the dental department, and the faculty administrative offices. The design of the remainder of the building had to be
finalized – the west wing, the north or museum wing, and the connecting
corridor. Before this could be done, the faculty executive had to decide
which subjects would be taught in the medical faculty and which ones in
the arts faculty. They referred the matter to the education and building
committees and then accepted their recommendations. The design of the
new Strathcona Medical Building included the central part between the
east and west wings (fig. 38) to house the library for sixty thousand volumes with a large reading room spanning the length of the top floor and
glass-floored stacks below. The three floors of the north wing were devoted to a spacious anatomical and pathological museum, (fig. 39) and
three large lecture rooms. The west wing included an assembly hall with
capacity for up to four hundred persons and accommodation for hygiene,

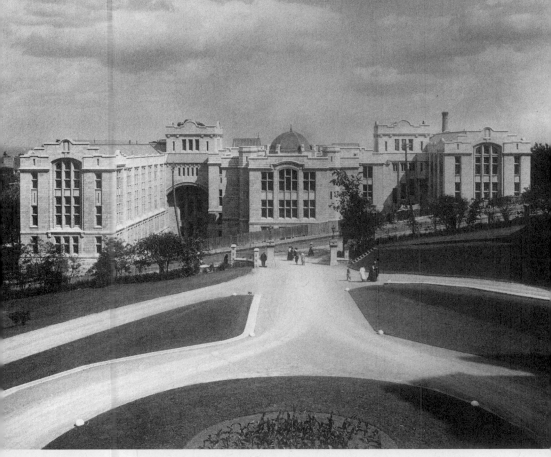

Figure 38
North side, Strathcona Medical Building from the front drive of the RVH.
Photo by William Notman, 1912

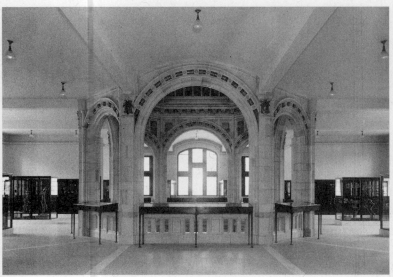

Figure 39
Strathcona
Medical Building,
one floor of the
Medical Museum
which occupied
three floors on
the north side of
the building.
Photo by William
Notman, 1911

pharmacology, and experimental medicine on the upper floors. In addition there was a facility for animals on the top floor of the west wing. Faculty approved the final design in February 1910 and the McGill governors approved the plans in April 1910. Construction started shortly thereafter and was completed the following year.

EXPERIMENTAL MEDICINE

One of the most important decisions during Shepherd's deanship was to establish a Department of Experimental Medicine, housed with hygiene in the west wing of the new Medical Building. This was the first formal recognition and support for the faculty's role in medical research.[55] In October 1912, J.C. Meakins was appointed secretary of the Committee on Experimental Medicine. In 1912 the faculty received an endowment of $60,000 to be known as the Cooper Fund.[56] Part of the interest from the fund was available to support the Department of Experimental Medicine. J.C. Meakins was appointed the department's director.[57]

Hardly had the department commenced activities when Meakins was granted leave of absence for the 1913–14 session in order to pursue further studies in Europe.[58] Shortly after his return to McGill, he went overseas again with the No. 3 Canadian General Hospital, so there was little activity in the Department of Experimental Medicine for the war years. Returning from overseas in 1918, Meakins reactivated the department, and several research projects were started, but then he resigned to accept a professorship in Edinburgh.[59] After the arrangements had been completed for the university clinic at the Royal Victoria, the faculty decided that John Tait, professor and chairman of physiology, would be the director of the Department of Experimental Medicine. In 1928 Tait and McNally started a research program on labyrinthine function. In May 1931 the medical faculty established a Department of Experimental Medicine and Surgery.

THE FLEXNER REPORT

The Flexner Report[60] (fig. 40) had its origin in an action taken in 1906–07 by the American Medical Association's (AMA) Council on Medical Education. Suspecting that some medical schools were "diploma mills" – more interested in financial gain for the directors of the medical school than in the quality of medical education – the council sponsored a survey of medical school education in the United States.

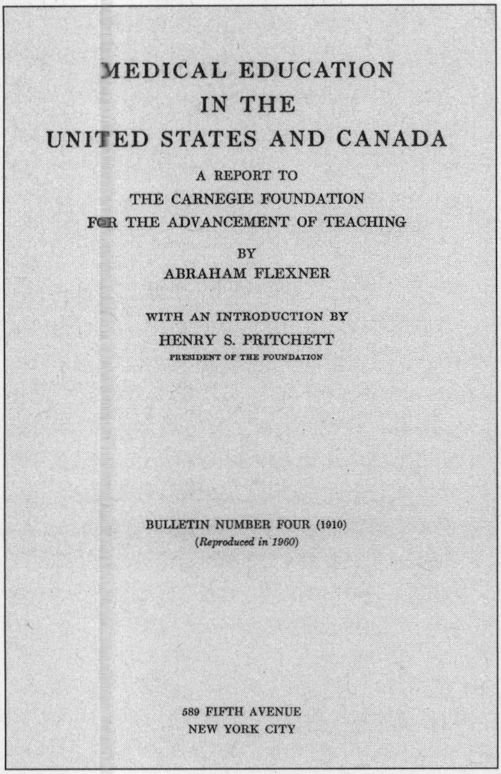

MEDICAL EDUCATION
IN THE
UNITED STATES AND CANADA

A REPORT TO
THE CARNEGIE FOUNDATION
FOR THE ADVANCEMENT OF TEACHING

BY
ABRAHAM FLEXNER

WITH AN INTRODUCTION BY
HENRY S. PRITCHETT
PRESIDENT OF THE FOUNDATION

BULLETIN NUMBER FOUR (1910)
(Reproduced in 1960)

589 FIFTH AVENUE
NEW YORK CITY

Figure 40
Title page of *Medical Education in the United States and Canada* by Abraham Flexner (NewYork, 1910)

The report of the survey was critical of many medical schools and had marked political overtones. In 1908 the council decided that it would be better if an independent organization published the report of the survey and approached the Carnegie Foundation. Henry S. Pritchett, president of the foundation, and the council agreed that in order to avoid claims of partiality, the report should not mention the AMA's findings or its role in the study. The Carnegie Foundation must make its own survey based on the AMA's findings.

The next step was for the Carnegie Foundation to appoint a qualified person to conduct the survey. The name of Abraham Flexner was suggested to Pritchett. Flexner was a schoolteacher from Louisville, Kentucky, who became disappointed with graduate education in the United States and went to Heidelberg in Germany to study science. His impressions of the intensity, emphasis, and quality of German science education influenced his opinions about North American medical education. One result was his book on American university education, *The*

American College: A Criticism.[61] The book came to Pritchett's attention. With Pritchett's support, together with the influence of Flexner's brother Simon (president of the Rockefeller Institute) and the president of Johns Hopkins University, Flexner was invited by the Carnegie Foundation to study medical education in the United States and Canada and to report to the foundation.

To determine what the ideal medical school was, Flexner went to Germany to visit schools there and studied the Hopkins program in the United States. He itemized positive features and established his criteria. To conduct the survey, Flexner visited a number of schools over the period of a week or two and then went home to write out the evaluations from his notes. He then sent letters to each of the deans for their corrections, which he included in his final report. Reading Flexner's sometimes searing condemnations, deans frequently complained to the Carnegie Foundation, mainly about the short time that Flexner had spent evaluating their facilities.

In making his evaluations, Flexner sat in the dean's office and asked for various records – such as financial, personnel, and student records, to which he applied his established criteria. These were:

1 the school's entrance requirements and their enforcement
2 the training and background of the faculty
3 the funds available from all sources to run the medical school
4 the number, quality, and adequacy of the student laboratories for pre-clinical training
5 the relationship between the medical school and its teaching hospitals, access to the hospitals, and the number of hospital beds available for teaching.

If the school did not meet his criteria in these five areas, Flexner said so in his report. As a result, the Carnegie Institute received many letters criticizing his attitude and his superficial evaluation of each school. Pritchett considered replacing him, but when Flexner's criteria for a good medical school were known, it was easy to see that, if he were given the required documents, it should take him no more than one or two hours to make his evaluation. In the end Flexner convinced Pritchett that he knew what he was doing.

Responding to harsh criticism of the Washington University School of Medicine in St Louis, Missouri, Robert Brookings, who was putting $15,000 to $20,000 into the medical school annually, demanded that Flexner come to St Louis to defend his report. When they met, Flexner asked if Brookings wanted to show him the medical school, or whether Brookings wanted Flexner to show him the medical school. Brookings agreed to let Flexner show him what the problems were. It took no more than two hours, starting in the dean's office where they looked at student qualifications, then going through and assessing various laboratories and other equipment, before Brookings conceded that what Flexner had written was correct. Brookings asked how to rectify the situation. Flexner's response was: "Close the medical school, get rid of the student body, build a new medical school on the Johns Hopkins model, get new chairmen and start over again."

Flexner surveyed 155 medical schools. Only sixteen required two or more years of college education as admission criteria. Only one, Johns Hopkins, required four years and a bachelor degree and completion of courses in chemistry, physics, biology, French, and German. About fifty medical schools had entrance requirements equal to high-school graduation. The remaining medical schools were proprietary, their only requirement for admission being the ability to pay the tuition fees.

The Flexner Report, published in 1910, established what medical education should be. Quoted widely by the press, it was an enormous public-relations success rather than an exposé of what was already known in 1906–07 by the AMA Council. The report produced prolonged debate and resulted in the closure of some seventy medical schools over the next five to ten years. Undoubtedly the report hastened the demise of the schools with the lowest marks in the AMA study – schools that would have been isolated by the AMA study anyway.

An important event during Shepherd's deanship was Flexner's visit to McGill in March 1909 and the receipt of his report in 1910. Flexner found a partially burned Medical Building, an energetic, scientifically oriented staff, ten of whom were full time, nineteen professors, an ample tuition income, good financial management from McGill University, advanced laboratories in all the subjects, plans for a new Medical Building, a large library, and ample hospital beds at the two teaching hospitals – all of which he considered evidence of advanced medical training. Flexner gave McGill an A-minus rating. The Toronto medical faculty also received an A-minus rating.

It is a misconception, however, that Flexner's visit stimulated changes at McGill because of his cryptic, irreverent comments on bad medical schools. What he saw at McGill had been developed before anyone had heard of Abraham Flexner, because of the influence of many previous members of the staff and the munificence of Sir Donald Smith, Sir William Macdonald, John H.R. Molson, Peter Redpath, and other benefactors.

What Flexner's report did not do for McGill was to seriously evaluate the clinical training at the Montreal General and Royal Victoria. The strong approval of the emphasis on the pre-clinical sciences only reinforced McGill's attitudes toward science training and probably delayed the concern for the quality of clinical training for at least a decade.

Although McGill fared well in the Flexner Report, many other schools did not. By 1930 most of the medical schools in Canada had obtained private funding to rebuild their institutions and were near the A level rating. Flexner went on to review medical schools in Britain and Europe.[62]

DEAN SHEPHERD'S RETIREMENT

Shepherd attended his last faculty meeting as dean in June 1914. At the first meeting for the session of 1914–15 on 28 September, the faculty executive approved a resolution:[63]

The members of the McGill Medical Faculty at this their first autumn session desire to place on record their high appreciation of the services rendered to the faculty by their retiring dean, Francis J. Shepherd, MD, LLD (Harvard and Edinburgh), FRCS (Edinburgh and England), whose term of office finished with the close of the last [1913–14] session. They recognize the high ideals that have always inspired his teaching during the 30 years he occupied the chair of anatomy. It was in a great measure owing to his zeal and earnest work that the museum was placed in the first rank of American medical museums connected with teaching schools. The library owes much to him – for years he acted as librarian and devoted time and energy to perfecting its arrangements, and through his influence many valuable donations have been received. During the term of his deanship the Faculty has made a steady advance in efficiency towards the attainment of which he has given much time and earnest thought. Dr. Shepherd's presence will be greatly missed by every member of the faculty.

Shepherd lived for fifteen years after his retirement from the deanship in 1914. He wrote his memoirs, held several administrative positions, and from time to time the medical faculty and the teaching hospitals sought his advice.[64] The McGill governors appointed Herbert S. Birkett to succeed Shepherd as faculty's seventh dean.[65]

3 World War I and the Early Postwar Years, 1914–22

> The question may be asked – whether as professors we do not
> stay too long in one place ... To a man of active mind too long
> attachment to one college is apt to breed self-satisfaction, to nar-
> row his outlook, to foster a local spirit, and to promote senility.
> WILLIAM OSLER[1]

THE CANADIAN OFFICER TRAINING
CORPS AND NO. 3 CANADIAN GENERAL
HOSPITAL (McGILL)

At the turn of the century, imperialism was a popular ideology, and
there were numerous imperialist spokesmen at McGill. Behind British
imperialism lay the belief that the moral, educational, and political development of Great Britain should be extended to the underdeveloped
world, including Canada. It was the justification for the colonial policies of Britain and was supported by two generations that flourished
during the second half of the nineteenth century and up to World War
I. (A similar situation was occurring in the United States at the time that
Theodore Roosevelt was president.) Kipling wrote about "the white
man's burden" – the duty to educate and protect the heathen from the
outside world.[2] This was certainly more than subtle racism. Victorian
morality became the focus of imperialists promoting dedication and
duty to the British Empire.

Lord Strathcona was a committed imperialist. He donated funds to
support military training at schools that prepared young men to be sent
to the corners of the world in the name of the empire. The empire was
felt to have a divine mission to Christianize and civilize the world and
to extend the concepts of freedom, justice, and peace by military means.
Imperialism stood for idealistic service and self-sacrifice in the name of
God, king and country. Stephen Leacock, Andrew Macphail, and John

McCrae – well known McGill imperialists – felt that Canada had taken the best of British values and adapted them for Canadian conditions. However, the horrendous casualties in World War I from infectious diseases, not from wounds, would raise serious questions about British imperialism.

In 1907 a McGill delegation – probably influenced by some of McGill's imperialist spokesmen – went to Ottawa to plead for federal government support for a rifle-training program that had been in operation at McGill for two years. The government's enthusiastic response was to ask Principal Peterson if McGill would be willing to sponsor a course of broader training designed for future officers in the military. McGill arranged such a course from 1907 to 1909. It was successful, and discussion continued towards establishing a government-sponsored officers training program at Canadian universities. The concept of a Canadian Officers' Training Corps (COTC) was conceived, and a course was established at McGill in 1912 – the first university officer training corps in North America. In November the armoury was the Joseph House at the corner of Sherbrooke and McTavish streets, a gift from Sir William Macdonald; the McGill campus was the parade ground.[3] The training was for command officers and not specifically for medical personnel; nevertheless, many McGill physicians and surgeons were associated with reserve military units in Montreal because of the imperialist tradition.[4]

Herbert Stanley Birkett (fig. 41), for example, retired in 1910 from a reserve unit of the Canadian Army Medical Corps (CAMC).[5] With the onset of the war in August 1914, he offered his services to the military and was reappointed lieutenant colonel in the Medical Corps and assistant director of medical services for No. 4 Military District (Montreal). Birkett saw the need for establishing a medical unit to support Canadian forces overseas. Consulting faculty members, he found that there was interest in a McGill medical unit if he would organize it. He obtained concurrence from Principal Peterson and then proposed his plan to form a medical unit to Major General Hughes, the minister of Militia and Defence. Hughes sent Birkett's plan to Sir Alfred Keogh, director-general of the British Army Medical Services. On 15 December 1914 Keogh agreed to accept the McGill proposal and suggested that a hospital unit of 520 beds be ready in the spring of 1915. Birkett would command the unit,[6] and Lt. Col. Henry Brydges Yates would be second-in-command. Other appointments were: Lt. Col. John McCrae in charge of medicine, with Majors Campbell Howard and Jonathan Meakins as assistant physicians; Lt. Col. John M. Elder in charge of surgery, with Majors Walter Henry P. Hill and Edward W. Archibald as

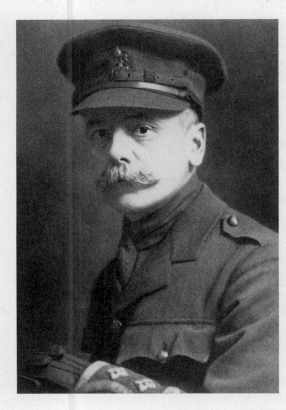

Figure 41
Herbert Stanley Birkett,
director of No. 3
Canadian General
Hospital (McGill),
1914–19. Photographer
unknown

assistant surgeons. These men had established reputations at McGill and a strong sense of duty. They were willing to spend an indefinite period of time overseas for the war effort. They were paid according to rank, and often that amounted to a reduction in income.

Extraordinary energy and organizational powers were necessary to get the medical unit together as quickly as possible. Unexpectedly, in January 1915 the War Office doubled the size of military hospitals to 1,040 beds. Birkett accepted the challenge, recruited more staff, and enlarged the McGill unit to thirty-five officers, seventy-three nurses, and 205 other ranks. The unit was ready by April 1915.

The logistics of getting seven Canadian general hospitals,[7] numerous field ambulances, and casualty clearing groups from Canada to Europe in 1915–16 was a tribute to the direction of the CAMC.[8] This involved transporting personnel and tons of materials – uniforms, tents, cots, bedding, bandages, ambulances, operating room facilities, solutions, x-ray and laboratory equipment, desks, chairs, cabinets, horses, and carriages – to England and then across the channel to France and Belgium.

Camp Valcartier[9] was the staging area for medical units from Quebec. From the hundreds of troops and units assembled there, the following emerged: three field ambulance units; one casualty clearing station; No. 1 and No. 3 Canadian General Hospitals, and No. 1 and No. 2 Stationary Hospitals. Medical supplies, uniforms, tents, and transportation arrived in chaotic order at Valcartier, often in insufficient amounts. Those items were shipped to Salisbury, England, where tons of equipment and supplies were spread out on the Salisbury Plain. Units took what was needed while they were training before they went to France.

On 6 May 1915 the McGill unit marched to the Montreal docks and embarked on the Canadian Pacific ship *Metagama*. After steaming through waters where the *Lusitania* had been sunk, the *Metagama* arrived at Devonport, England, on 15 May following an uneventful voyage. A special train transferred the men and goods to Shorncliffe where the unit trained.

On 14 June the unit received orders to embark for France. Personnel and supplies were loaded on the s.s. *Huanchaco* at Southampton, and on 17 June the ship took them across the English Channel to Boulogne, arriving the following day. After disembarking, the unit moved by train to a small town near the sea south of Boulogne – Dannes-Camiers – where there was a large tent camp of other hospitals, including No. 2 Canadian General Hospital. The McGill unit finally had a temporary location near the battlefront.

Once established, the unit rehearsed mock admissions of casualties. In August 1915 the first real patients arrived in small numbers. The first surgical operations were performed on 9 August. By 26 September the weather had changed to rain that leaked into tents and resulted in mud everywhere. Nevertheless convoys of motor lorries brought as many as 250 wounded soldiers from the battlefront a day. By the end of October 1,650 patients had been admitted, 450 operations performed, and twenty-one deaths had occurred. In spite of having to treat filthy, mud-caked troops with infected wounds, the results were satisfactory and survival rates high. Most operations were performed under chloroform anesthesia administered with a Vernon-Harcourt inhaler. Gas-oxygen mixtures (nitrous oxide) were used in short cases on the wards when painful dressings had to be changed. Spinal anesthesia with Stavarin, an anesthetic agent, was used in selected cases.

Cold weather and snow followed in November. Some tents collapsed or were blown down. Colonel Birkett closed the unit while he looked for more permanent quarters. He found them at an abandoned Jesuit

College northeast of Boulogne, where a small hospital was situated. After considerable renovation, the Jesuit College was made habitable, and on 11 January 1916 the McGill unit moved to the new site in eight hours – another remarkable feat. Within a few weeks the new hospital was ready for operation. On 15 February 1916, 144 wounded soldiers were admitted, and the work of the unit began in earnest.

Medical services at the battlefront were organized at different levels, depending upon what was needed, and were distributed at the front according to the battle conditions. The medical services were flexible, and the technical chain of command existed only for organizational purposes. Each regiment had its own stretcher-bearers stationed behind the front-line trenches, and they were called when needed. Wounded soldiers were removed to bearer posts where field ambulance stretcher-bearers picked them up and brought them to advanced dressing stations (ADS). From there, soldiers with trivial problems walked back to the trenches. Wounded soldiers with serious problems were taken by ambulance after first aid treatment to a triage centre. There the staff decided whether to send them to a casualty clearing station or to a regional general hospital located miles behind the front line. When there were a large number of wounded, they were moved down the line to a medical facility where they could be treated. Sometimes the front stations were overwhelmed, and the wounded were just taken to the next level. Organizational entities appeared and disappeared according to the need.

The fixed general hospitals such as No. 3 Canadian General Hospital were far enough behind the front lines to be secure and capable of handling thousands of patients per month. Because of the distance from the front, other entities existed to care for patients who needed emergency surgery that couldn't wait. Casualty clearing stations (CCS), of which there were only four, were large mobile surgical units where the wounded could be operated on to save lives. Otherwise wounds were cleaned and patients stabilized before moving them down the line to the nearest general hospital. Stationary hospitals were smaller than the general hospitals. The initial plan was that stationary hospitals would remain in England, but when requirements changed, some of them were sent to France as general hospitals.

What was important was proper medical care, not the chain of command. Patients were taken to wherever appropriate care was offered and available. Nationality was not considered when picking up casualties – at times the McGill unit treated German and other enemy wounded.

Large numbers of wounded were moved from the front during the Battle of the Somme in September and October of 1915.[10] Many were admitted to the McGill unit, and hundreds of operations were performed with a low infection rate.[11] Lt. Col. Elder, Major Hill, and Major Archibald performed most of the surgery, Captain W.B. Howell supervised the anesthesia, Cadets L.T. Black, L.H. McKim, and R.H. Malone ran the pathology laboratory, Captain A. H. Price and Captain W.A. Wilkins ran the x-ray facilities, and Lt Col. John McCrae, Major J.C. Meakins, and Major Campbell Howard, assisted by J.G. Brown, A.G. Henderson, and C.K. Russel, directed the medical department.

In 1916 and 1917 many patients were admitted to the McGill Unit and numerous surgical operations performed. In August 1917, 4,216 wounded were admitted and in September 4,192.[12] The original medical staff was eventually transferred, mostly to specialized medical hospital units. Birkett had to leave the unit in March 1917 for surgical treatment in England. John Elder then assumed command of No. 3 Canadian General Hospital, assisted by A.T. Bazin from the Montreal General. In 1917, 55,149 wounded were admitted, 3,383 operations were performed, and there were 301 total deaths, of which 102 were post-operative.

JOHN McCRAE

John McCrae[13] (fig. 42) had a reputation not as a practising physician but as a pathologist and later as a poet. After 1901 he was assistant pathologist at Montreal General and in his spare time wrote poetry, including this quotation from inside of the front page of the 1901 hospital Autopsy Record Book:

Here beginneth ye booke of yea deade wherein is fayrely set forth ye last state of four hundred seventeen persons that have departed from this lyfe; wherein be tabled diverse and strange and fearsome conditions that have led to ye same final end: God have them of His Grace.

And our Lyve is but a winter's day.
Some only breakfast and away.
Others to dinner stay and are fulle fedde.
The oldest men but supps and goes to bedde.
Large in his debt that lingers out the day.
He that goes soonest has the least to pay.

Twenty-eight of McCrae's poems were published between 1895 and 1917 in various magazines. There are contradictory stories about what

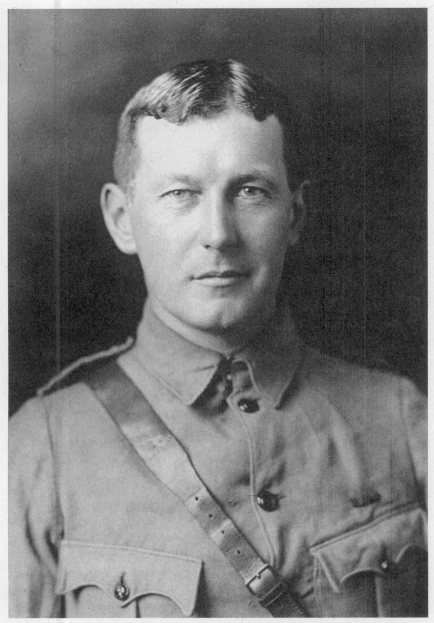

Figure 42
John McCrae, 1872–1918. Photographer unknown

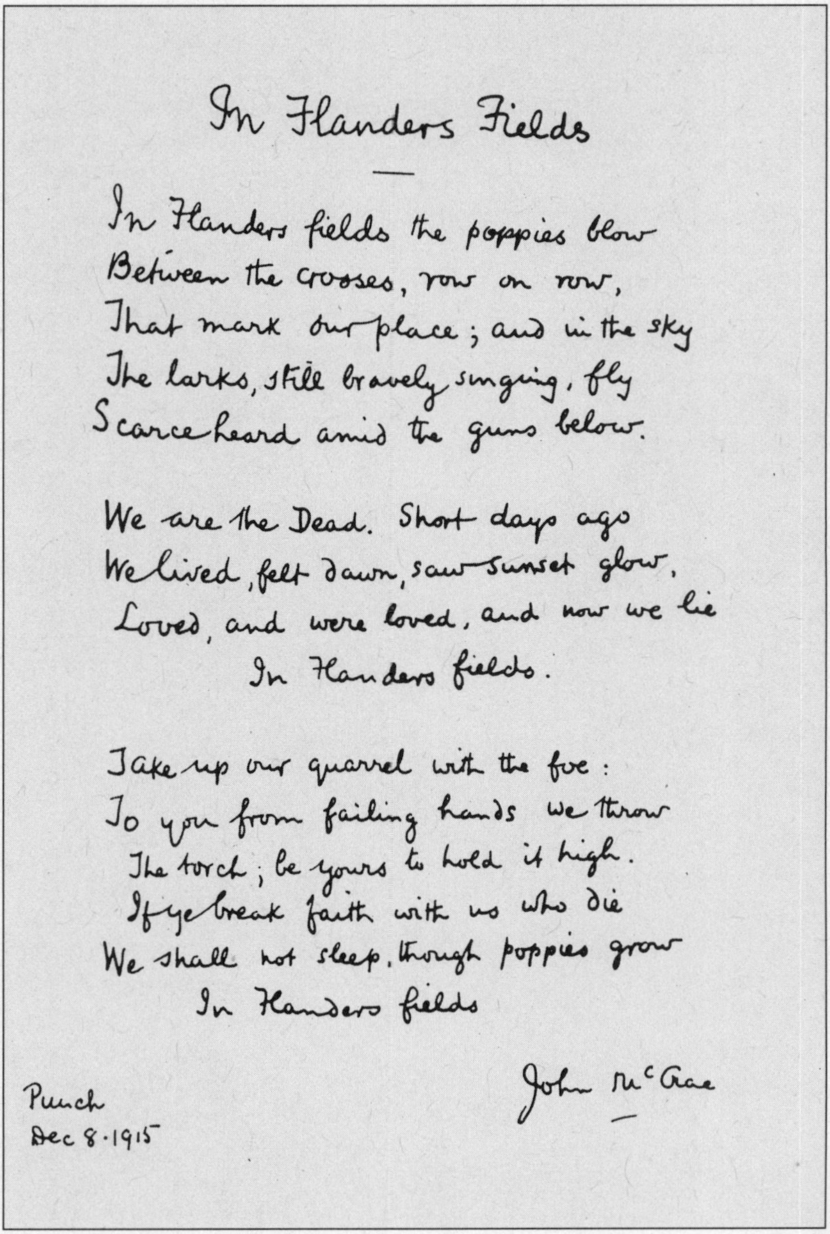

In Flanders Fields

—

In Flanders fields the poppies blow
Between the crosses, row on row,
That mark our place; and in the sky
The larks, still bravely singing, fly
Scarce heard amid the guns below.

We are the Dead. Short days ago
We lived, felt dawn, saw sunset glow,
Loved, and were loved, and now we lie
            In Flanders fields.

Take up our quarrel with the foe:
To you from failing hands we throw
The torch; be yours to hold it high.
If ye break faith with us who die
We shall not sleep, though poppies grow
            In Flanders fields

Punch
Dec 8·1915

John McCrae
—

Figure 43
John McCrae's poem "In Flanders Fields" in his handwriting. Osler Library

inspired him to write "In Flanders Fields" (fig. 43). Most likely he wrote the poem after the tragic death of his friend Lt. Alex Helmer by enemy artillery fire in 1915. McCrae's colleagues persuaded him to send the poem to the *Spectator,* but it was returned. He then sent it to *Punch* magazine with some other poems. "In Flanders Fields" was published at the bottom of a page in the 8 December 1915 issue of *Punch*. In a short time this poem made him famous throughout the British Empire.[14]

With the rank of lieutenant colonel, McCrae was officer in charge of medicine with the McGill unit from March 1915. He was serving in that capacity when on 23 January 1918 he became ill with a respiratory infection. In the next few days, despite his transfer to hospital and intensive care, his condition worsened to coma and death on 28 January 1918.

After the funeral, Lt. Col. J.M. Elder, commanding officer of No. 3 Canadian General Hospital (McGill) wrote to Col. H.S. Birkett, who was then in transit from France to Montreal, to describe McCrae's final days:

Army Post Office, B.E.F. France, 1 February 1918
Colonel H.S. Birkett c.b., a.m.s., 252 Mountain St, Montreal, Canada

My dear Birkett:
    This is the first letter I have written since McCrae's death and burial. I well know with what a shock you will get the news when you land; it will be more of a shock to you than it has been to all of us here, and I am sure you will want to know, in detail, all about it, as I was simply able to send a wire to [Principal] Peterson baldly stating the fact.
    On Wednesday [23 January 1918], he was as usual in the morning; in the afternoon, I found him asleep in his chair in the Mess Room. I asked if he was feeling unwell, and he replied, "I have a slight headache, and I think I must have eaten something that has disagreed with me". I advised him to go to bed if he was not feeling right, which he did; he never got up again. Saw him again at Mess time: said he thought he would stay quietly in bed, as he had a very severe attack of vomiting, and was sure he would be all right in the morning if he stayed quiet and ate nothing. He had no elevation of pulse or temperature at this time, and complained of nothing but soreness, like "La Grippe," in his legs. While he had his everyday cough, there was no increase in the respirations. I got the Night Supervisor to come in, sponge him off that night, take his temperature, which she found to be 99, with a pulse of 86.
    That night, the order came through to despatch him forthwith as Consulting Physician to the First Army. I read the order over to him, and told him I

should announce it at Mess, which I did in a nice little complimentary speech. He was very much pleased at the appointment; we discussed the matter at some length, as he expected to leave early the following week, and I got his advice upon what was best to be done on the medical side of the unit.

I looked in twice the next morning, early, but he was sound asleep, and remained so until I went down to the office. During the forenoon, I looked in on him once or twice, and he said he felt very much better, but still felt a bit sore, and did not feel like eating anything. He did not appear to be at all feverish, nor was his cough troublesome, nor did he have any special pain.

That afternoon he sent for me and said he feared he was in for pneumonia, because he noticed his sputum was rusty. I immediately had Rhea examine a slide of it, and Rogers go over his lungs. Rhea told me he thought that there were pneumococci in the slide, but Rogers could find no physical signs in the chest. His temperature, by this time, had gone up to 100½, but his pulse and respirations were normal. I saw he was worried a little about the possibility of pneumonia, so I put a nurse in charge of him in his own room, with instructions to take his temperature every two hours. As he was no better by evening, I phoned to Wimereux, and asked Sir Bertrand Dawson if he would be good enough to see him, telling him what we feared. I did this without McCrae's knowledge, as I knew he would protest. Like the good friend he has always been to us, Sir Bertrand came up at once. He, too, could find nothing in the chest, but agreed that he probably had an undiscovered patch of pneumonia somewhere, and that the best thing we could do would be to transfer Jack in the morning to No. 14 General Hospital, where he had been just a year before. That night, his temperature went up to over 101, but neither pulse nor respirations kept pace with it. He complained somewhat of headache and was restless till towards morning, when he fell into a calm untroubled sleep.

Next morning, Friday, the ambulance came up, and he left for No. 14 General Hospital, accompanied by D.S. Lewis. Dawson telephoned that night saying that Jack was considerably better. Saturday morning, the report was good, temperature had fallen, pulse and respirations were normal. Sir Bertrand told me he considered that it was a typical and probably an abortive attack of pneumonia. He was of the opinion that the vaccines which Rhea and Jack had been experimenting with for the cure of his asthma had influenced favourably the course of the disease.

By Saturday afternoon, he became worse, and developed symptoms of cerebral irritation. His pulse went up and his heart's action became irregular. I did not like his looks at all, but refrained from saying anything that would at all excite him. He seemed to me to be very heavy and stupid and not at all like his bright self.

That night, he had a good deal of cerebral irritation, and about 2:00 A.M., his temperature dropped suddenly to 97, and his pulse became weak and bad – a sort of pseudo-crisis. His pulse responded to cardiac stimulation. On Sunday morning Dawson 'phoned me that, in spite of his bad night, he thought his condition was not so bad, although he still dreaded some cerebral complication on account of the intense sleepiness which Jack showed. He suggested that Rhea and I should go down and do a blood culture and a lumbar puncture. We went down at once, but found a remarkable change. He had suddenly developed a right-sided hemiplegia, with a Bell's palsy, was quite unconscious, and was in fact dying with a pulse that I could not count. Needless to say, we did neither of the two things we went down to do, as it was quite hopeless. I had Cushing come down and see him with me that Sunday afternoon, as I thought it might be some comfort to Tom McCrae to know that Cushing had seen him. We both agreed that he could not go through another night, Dawson gave up all hope, and he died shortly after midnight at 1:30 A.M.

This is the correct diary of the awful tragedy that has come upon us, and I cannot, even yet, realize that I shall never see Jack again.

The funeral, which was held from No. 14 General Hospital to the cemetery at Wimereux (which you and I know so well), on Tuesday afternoon at 2:00 P.M., was by far the largest and most impressive military funeral I have ever seen anywhere.

Few deaths in the war caused greater anguish in Canada than this unexpected loss of McCrae, who had become a household legend because of his poem "In Flanders Fields." The medical faculty was so moved by his death that it memorialized him with a stained glass window (fig. 44) facing south on the second floor of the Strathcona Medical Building.

Elder was transferred in June 1918, having been chief of surgery at the McGill unit for three years and commanding officer from March 1917. L.H. McKim, the only one of the thirty-five original staff to remain with the unit after three years, was put in charge of surgery. D.S. Lewis replaced McCrae as acting chief of medicine. As reported by Fetherstonhaugh, from 7 August 1915 when the first patient was admitted at Dannes-Camiers until the McGill unit closed its doors in Boulogne on 12 May 1919, there had been a grand total of 143,762 admissions, 11,395 operations, and 986 deaths from all causes.[15]

Unfortunately a number of physicians and other personnel from the McGill Unit died during the war. These included, in addition to Lt. Col.

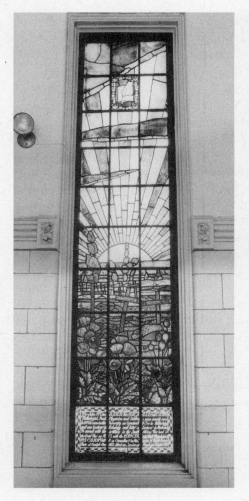

Figure 44
The centre of three memorial
windows in the Strathcona
Medical Building on the second
landing, facing south, dedicated
to members of the faculty who
died in World War. The centre
window for John McCrae depicts
a jewelled plaque in the upper
part bearing a book and quill, a
sunrise over Flanders fields with
crosses on the grass, and blood-
red poppies growing in the fields.
In the inscription below, McCrae
is described as "Pathologist,
Poet, Physician and Soldier. A
man among men." Photo by
Tom Humphry, 1994

John McCrae, Lt. Col. Henry Brydges Yates (second in command),
Maj. John Hamilton Adair, Sisters Jessie King and Evelyn McKay, and
Lance Corporal Harry Eaton.

The McGill unit was considered a model general hospital in France.
Numerous dignitaries visited it, including Queen Mary, Sir William Osler,
and McGill's principal, Sir William Peterson (fig. 45). When the unit
was demobilized in 1919, it was obvious that no one had anticipated
the magnitude of the hospital care that was to be delivered. Those who
went overseas had experiences in medicine and surgery that would not
be equalled in a lifetime.

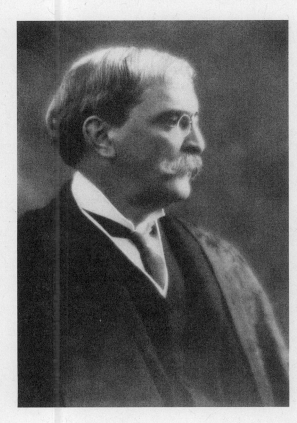

Figure 45
Sir William Peterson,
1859–1921.
Photographer unknown

F.A.C. SCRIMGER AND THE VICTORIA CROSS

Many McGill physicians were decorated for their war efforts. Francis Alexander Carron Scrimger (fig. 46),[16] a junior medical officer, was awarded the Victoria Cross, the highest military award for valour given in the British Empire, for acts of heroism on 25 April 1915.[17]

At the onset of hostilities Scrimger felt an urgent need to join the military. In 1914 he was appointed captain in the Montreal Heavy Brigade of the Canadian Artillery and sent to France in 1915. The trim, mild-mannered doctor's devotion to duty and to his fellow men propelled him to national renown when he was faced with a perilous situation at the front on the afternoon of 25 April in a small town in Belgium. Scrimger was tending to wounded soldiers approximately two miles north of Ypres[18] in a farmhouse being used as an observation post, medical station, and headquarters. About 5:00 P.M. a German airplane

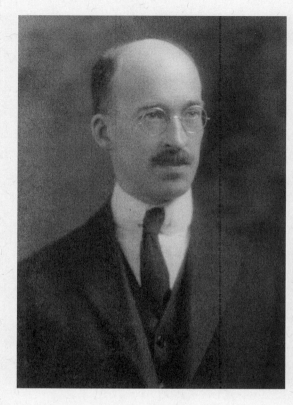

Figure 46
Francis Alexander
Carron Scrimger, vc,
1876–1937. Photo by
William Notman, 1922

with British markings flew over and bombed the house. Capt. Harold
McDonald[19] was struck in the left side of his neck, face, and shoulder
and was bleeding and not expected to survive. Further shelling forced
the other officers to abandon the farmhouse, along with all the wounded soldiers who could walk.

Scrimger knew that McDonald could not get away in the face of a
German advance. After shielding him with his body when there was a
direct hit on the roof, he then carried the helpless officer on his back
about twenty-five metres from the farmhouse, dropping into a shell
hole and shielding him once again while the Germans lobbed seventy-
five shells into the area.

After the shelling, the nearby German infantry began to advance.
Fate was with Scrimger and McDonald, however, because of 350,000
rounds of small-arms ammunition in a storeroom that had caught fire.
When these rounds began to go off with the heat, the advancing Germans, approximately 250 metres away, thought that this represented
more resistance and halted to dig in. The shelling ceased soon after.

Scrimger returned to the stable where there were about twenty men unevacuated. With the help of bearers, he moved them together with Capt. McDonald to safety further down the road. Later he walked to a nearby town, Wieltje, which was in allied hands, to mobilize more help. Scrimger and other men brought the wounded soldiers down the line and arranged for their transfer where necessary to base hospitals in England.

At the second Battle of Ypres in April 1915 Canadian troops that had trained for only a few weeks at Camp Valcartier and a month or two in England met their first test. Canadian, British, and French troops were defending Ypres in southern Belgium. During this battle the Germans experimented with the use of chlorine gas. The Canadians, despite being untrained in trench warfare, outnumbered, equipped with inferior rifles, and suffering from the gas attacks, held off German counterattacks from 22 April to 3 May 1915 using makeshift gas masks. Out of 18,000 Canadian troops involved in this campaign, there were 5,975 casualties and 1,000 deaths. Most of these casualties were received and treated at the McGill Unit.

For his actions above and beyond the call of duty, Scrimger stepped into the pages of Canadian military history. He was one of the first Canadians to be awarded the Victoria Cross. After a short rehabilitation leave, he returned to the front for the remainder of 1915. In December he developed an infected finger on his left hand from a scalpel wound and was evacuated to England. Recovery took almost a year and required partial amputation of the infected finger.

THE McGILL FACULTY OF MEDICINE DURING WORLD WAR I

On the home front, the medical curriculum and the five-year course did not change during the war. With many physicians and surgeons in Europe, the remainder of the teaching staff carried on as best they could. They had a double load – increased teaching assignments and added patient loads from the medical practices of the absent doctors. They continued to teach students in the traditional way because it was not the time to make changes. Interest in research at the medical school, despite the war, was conspicuously lacking. On the other hand, in the undergraduate McGill faculties, research in physics, chemistry, and metallurgy was prominent. Of particular note was the work done on sound localization, acetone, and magnesium production. The medical faculty was content to keep up the established teaching program, finally lengthening the curriculum to six years in 1919 to provide another clinical year for all students, most of whom still did not get house-officer training on graduation. There was a complacency in the faculty that had been given an A-minus rating by Flexner in 1910. With so many of the teaching staff overseas, it was in a holding situation.

Applications to the medical faculty had decreased during the war as many young men enlisted for overseas duty. Clinical training had improved a little with an increased number of house officers at the hospitals but only the best students were accepted. Students in the fifth (from 1907) and sixth (from 1919) years were taking on more duties on the wards, but a Hopkins-style clerkship was still lacking because of the restrictions imposed by the boards of governors of the two hospitals.

CONVOCATION CEREMONY, 1916

The bubble of complacency burst in 1916 at the spring convocation ceremony during a speech given by Harry Goldblatt, the class valedictorian. Goldblatt, a graduate of the five-year course, was one of four extraordinary Jewish students whose names began with G: Harry Goldblatt, Louis Gross, Alton Goldbloom, and Sy Greenspoon. "The four Gs" were class leaders. Goldblatt, Gross, and Goldbloom rotated between first and fourth places in the class throughout the five years of the medical course.

Goldblatt was the most popular student and first in the final year. He later achieved fame for discovering renin and delineating the relationship of the kidney to hypertension.

Gross was the youngest, graduating just before his twenty-first birthday. He was recognized as the number-one student in the class and was awarded the Holmes Medal. Research oriented, he developed a reputation in the area of arteriosclerosis. Well into a promising career he died in an airplane crash in 1937 at age forty-two. Three thousand attended his funeral service, including Paul Dudley White, the famous Harvard cardiologist, and C.F. Martin (fig. 47),[20] former dean of the medical faculty.

Goldbloom was fourth in the class and won a graduation prize. He became a well-known pediatrician and was the third chairman of McGill's department of pediatrics.

Sy Greenspoon was also an excellent student. He was an extern at Johns Hopkins Hospital and an intern at Peter Bent Brigham Hospital in Boston. When he returned to Montreal, he was active in founding the Jewish General Hospital. Later he moved to England.

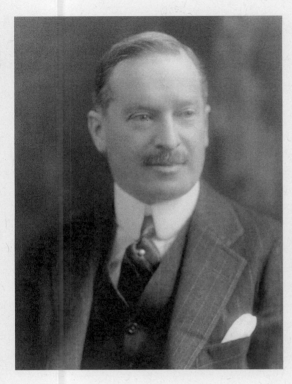

Figure 47
Charles Ferdinand
Martin, 1868–1953.
Photo by William
Notman, 1922

These brilliant students went through the five-year medical course working hard and observing everything, good and bad, about the faculty.[21] Although he was known as a gentle and tolerant person, Goldblatt decided that he couldn't miss the opportunity at the convocation ceremony to relate an honest assessment of the medical school's problems. The prizes were awarded and the graduates were capped, and then Goldblatt took the podium to deliver his valedictory address.

After the usual platitudes, Harold Segall reported, Goldblatt exploded a bomb. He stated that McGill's reputation in medicine was in serious jeopardy, and in its present state it was becoming a second-rate school. He even mentioned that the Carnegie Foundation might lower McGill's classification to a B level. He enumerated the deficiencies, stunning the professors by citing the lack of research in medicine as a major problem. McGill had lived too long on the reputations of Howard, Roddick, Ross, Osler, and Shepherd in the 1880s and 1890s.

The senior members of the faculty at the convocation sat fuming at the unprecedented criticism from this seemingly ungrateful Jewish student. In response, Professor C.F. Martin stood up to placate the audience. The situation was not as bad as described, he said, and there were plans to expand the research program. However, Martin and other thoughtful faculty members, including Acting Dean Blackader, knew that what Goldblatt had said was true. Resting on past laurels, McGill had slipped from what Flexner had reported in 1910. The practical problem was that Canada was involved in a war, and until it ended, there was little that could be done to change the programs. Goldblatt's courageous speech called attention to a situation that no one wanted to discuss. The elusive text of the speech has never been found, and Goldblatt later denied that he gave it. But thanks to his sister and the late Harold Segall, both of whom were present, a first-hand description of the event has been recorded.[22]

REFORM AND REORGANIZATION OF THE CLINICAL DEPARTMENTS

Following the valedictory address at the convocation in May 1916, members of the faculty began to consider reform in the clinical departments where Goldblatt had directed his criticisms. Martin, despite his statement at the time that the situation wasn't as bad as described, had already been thinking of reform. He was not in a position of real influence, however, until 4 November 1916 when he was elected chairman of the Education Committee, one of the standing committees of the faculty.[23]

Martin was endowed with a number of traits, amongst them foresight and leadership, that made him the right person to lead McGill out of its wartime doldrums. The Education Committee, with Martin as chairman, continued its deliberations throughout 1917. In December 1917, Acting Dean Blackader received a letter from Walter Vaughn, secretary of the university board of governors, in which he suggested that the medical faculty consider a more formal organization of the clinical departments by appointing a single university head for each department.[24]

On 5 January 1918 the Education Committee submitted a three-page report to the medical faculty with recommendations:[25]

1 a full-time dean of the medical faculty (with appropriate salary)
2 a single chairman of each of the university clinical departments
3 the chairmen of the clinical departments responsible for appointments, teaching assignments, and coordination of teaching schedules amongst the hospitals
4 mandatory retirement from the university at age sixty-five.

In April 1918 Martin called a meeting of the hospital directors and other representatives of the clinical departments to discuss a more detailed proposal. This was the formation of a joint university-hospital committee to judge all senior academic appointments to the teaching hospitals and the university. It was also proposed that the members of the teaching staff should be limited to teaching in their own specialty fields – a move to limit teaching to specialists. The faculty adopted the proposals and the Education Committee's recommendations of January 1918, unanimously. In June 1918 H.A. Lafleur, chairman of the Committee for Reorganization of the Clinical Departments, submitted a report to the university board of governors. It was adopted with minor changes from the January 1918 recommendations.[26]

Regarding the reforms at McGill, we must digress to Osler's activities in England. After Osler left Hopkins in 1905 to be Regius Professor of Medicine at Oxford, he was initially opposed to the full-time concept in clinical medicine – that is, having clinicians who were paid a salary by the medical school to practise medicine in a limited way. As chief of medicine at Hopkins, Osler made a great deal of money from private consultations outside the hospital and medical school.

However, Osler became aware of the poor medical education in London hospital-based medical schools, where part-time teachers taught both the pre-clinical and clinical subjects. In 1913 he testified before the Haldane Commission that was convened to investigate the quality of medical education in London hospital-based medical schools.[27] He proposed that the ideal medical school should follow the German model, with full-time pre-clinical teachers as well as full-time clinical professors whose role was to teach students and to see patients with remuneration by salary. In this way Osler acknowledged the value of the full-time system, although he was never wholly converted to the concept.[28] There was a sharp contrast between McGill as a university-based medical school and the typical London hospital-based medical school. McGill had a far superior school in pre-clinical subjects. To improve both McGill and the London hospital-based medical schools, Osler saw the value of full-time clinical teachers whose duty was to teach, perhaps conduct clinical research, and see patients in the clinic setting.

After McCrae's death in January 1918, D.S. Lewis was acting chief of medicine at the McGill Hospital Unit in Boulogne. On 15 February 1918 C.F. Martin was appointed provisional lieutenant in the CAMC, and in July 1918 he went to France with the rank of lieutenant colonel.[29] He replaced Lewis as chief of medicine at the McGill unit until November 1918 when he was transferred to Canadian Army

Headquarters in England as a medical consultant in the London area. In that capacity he had many opportunities to see Osler and to speak to him about conditions in Montreal.[30] They discussed the situation at McGill with its stagnant clinical services. We have to assume that Martin and Osler discussed the idea of applying the full-time system to McGill and getting foundation money to bring Jonathan Meakins to McGill from Edinburgh as director of the department of medicine and a McGill-RVH clinical research unit.[31]

Apparently Osler was in agreement with Martin's ideas that had been adopted by the Faculty Education Committee in 1918. In July, August, and September 1919, Osler sent letters and telegrams about the situation to a number of people at McGill and other medical schools – to Dean Birkett; to George Armstrong, professor and chairman of surgery; to the MGH and RVH medical boards, to his old friend William Welch, chief of pathology at the Johns Hopkins University; and to John D. Rockefeller Jr.[32] To Dean Birkett he wrote

From the Regius Professor of Medicine, 13 Norham Gardens, Oxford, U.K.
29 July 1919

To the Dean of the Medical Faculty, McGill College

Dear General Birkett:
   The situation is this – McGill simply cannot afford to fall behind other first-class schools in the development of modern clinics in medicine, surgery, and obstetrics and gynecology. New conditions have arisen and to meet them it is essential to have sympathetic and active co-operation of university and hospitals.
   Medically Montreal occupies a unique position – a school with a record of splendid work and two of the best equipped hospitals on the continent; but a new departure is needed which will involve change of heart as to methods, etc. and a realization of the full responsibility of the hospitals in this matter. It is their job quite as much as that of the university; and the clinics should be under the joint control of both bodies.
As to the details:
   1 The establishment of two clinical boards, one of the MGH and the other of the RVH to control all arrangements relating to the hospital side of the university work. The Principal, the President of each hospital, with two collegiate and two hospital representatives to form each board, which would be separate and independent and would control the appointments of the heads of the clinics.
   2 The clinics: A. 80 to 100 beds in each hospital for each medical and surgi-

cal clinic. B. An outpatient department associated with each clinic. C. Ample clinical laboratory facilities. D. Specific budgets for each clinic.

3 Personnel: A. Professor in charge of each clinic, appointed by the clinical board or by an *ad hoc* committee named by them for the purpose. A whole-time man, or if thought wiser, largely so. Salary $10,000 paid partly by the university and partly by the hospital. B. Assistants, whole and part-time named by the professor and appointed by the clinical boards, with salaries ranging from $1,000 to $ 3,000.

4 Teaching: The complete control of the teaching of medicine and surgery would be in the hands of the two professors in each subject. Others would receive clinical professorships and help in the ward and other teaching.

5 The obstetrical and gynecological clinics could be organized on similar lines, in connection with the hospitals and the university maternity.

6 Throw the appointments open to the best men available.

Now, Birkett, three things are necessary to carry out such a scheme;

1 A realization on the part of all concerned that we are at the parting of the ways, and that a new deal is a necessity.

2 A self-denying ordinance on the part of men at present in charge.

3 Money – for which an appeal should be made to the public. Possibly the Rockefeller Board might help, but this is a citizens' affair which should appeal to all who are anxious to see Montreal keep in first rank as a medical centre.

Yours sincerely,

W. Osler

Osler's letter stressed the need for outside money to accomplish the proposals, and he followed up on his letters by writing to John D. Rockefeller Jr to describe the plight of McGill and Canadian medical schools in general and their need for money. His letter caused a great stir in the medical faculty. Unfortunately, Osler died of complications of pneumonia and septicemia on 29 December 1919.

Birkett meanwhile sent copies of Osler's letter to all department heads. This stimulated discussion and meetings. In January 1920 a special session of the faculty executive was called to discuss Osler's letter. The faculty adopted his recommendations with minor changes. A joint university-hospital board would have as members: the principal, the presidents of the MGH and the RVH, and two members of the medical board of each hospital; it would have a mandate to make senior appointments to the medical faculty and the teaching hospitals.

The university board of governors, supporting the reform in the medical faculty, finally acted on the faculty's suggestions of 1918. In early 1921 the university governors approved the following list of single heads for the clinical departments:[33] F.G. Finley in medicine (he resigned to become dean 1921–22); G.E. Armstrong in surgery (he was dean 1922–23, and then retired in 1923); W.W. Chipman in obstetrics and gynecology; J.W. Stirling in ophthalmology; and H.S. Birkett in otolaryngology.

THE ROCKEFELLER FOUNDATION GRANT TO CANADIAN MEDICINE, 1921

Osler's correspondence in the fall of 1919 was the impetus behind John D. Rockefeller Jr's decision in December 1919 to provide $5 million to support Canadian medical education.[34] Shortly before the formal announcement of the funds to be made available, two Rockefeller representatives, Richard Pearce and George Vincent,[35] came to Montreal in March 1920 to visit McGill and the teaching hospitals. After negotiations with McGill's acting principal, Frank Adams,[36] in the summer of 1920, the foundation promised a grant of $1 million to support research in a pathology institute on Upper University Street (opposite the Royal Victoria), and in a new and renovated building for the basic science departments of physiology, biochemistry, pharmacology, biology, botany, and experimental medicine and surgery.[37] McGill had to raise $900,000 to construct the Pathological Institute (fig. 48)[38] and to renovate the old Medical Building so that it would become the Biology Building. Members of the Royal Victoria's board of governors purchased the property on Upper University Street from McGill University to secure the placement of the Pathological Institute adjacent to the hospital. The Rockefeller Foundation would endow the departments.[39] The Rockefeller grant in 1921, the year of McGill's centennial, was mainly a response to Osler's communications in 1919.

Martin was able to meet with Pearce and Vincent and gleaned important information about their attitude towards funding university projects. In a letter written to Pearce on 16 March 1920, Martin expressed his personal appreciation for their very kind and frank suggestions for his future proposal to support a full-time professorship in medicine and a clinical research unit at the Royal Victoria.

GENERAL SIR ARTHUR WILLIAM CURRIE

Along with C.F. Martin, the recently appointed principal, General Sir Arthur William Currie (fig. 49), began to play an important role in di-

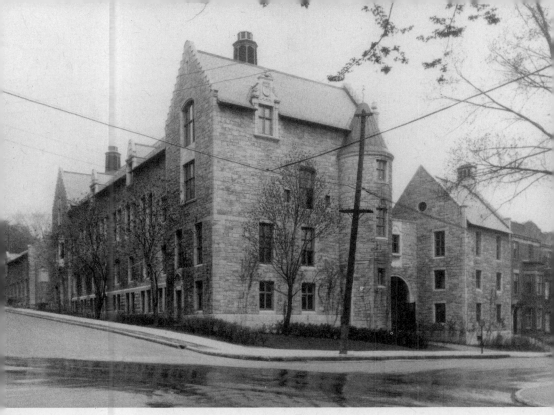

Figure 48
McGill University Pathological Institute, opened 1924.
Photo by William Notman, 1924

recting the destinies of McGill. Arthur Currie was born in Adelaide, a small town in rural southern Ontario, on 5 December 1875. He grew up in Napperton between Sarnia and London and attended the Strathroy Collegiate Institution. After a stint at teaching, he moved to Victoria, British Columbia, to go into real-estate with a partner. Although he did not have much military training, Currie developed a strong interest in the local militia. His extraordinary organizing skills and ability to instil loyalty in his troops helped to develop his reputation for leadership. He was promoted to the rank of lieutenant colonel.

When the depression of 1913 came, Currie's real-estate business suffered, and he was in serious financial trouble. At the point of bankruptcy, he decided to use some of the local militia's funds that were earmarked for uniforms for his regiment to pay his debts. Of course, he planned to repay the loan as soon as business improved. How was he to know that war would be declared in August 1914 and that he would be offered a command in the Canadian Army Corps? Currie was aware of the possibility of being exposed for embezzlement of government

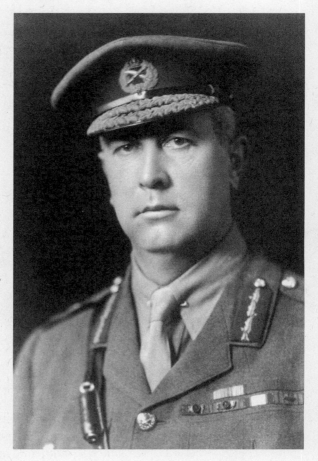

Figure 49
General Sir Arthur
William Currie,
1875–1933. Photo
by William Notman,
date unknown

funds, but he accepted the commission. Even though he repaid the loan, it remained the source of serious worry for him throughout the war.

Events moved quickly in the Allied Command due to the progress of the war. Currie proved that he and the Canadian Forces were capable of planning and carrying out well-coordinated attacks on the enemy. After a period of trench warfare, increased hostilities began on both sides. The Germans mounted an offensive on 22 April 1915 attacking Ypres, a small town in Belgium. As commander of the Second Brigade, Currie was requested to send the troops northward to fill in a gap when the Allied high command prepared for a counterattack.

Currie was considered a cool-headed and sensible leader and was the one above all others who was given credit for holding back the Germans at Ypres. King George showed his appreciation by decorating him with the Order of the Bath. The French gave him the Légion d'Honneur. In June 1917 he became General Sir Arthur Currie and commander of the Canadian Corps in France.

After the war ended in November 1918 and Currie had been discharged from the army, he spent some time in London doing army business and while there received many honours.[40] While he was in London, Major-General Sam Hughes (1853–1921) in Ottawa began to accuse him of negligence during the war for allowing excessive loss of lives of Canadian soldiers. Hughes had been a member of the Canadian Parliament from 1892 to 1916 and minister of Militia and Defence from 1911 to 1916, and he was incensed that Currie had not supported a senior promotion for his son, Garnett Hughes. Currie finished his military reports in London and did not pay much attention to Hughes because military records were available for anyone to see. Hughes, malicious and vindictive, had threatened both General Byng and General Currie. He spoke to the press so that when Currie came back to Canada, there was no reception for him as a war hero at Halifax or Ottawa. Currie still refused to challenge Hughes. He settled in Ottawa and was appointed inspector general of the Militia Forces of Canada with a mandate to begin a peacetime reorganization of the military.

Currie was not happy in Ottawa because of the slanderous Hughes and was looking for a start in a new career elsewhere. Fortunately on 12 April 1920, Frank Adams, acting principal of McGill, proposed to confer an honorary degree on Currie and had an opportunity to talk with him. In 1919 the post of principal of McGill had been awarded to Sir Auckland Geddes to succeed Sir William Peterson, but Geddes requested leave of absence for 1919–20 and then resigned as principal in March 1920 to become British ambassador to the United States. Geddes was asked to name a successor, and when Currie's name was suggested, recommended him. At first Currie hesitated to accept the appointment because he had not attended college, but McGill made him an offer that he could not refuse, which he accepted. He became the eighth principal and vice-chancellor of McGill University on 31 May 1920.[41]

Aware of his shortcomings, Principal Currie overcompensated by involving himself in every sphere of administration at McGill.[42] He was a decision-maker and a loyal supporter of the university, and soon became aware of the problems and plans of the university and its professors. His devotion showed so much human earnestness that he gained the loyalty of his colleagues and eventually achieved a healthy growth of the university. One of his first major accomplishments was to direct a fund-raising campaign in 1920 to resolve McGill's financial problems. The campaign raised more than $6 million in a short time – $900,000 of which went for construction of the Pathological Institute and the Biology Building.[43]

WOMEN IN THE MEDICAL FACULTY

In 1888 Octavia Ritchie was one of the first women to apply for admission to McGill Faculty of Medicine.[44] The faculty was not the least bit interested and rejected her application.[45] Maude Abbott applied for admission the following year and received the same negative response from the registrar.[46] Rejection made the two women more determined to fight. Octavia Ritchie went to the Women's Medical College in Kingston,[47] while Maude Abbott, valedictorian of the class of 1889, was determined to remain in Montreal.

A women's support group was founded in 1889 in Montreal called the Association for the Promotion of Special Education of Women (APSEW). Many influential women were members; Octavia Ritchie was secretary. APSEW drew up a formal petition and sent it to McGill calling for women's professional education to be equal to men's in all respects. They requested co-education, separate education, or a mixture. As expected, in 1889 the medical faculty rejected the petition. The opposition hadn't changed: once again it upheld the Victorian image of women as feminine, maidenly, charming creatures not suited for public life or the rigours of medical training or practice. Women were best suited as mothers, sympathetic companions, or house servants. APSEW was thwarted for another year.

In 1890 the medical faculty at Bishop's University decided to admit women and invited Octavia Ritchie to transfer from Kingston and Maude Abbott to enrol. Octavia Ritchie graduated M.D., C.M. from Bishop's in 1891; Maude Abbott, a senior prize-winner, graduated in 1894. The McGill faculty considered that the problem had gone away because the two main activists had gone elsewhere. Occasional applications from women were submitted and rejected over the next twenty years. They either went to Bishop's medical faculty until it closed in 1904 or to Toronto.

In 1898 Maude Abbott was appointed assistant curator and in 1899 curator of McGill's Medical Museum. In 1901 the faculty determined that she was not a regular member of the teaching staff and that any demonstrating or teaching that she did at the museum was incidental to her post as curator.[48]

In 1905 Adami and Shepherd supported Abbott for an appointment as Governors' Fellow in Pathology.[49] They also were helpful in arranging increases in her stipend as curator. In 1910 they proposed that as a Bishop's graduate she be granted a McGill M.D., C.M. *ad eundem*. At the following faculty meeting she was recommended for a McGill M.D., C.M. *honoris causa*.[50]

In 1913 the faculty recommended that women should be admitted to the study of medicine at McGill on the same basis as men, providing that the teaching hospitals agreed.[51] The medical boards of Montreal General and Royal Victoria replied that they were unwilling to accept female medical students on the hospital wards, so the policy of not admitting women continued.[52]

During the war the question of female admissions to the faculty was again raised because of the decline in the number of male applicants. The Montreal Council for Women in 1917 sent a resolution to McGill requesting it to open its doors to women in all professional faculties. The resolution went to the medical faculty and was rejected. In the summer of 1917, undaunted, Mary Christine Childs and Lillian Doris Irwin requested permission to be accepted into McGill's first year medical class as special students to qualify for transfer to the second year of the Toronto medical school where women were admitted. Robert Ruttan, professor of chemistry, had tutored them along with Jessie Marion Boyd and Eleanor Susan Percival. All four were registered as partial B.SC. students. It was made quite clear, however, that their admission as special students in no way constituted regular admission to the medical faculty.

With their toes in the door, the four women continued to agitate for regular admission to the faculty. Considerable lobbying having been done, at a special meeting of the faculty executive on 16 April 1918, Professors Blackader and Ruttan moved "That the Faculty recommend to the Corporation that women be admitted to the study of medicine, provided that they have taken a degree in Arts from a recognized university, or that they take a double course of BA, MD, CM, or BSc, MD CM, at McGill University and thus give evidence that they are sufficiently mature and otherwise qualified to take up the study of the professional branches."

The motion was amended to allow for entry only after two years in the arts faculty, which did not put them on the same basis as men candidates. The amended motion carried. The faculty executive hoped that the teaching hospitals would cooperate and assist with this endeavour. Thus, bowing to the changing times, to women's groups, the press, and

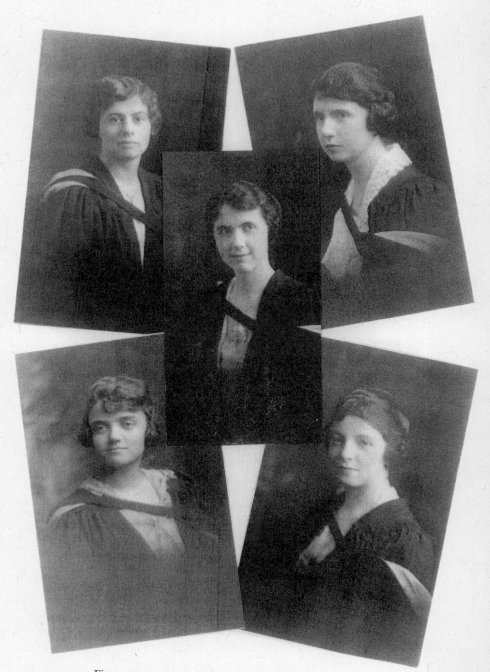

Figure 50
First women graduates of McGill Faculty of Medicine
1922. *Left to right, upper row*, Lillian Doris Irwin,
Jessie Marion Boyd; *middle row*, Eleanor Susan
Percival; *lower row,* Mary Christine Childs, Winifred
Alice Blampin. Photos by William Notman, c. 1919–22

sympathetic faculty members, women were admitted to the McGill Faculty of Medicine in the fall of 1918. Childs, Boyd, Irwin, and Percival (fig. 50) bravely came on the first day as women pioneers in the regular course of medicine, with some special concessions for the anatomy laboratory. Winifred Alice Blampin joined the group in second year as a transfer student.

As expected, they were on trial and had to endure discrimination from the men. The height of this was a self-appointed delegation of men who went to the home of Jessie Boyd one afternoon in the fall of 1918 to ask her and the other women to resign. This astounding affront had the reverse effect, convincing the women to work harder to prove themselves, and prove themselves they did. At convocation in the spring of 1922 Jessie Boyd was second overall in the class of 126 and won the Wood Gold Medal for excellence in clinical medicine. Winifred Blampin won the first Senior Medical Society prize. Boyd and Mary Childs were admitted to Alpha Omega Alpha, the National Honour Medical Society. Thus, two of the five senior prizes went to the women.

Although this was a milestone in McGill's educational history, the women had to be overqualified to survive. All were victims of the traditional minority group mentality that they had to excel to be equal. To celebrate, Maude Abbott, who had endured discrimination at McGill for years, proudly took the five women to the Ritz-Carlton Hotel[53] for a special reception to honour their graduation. Jessie Boyd went on to become a distinguished professor of pediatrics at McGill. In 1979 her alma mater honoured her with D.SC. *honoris causa*.[54]

4 The Charles F. Martin Years, 1923–36

The second, and what is the most important reform, is in the hospital itself. In the interests of the medical student, of the profession, and of the public at large we must ask from the hospital authorities much greater facilities than are at present enjoyed, at least by the students of a majority of the medical schools of this country. The work of the third and fourth year should be out of the medical school and transferred to the hospital...which is the proper college for the medical student, in his last years at least.
WILLIAM OSLER[1]

REFORM IN THE DEPARTMENT OF MEDICINE

In June 1923 the university governors appointed Charles F. Martin as the first full-time dean of the medical faculty and put him in a position of power so that he could get his projects done.[2] Martin and Principal Currie were leaders and decision-makers, and their combined efforts brought a great deal of progress to the medical school. One of their first projects was to negotiate funding for reform in the Faculty of Medicine.

Jonathan C. Meakins (fig. 51) had been a promising resident under Martin at the Royal Victoria Hospital and was appointed to the McGill teaching staff in 1911. During World War I he developed a reputation for pulmonary research. In 1919 he was offered and accepted the position as Christison Professor of Medicine and Therapeutics at Edinburgh University for a five-year term. The Edinburgh medical faculty had just revised its curriculum with funds from the Rockefeller Foundation and wanted a prestigious figure to start a research program on a full-time basis with a five-year contract. This arrangement gave Martin time to develop a McGill program that would include Meakins. Martin and Currie corresponded with Meakins about the plans to have a single chairman of medicine and to develop a clinical research unit at the Royal Victoria. While Martin was manoeuvering and negotiating for the reform, he regularly consulted Principal Currie as a formidable

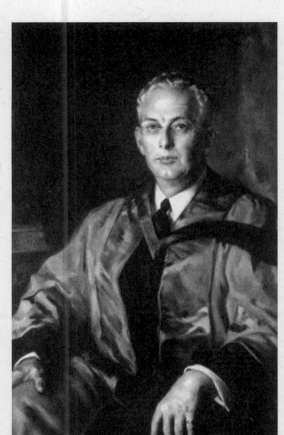

Figure 51
Jonathan Campbell
Meakins, 1882–1959.
Portrait by Alphonse
Jongers. Currently at
College Headquarters,
Royal College of
Physicians and Surgeons
of Canada, Ottawa

ally for his ideas. Currie had gained a reputation for forethought, deci-
siveness, and loyalty and for not shrinking from confrontation.

In 1923 Martin stepped up his plans by again discussing the need for
a full-time professor and chairman of medicine of the McGill faculty.
He contacted Alan Gregg, who had replaced Richard Pearce as medical
director at the Rockefeller Foundation, concerning the McGill project.
In October 1923 Martin proposed to Gregg and George Vincent, general director of the foundation, the appointment of a full-time professor of medicine who would be the McGill chairman of medicine,
physician-in-chief, and director of a clinical research unit at the Royal
Victoria. The hospital would provide the space and the local support
while the Rockefeller Foundation would endow the professorship and

funding for the research clinic to a minimum of $25,000 a year. Martin wanted Meakins to head McGill's department of medicine and make the Royal Victoria McGill's major teaching hospital.

Although the Rockefeller Foundation had planned to fund the program at Edinburgh to keep Meakins in Scotland, it did not interfere with McGill's attempts to bring him back to Montreal. Plans were finalized with McGill and the Royal Victoria authorities by 22 May 1924. Currie and Martin cabled Meakins that the way was clear for his appointment as chairman of medicine, physician-in-chief at the Royal Victoria, and director of an RVH clinical research unit, later known as the University Clinic. On 26 May 1924 the Rockefeller Foundation wrote to Martin giving official notice of the gift of $500,000 for the development. Meakins returned to Montreal in September 1924 to supervise the renovation of Ward K at the Royal Victoria for the University Clinic and to make staff appointments.

Martin saw the Royal Victoria as an easier institution in which to introduce the full-time concept than the tradition-bound Montreal General. His overall plan for reorganization of the university medical faculty did not include support from the Rockefeller Foundation for a full-time position in the department of medicine at the Montreal General. This did not pose a problem, because Campbell Howard (fig. 52) had already been approached for the position of MGH's physician-in-chief. He preferred instead to be paid a nominal salary from McGill, and his income would come mainly from private practice. He undoubtedly had been influenced by Osler regarding private practice, but the decision turned out to be a blunder. He also wanted to be a full professor at McGill, which was readily accepted since he had developed a great reputation at the University of Iowa.[3]

THE SIR HENRY GRAY AFFAIR

In the midst of the delicate negotiations with the Rockefeller Foundation, Sir Henry Vincent Meredith (fig. 53), the RVH president, almost scuttled the relationships between McGill and the foundation by acting in an arbitrary and unprofessional manner regarding the appointment of a surgeon-in-chief at the Royal Victoria.

In 1923 George Armstrong (fig. 54)[4] was professor of surgery and the RVH's chief surgeon. With his reputation he filled the Ross Pavilion with private patients. In the fall of 1923 he announced plans to retire from his university and hospital appointments. Meredith, who saw a busy surgical practice as a way of keeping the Royal Victoria financially

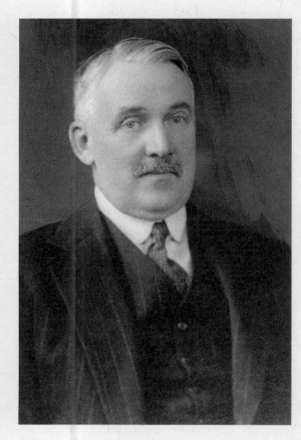

Figure 52
Campbell Palmer
Howard, 1877–1936.
Photo by William
Notman, 1929

solvent, moved quickly to find a successor to Armstrong. He sent Horst
Oertel, professor of pathology, to New York City to interview Alan
Whipple, the famous Columbia University surgeon, for suggestions for
the position at McGill. Whipple gave Oertel two recommendations:
Wilder Penfield, a neurosurgeon and assistant director of the New York
Neurological Institute, and Fordyce St John, a general surgeon in Columbia's department of surgery. Both doctors, however, refused Oertel's
invitation to visit Montreal. Armstrong then suggested that Meredith
approach Sir Henry Williamson Gray, an outspoken general surgeon
from Aberdeen, Scotland.[5] Armstrong had met Gray in France during
World War I and admitted that he did not know him well.[6] Gray had
never held an academic position although he had been knighted during
the war for his surgical contributions.

Meredith was determined to find a surgeon-in-chief for the Royal Victoria as soon as possible, and he ignored the protocol for appointments to

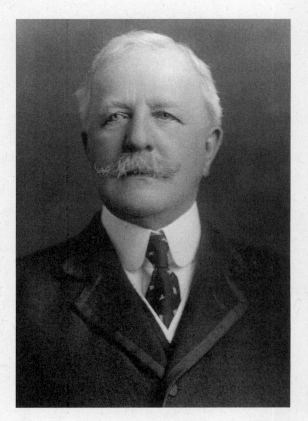

Figure 53
Sir Henry Vincent
Meredith, 1850–1929.
Photo by William
Notman, 1910

McGill teaching hospitals – the Joint University Hospital Board chaired
by Principal Sir Arthur Currie. Meredith invited Gray to visit Montreal in 1923 but did not acquaint him with the underlying dynamics of
the situation. Essentially Meredith promised him an appointment as
surgeon-in-chief at the Royal Victoria and then convinced the RVH
board of governors to ratify the appointment.

Since Henry Gray would be succeeding George Armstrong, Meredith presumed that he would have similar appointments. Meredith also
felt that he could persuade Principal Currie to give Gray a university
appointment as professor of surgery. However, Meredith greatly over-
estimated his own position. The first setback came when Armstrong
took Gray to meet Currie to discuss the McGill appointment. Currie,
who had no idea who Gray was or why he was in Montreal, was incensed that the protocol for making university appointments had been
bypassed. He told Gray in no uncertain terms that there was no senior
position at McGill available for him without a thorough investigation

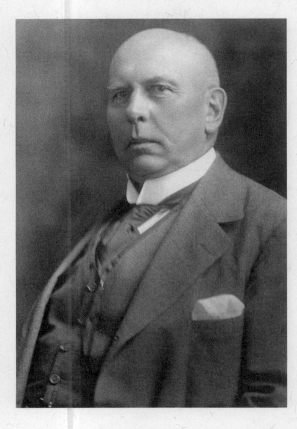

Figure 54
George Eli Armstrong,
1855–1933. Photo by
William Notman, 1920

by the Joint University Hospital Board. Currie did not back down.[7] Subsequent inquiry about Gray in the United Kingdom was unfavourable and revealed that he was not qualified for the McGill position. No one knew why he had been knighted.

At the same time, Martin and Currie were negotiating with the Rockefeller Foundation for support of the full-time professorship in medicine and the establishment of a university clinic at the Royal Victoria. When the Rockefeller executives heard that Meredith had unilaterally ignored McGill's policies and appointed a surgeon-in-chief to one of the teaching hospitals, negotiations were put on hold until the university asserted its policies.[8] Martin went to New York to assure the foundation that McGill would rectify the situation created by Meredith. He was astounded to hear that Meredith had preceded him and had said that Currie knew about Gray from the beginning – which was a fabrication.

The first move by the university was to appoint Edward W. Archibald (fig. 55) chairman of the McGill department of surgery.[9] The

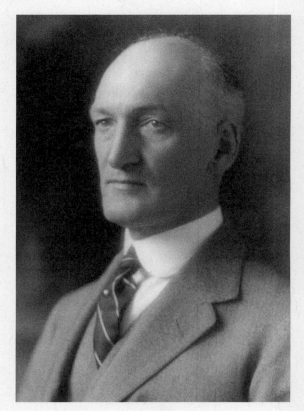

Figure 55
Edward William
Archibald, 1872–1945.
Photo by William
Notman, 1920

Rockefeller Foundation liked Archibald and was pleased with his appointment. However, a difficult situation had been created with Archibald as professor and chairman of surgery at McGill but with no control of surgery at the Royal Victoria, and Gray as surgeon-in-chief of the Royal Victoria with a junior faculty position and no control over student teaching or policy. The second move by McGill was to remove Gray from the student surgical lecture rotation after a trial year because he was a poor and disorganized teacher. This move was calculated to humiliate him, and it did just that.

The final challenge to the beleaguered Gray (an insensitive man who did not care for McGill tradition) concerned a patient in the Royal Victoria. The patient's family wanted the attending physician to consult Gray for his opinion. Gray recommended a surgical procedure. The attending physician did not trust Gray and asked Martin to give a second opinion. Martin disagreed that surgery was indicated, contradicting Gray's opinion.[10] Gray, again humiliated, called for an investigation of Martin by the CMA[11] and wrote a long, rambling, paranoid letter to the CMAJ saying that his programs were being interfered with and that there was a plot against him.[12] The editor refused to publish the letter, realizing that there was no proof of Gray's allegations. When the information got back to McGill about the bad publicity Gray was producing, Principal Currie demanded Gray's resignation in 1925 as the only solution for the problem. Meredith acknowledged that he had made a mistake in appointing Gray.

After nearly losing the Rockefeller Foundation's grant for a full-time program in medicine, McGill now moved to take control of its appointments. This convinced the foundation that an investment in McGill's medical faculty was safe. Meredith had been beaten by Currie and Martin and was no longer a problem.

The Gray affair ultimately strengthened McGill's resolve to tighten its policies on appointments. The reputations of Currie and Martin were also strengthened as they began to plan for the funding of a new McGill facility for surgical research.

THE UNIVERSITY CLINIC, 1924–36

The McGill University–Royal Victoria Hospital Medical Research Clinic directed by J.C. Meakins – or the University Clinic, as it was usually known – was the brain child of C.F. Martin in 1918. Located in Ward K at the Royal Victoria, it was dedicated to research in several areas: metabolism, pulmonary function, neuropathology, neurology and neurosurgery, allergic disease, and endocrine and cardiac diseases. The clinic had a major commitment to pulmonary physiology and medicine because of Meakins's focus; it trained many scholars in various fields.[13]

Meakins saw an opportunity to study a broad spectrum of cardiac, respiratory, endocrine, and muscle diseases. When making appointments to the clinic, he was not constrained to M.D. degrees. A small metabolism service at the Royal Victoria was taken over by the clinic, with E.H. Mason in charge. He studied various aspects of diabetes and other endocrine disorders, and played an important role in developing a diabetic service and clinic at the RVH. In 1928 he started a private practice but still taught on the diabetic wards. Maude Abbott was a research associate at the clinic. She was interested in pulmonary function in congenital heart disease. Ronald Christie, a fellow under Meakins, studied pulmonary function in health and disease.

In 1926 G.R. Brow studied the physiology of cardiac muscle function and its relation to the sympathetic nervous system. C.N.H. Long and T.R. Parsons were interested in the chemistry of muscle function in heart disease and anesthesia. Long later went to the University of Pennsylvania, then to Yale Medical School as professor of physiology and finally as dean of medicine.

J.B. Scriver studied calcium metabolism and sickle cell disease. C.J. Tidmarsh studied gastrointestinal diseases. J.S.L. Browne (B.A. 1925, M.D., C.M. 1927, Ph.D. 1932) was a brilliant but eccentric endocrinologist who had been trained by J.B. Collip. Browne and Eleanor Venning (Ph.D. 1933) studied the hormones of pregnancy and made major contributions to the understanding of fertility and sterility. Kenneth Evelyn, a Ph.D. physicist and later an M.D., invented a photoelectric colorimeter in 1936 that could determine haemoglobin and other components of blood.

Wilder Penfield and William Cone, both neurosurgeons, joined the University Clinic in 1928 and began studying the development of glial scar tissue in the brain using special stains in preparing tissue samples. Penfield became interested in epilepsy and in 1934 founded the Montreal Neurological Institute (MNI) across University Street from the Royal Victoria Hospital. The MNI was dedicated to treatment and research of neurological diseases.

The University Clinic attracted talented young scientists to work along with clinicians to study human physiology in health and disease. The work done there in many fields provided an exciting background for resident training in medicine. Medical graduates from across the country sought positions on the Royal Victoria's house staff because of Meakins's research unit.

REFORM IN THE DEPARTMENT OF SURGERY

Gray had completely disrupted the RVH department of surgery by attempting to reorganize hospital systems, failing to promote research, refusing to wear gloves in the operating theatres (the hospital standard required of all other surgeons), and refusing to cooperate with teaching rotations for third and fourth year medical students. As a result the morale in the RVH department of surgery in 1924 had been extremely low.

After Gray was forced to resign the following year, Meredith's control of affairs at the hospital declined, but he still blocked Archibald's appointment as surgeon-in-chief. Archibald, however, as professor and chairman of surgery at McGill, informally assumed the position of surgeon-in-chief while making departmental decisions and preparing the annual report. Meredith did not approve of Archibald because he was not interested in full-time private practice, but after the Gray affair, he was not going to confront Martin or Currie again.

Following Gray's departure, there were two surgical services at the Royal Victoria, one under Archibald and the other under C.B. Keenan. F.A.C. Scrimger worked with Archibald, F.E. McKenty with Keenan. The Archibald service was involved in research – surgery for tuberculous and nontuberculous lung disease, and surgery and treatment for pancreatitis and other gastrointestinal conditions.[14] Archibald published regularly and had an international reputation. Keenan was a practical, experienced, and able surgeon who ran a busy surgical practice but was not interested in research.[15]

By tradition the Royal Victoria's annual reports were statistical accounts of admissions, outpatient visits, operations, and diagnoses. After he arrived in 1924, Meakins changed the annual reports; in 1925, the report from the RVH's department of medicine also stressed the department's activities. After 1926 reports included detailed accounts of research performed by members of the department as well as a list of publications. Meakins also changed the form of reports from the McGill medical faculty, and Archibald followed his example with the reports from the McGill department of surgery.

Meredith began to withdraw from his duties as president of the Royal Victoria and no longer had absolute control over all aspects of RVH life. He declined mentally and by 1928 showed definite signs of senility.[16] Resigning late in 1928, he was succeeded by Sir Herbert Holt,[17] who was willing to work with Martin and Currie and changed the direction of the hospital. Martin thought that a research clinic arrangement similar to the department of medicine would give a boost to the department of surgery and might help to reverse the loss of morale following Gray's resignation.

With no official surgeon-in-chief at the Royal Victoria, the Rockefeller Foundation was not interested in funding a proposal for surgical research as long as the unstable situation existed at the hospital and as long as Meredith was president. Martin knew that without Archibald's appointment as surgeon-in-chief and without the approval of the chairmen of the basic science departments of anatomy, physiology, biochemistry, and pharmacology, he was not going to be able to convince the Rockefeller Foundation to fund a basic surgical research program.

Martin knew that Archibald could rehabilitate the dispirited department and build the RVH into a leading centre for training young surgeons. In an incredible effort in 1928, Martin put all his negotiating skills to the test to approach the Rockefeller Foundation again for funds to establish a surgical research program. Currie also had an influence in these negotiations. After persistent work with the foundation and the RVH board of governors, a workable plan was proposed: the foundation would support surgical research and training at the hospital for five years, providing that the hospital's board of governors made an equitable contribution and appointed a prestigious surgeon-in-chief.[18]

To assure success, Martin devised some academic choreography in which the various participants were to play their independent parts. Timing was also an important element. Once Martin had obtained conditional consensus from the various participants in this academic play, it was mid-December of 1928. His original plan had not included the ebullience of the holiday season, which could now be used to add a positive element to the proceedings. With a conditional promise of a grant from Rockefeller, he obtained agreement from the university governors to appoint a surgeon-in-chief for the Royal Victoria. Bearing in mind the Gray experience, the governors deferred the decision to the RVH medical board. Martin received the board's recommendation to appoint Archibald on 19 December, and Archibald accepted the appointment on 21 December. The university governors met at Chancellor Sir Edward Beatty's[19] office in Montreal's Windsor Hotel on Monday, 24 December 1929, at 3:00 P.M. Martin carefully presented the required documents, and Archibald was appointed RVH surgeon-in-chief. The performance was completed as darkness fell and Montrealers rushed home for Christmas Eve festivities. Martin was ahead of Santa Claus by only a few hours.

The Rockefeller grant would help to establish a surgical clinic at the RVH, with annual support provided for five years. The McGill departments of anatomy, physiology, biochemistry, and pharmacology agreed to participate with the surgical research program. To reassure the Rockefeller people, Sir Edward Beatty and Sir Herbert Holt went to New York to confer with the directors, telling them that that the hospital's stability had been restored and that McGill and the Royal Victoria supported the program. The foundation agreed to fund the surgical research clinic, provided that McGill and the Royal Victoria met their commitments.

Rockefeller provided $85,000 from 1929 to 1932 and later an additional $30,000 as extensions of the original grant. The hospital and McGill provided matching funds. Many prominent names arose from the McGill-RVH surgical research unit, including Arthur Vineberg for pioneer work on cardiac revascularization, Donald Webster for contributions in gastro-intestinal physiology, and Stewart Baxter for contributions in thyroid and pediatric surgery.

RETURN TO THE FOUR-YEAR COURSE

Martin had graduated M.D., C.M. in 1892 after completing the four-year medical course. He was professor of medicine when the five-year course was started in the 1908–09 session and the six-year course in the 1919–20 session, so he was familiar with the arguments about the length and content of the medical school curriculum. Those topics occupied a great deal of time during his deanship from 1923 to 1936. In the closing years of Martin's term, the faculty took important decisions regarding the medical course that stayed in force for many years thereafter.

Most of the faculty agreed about instruction in the pre-clinical and clinical subjects. There were two controversies, however. First, should the basic subjects – chemistry, physics, and biology – be taught in the medical school, or should they be part of a pre-medical course and the entrance requirements to the medical faculty? Second, should the students' practical work in the teaching hospitals be under the direction of the medical faculty and included in the medical school curriculum? That was the objective of the fourth and fifth years of the five-year medical course and the fifth and sixth years of the six-year course.

Some members of faculty – particularly S.E. Whitnall, professor of anatomy, and J. Tait, professor of physiology, both with British backgrounds – felt that the curriculum should include the basic subjects and the final years of practical training. They proposed lengthening the medical course to seven years.

By 1923 the faculty realized that many students in the first-year class had studied chemistry, physics, and biology in an arts or science faculty, either at McGill or another university. The first year of the six-year course included instruction in those subjects, and for many this was repetition. The solution was to define the entrance (matriculation) requirements to include successful completion of instruction in chemistry, physics, and biology in a pre-med course.[20] Starting in September 1924 the medical curriculum reverted to five years for first-year students who fulfilled the new entrance requirements. In 1931 there was a further revision of the curriculum: the first two years of the five-year course comprised the pre-clinical group of subjects; the final three years included the clinical group of courses including both required and elective subjects.[21]

Having dealt with the entrance requirements and the first-year curriculum, Dean Martin appointed a special committee of faculty to study the second problem. After the experience of several decades, the faculty realized that it had little control over what medical students were allowed to do in the teaching hospitals. Some graduating students were appointed as interns or house officers and had valuable practical experience treating patients before entering practice. Most graduating students, however, were eligible for a licence after graduation, and they started medical practice with minimal practical experience.

The special committee reported to the faculty in April 1934 recommending that all graduating students should have a hospital internship after graduation before receiving a licence to practise medicine. The medical curriculum would be reduced to four years – four sessions of thirty-six weeks instead of five sessions of thirty weeks. This amounted to a reduction of only six weeks of instruction, but the students would graduate a year earlier. The committee suggested that the new curriculum should start with the 1934–35 session. However, this change required the approval of the university governors and the McGill Corporation, and the cooperation of the teaching hospital and the provincial medical licensing boards.[22]

The hospitals had to develop programs and facilities to accommodate an increased number of interns. They would receive room, board, and uniforms but no stipend.[23] In February 1935 the faculty confirmed that the minimal entrance requirement for the four-year course would be three years of a B.A. or B.Sc. course to include chemistry, physics, and biology, but otherwise pre-med students could take additional courses according to their interests.[24] All approvals and arrangements were completed, and the four-year course started with the 1936–37 session. That class graduated M.D., C.M. in May 1940, and graduates were eligible for licensure after an internship of one year. In 1940 there were two medical graduating classes at McGill – the last class of the five-year course and the first class of the four-year course. By the mid-1930s most medical schools had four-year courses – generally two pre-clinical years followed by two clinical years. This pattern has continued since, with many revisions of the four-year curriculum.

THE MONTREAL NEUROLOGICAL INSTITUTE

In the early 1900s neurosurgery was in its infancy and was done around the world by general surgeons who either taught themselves or had a short stint in London at the National Hospital for the Paralysed and Epileptic at Queen Square. Sir Victor Horsley (1857–1916) was director of neurosurgery at that hospital from 1886 until World War I. He was the first major figure with a scientific background to commit himself to surgery in a neurological institution where he had considerable help from neurological associates. Montreal was no exception to the general rule. James Bell, the second chief surgeon at the RVH,[25] and James Stewart, physician-in-chief, were interested in neurological disease. Without specific training, by default they acted as neurologists. Initially, neurosurgical procedures were performed only for head trauma. Gradually, as neurological diseases began to be understood better, elective procedures were performed when a diagnosis could be made with some localization – not always precise. At the time only skull x-rays were available.

Bell taught Archibald his neurosurgical techniques, and Archibald gradually took over most of the neurosurgical cases. To gain more experience, he went to London to work with Sir William Gowers and Sir Victor Horsley for three months in 1906.[26] When he returned to Montreal, he assembled material and published a monumental chapter in a surgical compendium on neurosurgery.[27]

Stewart died in 1906, and his replacement in neurology was Colin Russel (fig. 56), the first well-trained neurologist at McGill. After Bell died in 1911 from acute peritonitis,[28] Archibald agreed to continue his surgical practice. Although he performed neurosurgical procedures after Bell's death, his interest and support for neurosurgery decreased because of his competing interests in pulmonary, gastro-intestinal, and pancreatic diseases.

After the interlude with Sir Henry Gray from 1923 to 1925, the gradual reorganization of the Royal Victoria's department of surgery, the establishment of a surgical research unit, and the two surgical services run by Archibald and Keenan, each service had to deal with head trauma. Neurologists at both the Montreal General and the Royal Victoria referred patients with complex neurological diseases that required elective surgery to Harvey Cushing in Boston. Unhappy with this system, Archibald and Keenan in 1927 proposed that the RVH governors establish a sub-department of neurosurgery and appoint a full-time neurosurgeon. Determined to find a candidate, Archibald mentioned his problem when visiting an old friend, Archibald Malloch, in New York City. A medical historian and bibliophile formerly from Montreal, Malloch had been greatly influenced by Sir William Osler at Oxford. He suggested Wilder Penfield, assistant director of neurosurgery at New York Neurological Institute. Penfield had been a Rhodes Scholar

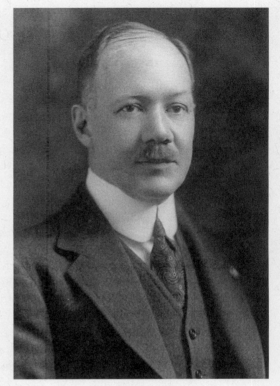

Figure 56
Colin Russel, 1877–1956.
Photo by William Notman,
1920

at Oxford where he too had come under the influence of Osler. This chance introduction changed the history of neurosurgery in Canada.[29]

Archibald wrote to Penfield that he wanted to come to New York to watch him operate. On 25 June 1927 he arrived at the Presbyterian Hospital where Penfield, assisted by William Cone, was operating on a patient with a pontine angle tumour. At lunch after the surgery, both men discussed their ideas – Archibald's for developing a neurosurgical program at the RVH, and Penfield's for forming a team to investigate neuropathological and neurosurgical problems. Penfield charmed Archibald, and just before leaving, Archibald invited him to come to Montreal to consider appointments at McGill and the Royal Victoria in neurosurgery.

On 12 January 1928 Penfield arrived in Montreal, beginning his visit with a lecture to medical students on the diagnosis of brain tumours. The dean and Professor Jonathan Meakins attended the lecture. Then Martin, Archibald, and Penfield went to the Pathological Institute to talk with Horst Oertel, chief of pathology. They asked him for space in

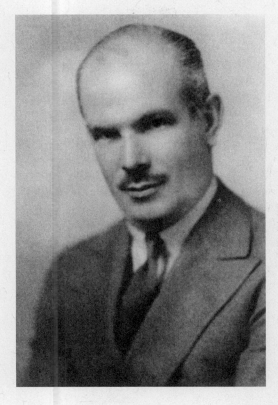

Figure 57
Horst Oertel, 1873–1956.
Photo by William Notman

his institute. Oertel (fig. 57), who did not like clinicians dabbling in pathology, offered two small rooms, one already occupied.

This arrangement was unsatisfactory for Penfield. Meakins, however, saved the day. After hearing this story, he offered three rooms in the University Clinic, which were being used for hospital and clinical research. Subdividing the rooms would provide sufficient space for what Penfield wanted, so the agreement was sealed. In October 1928 Penfield would come to Montreal with a team including his assistant, William Cone (fig. 58), his resident, Joseph Evans, and his chief technician.

After a year Penfield told Martin and Archibald that he needed more space and wondered if the Rockefeller Foundation might be interested in supporting a program to expand the neurosurgical facilities. Martin was reluctant to become involved, because he had just completed negotiations with the foundation for the department of experimental surgery under Archibald the same year, but he told Penfield that he was free to approach the foundation independently. Penfield did so, corresponding with Pearce, whom he had already met in New York City.

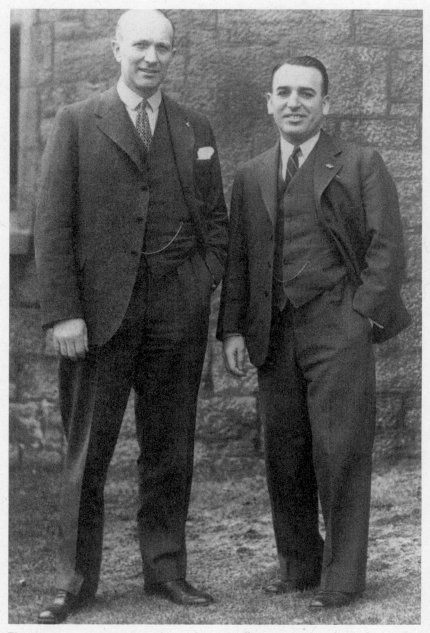

Figure 58
Wilder Graves Penfield, OBE, 1891–1976 and William Vernon Cone,
1897–1959. Photographer unknown, c. 1928

Pearce expressed interest in his idea; the foundation, he said, was considering other proposals in neurosurgical research. Pearce, however, felt that this was not the time for Penfield to apply for funding, because McGill had just received a grant. Penfield stated that he was still interested in founding an institute for neurological research and that he did not care where it was situated. A wealthy benefactor from New York had given him $10,000 in 1929 and 1930 and a bequest of $50,000 a little later. These funds enabled him to keep his McGill laboratory functioning for the present, but he was thinking of the future.

The plans were put aside when Pearce died suddenly. Penfield's three-year contract at McGill was drawing to an end in 1931, and because there was no action to renew it, there was a strong possibility that he and Cone would leave McGill. The University of Pennsylvania was at this time actively recruiting them. Martin saw the threat of losing Penfield and alerted the Royal Victoria's board of governors. He suggested going again to the Rockefeller Foundation with a proposal for expansion of the neurosurgical clinical and research facilities. Meanwhile, Penfield was offered Wards A and K at the RVH, which would give him a total of forty-two beds, but they were in different parts of the hospital, and this really was not what he wanted.

Dean Martin sensed the urgency of the situation. Hearing that the University of Pennsylvania had made a proposal and had invited Penfield to consider directing a funded neurological institute, it did not take Martin long to figure out that the funding was coming from the Rockefeller Foundation. In a bold move, he called Alan Gregg, Pearce's successor at the foundation, and explained the impasse they were facing in Montreal. He asked that before any decision was made about Philadelphia, Gregg should come to Montreal to hear McGill's proposal for a neurological centre. This call typified Martin's belief in McGill and his focus on improving clinical research at the medical school.

Early on 10 October 1931 Gregg arrived in Montreal. Penfield met him at the Westmount Railway Station and took him to his home on Montrose Avenue. After breakfast the two men got to know each other. Gregg had read the proposal for support of a neurological unit that Penfield had sent to Pearce in 1929. Gregg was interested in supporting a focused and collaborative scientific effort for a dedicated centre for diseases of the nervous system. Penfield was quite taken aback by Gregg's candid statement; it was more than he had hoped.

Later that day Gregg met with Martin and Archibald to discuss Penfield's proposal. The following day Gregg came to the point with Penfield and asked him for the background for his proposal of a clinical research centre for neurological diseases. What team had he put together, and was there local support for building a separate centre? He wanted a man with a "germinal idea" who could carry his ideas to completion. The fact that Penfield had just such an idea appealed to him. When he left Montreal, Gregg said that the Rockefeller Foundation wanted to fund a neurological institute somewhere – either in Philadelphia, Boston, or Montreal – and wanted Penfield to make a formal proposal and decide where he wanted it to go.

Penfield probably had already made up his mind to stay in Montreal; however, he had to wait for William Cone to agree to stay with him. When Cone decided against Philadelphia, Penfield sent a telegram to Gregg on 23 November 1931 stating that he had thrown in his lot with McGill. Shortly thereafter Martin and Penfield took the formal proposal for a Montreal Neurological Institute (MNI) to the Rockefeller Foundation in New York.

When it became certain that the foundation would support Penfield's proposal, Principal Currie then stepped in as McGill's official representative to take charge of the building program and kept a tight rein on the available funds. Rockefeller gave McGill $1 million as an endowment for the neurological institute and $230,000 for half of the building cost, the remainder to come from local donors. J.W. McConnell and Sir Herbert Holt gave $100,000 each, and other donors gave the rest. A later request to the Rockefeller Foundation for more funds to make up a shortfall was refused, even after Currie and Penfield visited New York. However, the foundation did provide the money when it was realized that salaries for the first year of the centre's operation had not been factored into the original request.

The Montreal Neurological Institute was formally opened on 27 September 1934 with "that observance of ceremony and dignity" that became the trademark of all MNI formal developments. Many famous and influential people were in attendance, including the mayor of Montreal, Camilien Houde, the Quebec minister of Public Health, Athanase David, Dean Charles Martin, the president of the Royal Victoria, Sir Herbert Holt, chairman of surgery at McGill, Edward Archibald, the chairman of neurosurgery at Harvard University, Harvey Cushing, and Gordon Holmes (later Sir Gordon), who was senior staff member of the National Hospital at Queen Square London.[30] Principal Currie died shortly before the MNI opened.

Once again Dean Martin had played a major role in establishing a funded clinical research centre at McGill. Principal Currie, however, played an equally important role. A tough, decisive ex-commander of the Canadian Army in Europe in World War I, Sir Arthur provided formidable support in these endeavours as McGill's chief administrative officer. It is easy to understand why the word at the Rockefeller Foundation was that, when Martin and Currie were coming to New York, the chequebook was to be locked away because two men were so persuasive.

THE RODDICK MEMORIAL GATES

Sir Thomas Roddick was obsessed with punctuality to the point where he would arrive at the front entrance to the McGill campus, drive to the Medical Building, and walk into the lecture room at the exact time his lecture was scheduled to begin. Punctuality was so much a part of his life that he and his wife, Lady Amy Redpath Roddick, discussed the need for a central clock at McGill to serve as a guide for the students. After Sir Thomas died of complications of pernicious anemia on 20 February 1923, Lady Roddick offered to contribute money for the construction of formal gates and a clock tower at the Sherbrooke Street entrance to the McGill campus to replace an earlier wooden structure. She wanted McGill to arrange the design of the gates in the style of the Arts Building. Her only requirement was that the design of the gates should include a clock tower.

Sir Herbert Holt, reputed to be the wealthiest man in Canada, was chairman of the Roddick Memorial Gates Committee. Other committee members were Principal Sir Arthur Currie, Mrs Aps Glasco, Dr Harrison, W.R. Miller, Cleveland Morgan of Morgan's Department Store, professor of architecture R. Traquir, and the Honorable George Foster, who represented Lady Roddick. Designs were submitted, and in February 1924 the committee chose the one that was in keeping with the portico of the Arts Building. The architect wanted the gates to frame the front of the Arts Building from Sherbrooke Street and McGill College Avenue and to be a grand opening into the McGill campus. The stone for the gates, except for the columns and the capitals, was hand-carved Indiana limestone. The clock tower was on the west side of the gates when entering the McGill grounds, with clock faces on three sides. The clockworks were accessible by a small bronze door at the back of the tower. Construction started in 1924 (fig. 59) and was completed in time for the June 1925 convocation, when the gates were officially opened (fig. 60). The plaque on the west side of the clock tower reads

These Gates were erected in memory of
Sir Thomas George Roddick MD LLD FRCS LMCC
MCMXXIV

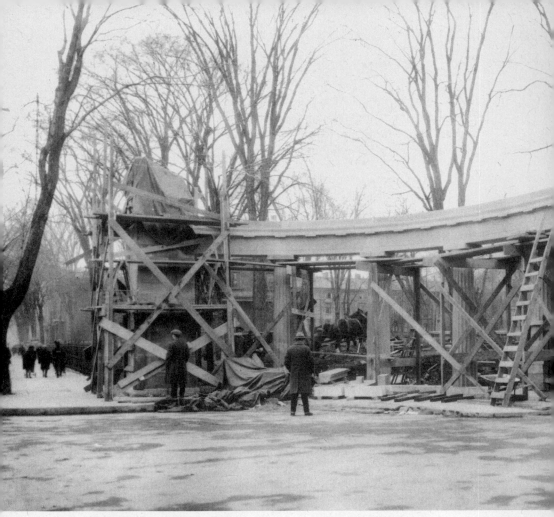

Figure 59
Roddick Memorial Gates under construction. Photo by William Notman, 1924

Left: Figure 60
Roddick Memorial Gates, completed. Officially opened June 1925.
Photographer unknown. The elm trees planted by Sir William Dawson in 1855
died of Dutch elm disease in the 1970s.

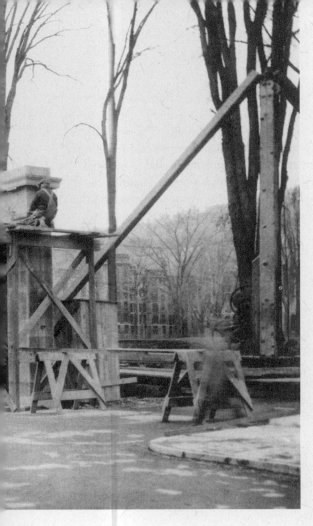

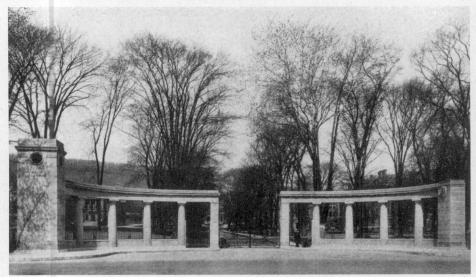

In 1925 the chimes in the clock tower sounded on the hour, day and night. When this annoyed people living on McGill College Avenue and along Sherbrooke Street, the clock's chimes were silenced as a community gesture for almost forty years. After 1960, commercial buildings replaced the houses and apartments in the neighbourhood. The clock's works were repaired, and for a while the chimes of the Roddick Gates rang out. At the time of writing, the chimes have again stopped, and the three faces of the clock tower seldom manage to tell the same time.[31]

THE OSLER LIBRARY

An important event during Martin's deanship was the official opening, after years of planning, of the Osler Library in the Strathcona Medical Building on 29 May 1929.

From student days Osler had been a bibliophile and a collector. His literary activities had increased after he moved to Oxford in 1905 and with his appointment as a curator of the Bodleian Library. He spent his own money and gifts from his brother Edmund to collect rare books including first editions and incunabula. For a decade his home at 13 Norham Gardens was overflowing with books and manuscripts.

After 1910 Osler began to organize under eight headings the catalogue that would become the *Bibliotheca Osleriana*.[32] So that it would not be broken up on his death, he decided to bequeath his library to his alma mater, McGill – but with one caveat: the *Bibliotheca* had to be completed before the collection would be moved from 13 Norham Gardens. Osler had made substantial progress on the *Bibliotheca* before his death in December 1919, but it was far from complete; his library remained at 13 Norham Gardens for a decade.

In 1920 McGill received official notification from Lady Osler about Osler's bequest.[33] S.E. Whitnall, the recently appointed professor of anatomy, was authorized to visit Oxford as the official representative of the McGill's medical faculty to make arrangements for the library's transfer to Montreal. Whitnall was a logical choice, since he had been a student and teacher at Oxford.[34] In 1922 Osler's nephew, William Francis, moved into Norham Gardens to complete the cataloguing. At McGill there was a debate whether the Osler collection would be part of the University Library, the Medical Library, or a separate collection. It had been Osler's wish that his bequest would form the basis of a library that would educate students in the history of medicine and science and be a centre for research in those areas. The medical faculty decided that the Osler Library, defined as "a collection of books donated by William

Osler," would be a separate entity.[35] McGill received an endowment of $27,000 for its support.[36]

Percy Nobbs designed elegant rooms for the library – described by Michael Bliss as "a mixture of shrine and mausoleum," on the third floor of the Strathcona Medical Building. The university governors approved his plans. The faculty appointed Whitnall, Macphail, and Birkett to oversee the transfer of the books from Oxford to McGill.[37]

As chief editor of the *Bibiliotheca Osleriana*, Francis made slow progress with the cataloguing, in spite of help from Archibald Malloch, Ramsay Wright, and R.H. Hill from the Bodleian Library. Francis was an inexperienced bibliographer. Osler was his hero, and he wanted perfection in every citation. At times he delayed decisions for days while considering grammatical and bibliographical construct. Lady Osler became frustrated with the slow progress and Francis's custom of working late at night and rising at 10:00 A.M. Unfortunately, she died 31 August 1928 before the *Bibliotheca* was completed. Oxford Press finally took over the project and forced its completion. Oxford Clarendon Press published the 786-page *Bibliotheca Osleriana: A Catalogue of Books Illustrating the History of Medicine and Science Collected, Arranged and Annotated by Sir William Osler, Bt., and Bequeathed to McGill University* in 1928.

The eight thousand books were packed in eighty-six huge cases for shipment to Montreal. When they arrived on 4 February 1929, Francis – who had been appointed Osler Librarian – began unpacking, sorting, and placing the books on the library shelves. Until his death in 1959, he continued in the position, providing a consulting service for a wide audience and establishing the library as an outstanding resource centre for the history of medicine.

In 1966 the Osler Library was moved intact to the new MacIntyre Medical Building. Later the Wellcome Camera, the W.W. Francis Wing, and the Robertson Rare Book Room were added.[38]

DEAN MARTIN'S RETIREMENT

In 1935 the McGill governors decided that sixty-five was the age for mandatory retirement for academic staff. In 1936 Martin was already three years beyond retirement age. Although he had been a member of the teaching staff since 1894, professor of medicine from 1907 to 1936, and full-time dean from 1923 to 1936 and was still in vigorous health, the regulation applied to him as well as to Stephen Leacock, Maude Abbott, and ten other members of the McGill teaching staff.[39]

For years Martin, his wife, and her relatives had been generous in their support of the Art Association of Montreal, later renamed the Montreal Museum of Fine Arts and then the Musée des Beaux Arts. After retirement Martin transferred his energy and administrative talents to the Art Association, which was desperately in need of help. He served as president from 1938 to 1947 and from his efforts the Art Association achieved financial stability and continued an active role in the cultural life of the community. Martin died in Montreal in 1953.[40]

5 Pre-Clinical Subjects

To the physician particularly a scientific discipline is an incalcula-
ble gift, which leavens his whole life, giving exactness to habits
of thought and tempering the mind with that judicious faculty
of distrust which can alone, amid the uncertainties of practice,
make him wise unto salvation.
WILLIAM OSLER[1]

ANATOMY[2]

As professor and chairman of the anatomy department from 1883 to
1913, Francis Shepherd lectured to the medical students from 9:00 to
10:00 A.M. five days a week throughout the academic year. He stressed
the importance of dissection, and after his lectures he visited the dissection room with his demonstrators. In the 1880s the medical students spent up to five hours a day in the dissecting room, including
evening sessions. In 1894 when the academic year was lengthened
from six to nine months, the evening sessions in the dissection room
were discontinued.[3]

After 1880 when Shepherd gained surgical experience, he adopted a
practical approach to anatomy, including in his lectures examples of the
importance of anatomy in medical and surgical practice.[4] At the turn of
the century, however, he recognized that anatomy could no longer be
emphasized as much as it had been because of progress in physiology,
chemistry, and pharmacology – all requiring more time in the curriculum. Although anatomy was important, it was no more important than
the other subjects.[5]

For the 1907–08 session, anatomy was taught in the first and second
years of the four-year course, and the faculty introduced a course in
practical anatomy for fourth-year students on Saturday mornings, for a
total of 450 hours.[6] Most medical licensing authorities required a

minimum of two hundred hours of combined lecture and laboratory instruction in anatomy for registration.[7]

In 1908 Shepherd became dean, and he had assistants to share the teaching load in anatomy.[8] When the east block of the SMB was completed in 1910, the anatomy department moved into spacious quarters on the third floor. There was a large dissection room with good ventilation and lighting, preparation and storage rooms, a nearby lecture theatre, and offices for the professor and junior teaching staff.[9]

Shepherd chose his demonstrators carefully, and several went on to illustrious careers – A.T. Bazin, H.S. Birkett, J.M. Elder, A.M.T. Forbes, R.L. MacDonnell, and R.T. McKenzie. But in his many years as professor of anatomy, none of his students had chosen anatomy as a career.[10] A possible explanation was Shepherd's attitude that the subject was a means to an end – an essential training for practice, especially for surgery, not an end in itself. For years he was the leading Canadian anatomist, with an international reputation. Later, J.C. Boileau Grant (1886–1973) of Winnipeg and Toronto eclipsed his reputation.[11]

When Shepherd retired as professor of anatomy in June 1913, the faculty minutes included a tribute:[12]

Members of the Medical Faculty have learned with the greatest regret that Dr. Shepherd has tendered his resignation from the chair of anatomy to the Governors of the University. From the time of his appointment in 1875 to the post of demonstrator of anatomy, Dr. Shepherd has spared no effort in the building up and organization of his department so that today McGill has a department of anatomy which is recognized and appreciated all over the world. As a teacher Dr. Shepherd has emphasized the importance of human anatomy. His lectures, always forceful and interesting, have been made doubly attractive by his free and artistic use of the blackboard, while his thorough method of dissection-room instruction has never failed to make a lasting impression on his students. Apart from his work as a teacher Dr. Shepherd has taken an active interest in the Medical Museum and more especially in the anatomical section, which although it suffered greatly during the [Medical Building] fire [15 April 1907] it has again been brought up to the highest standard. In his field of research Dr. Shepherd has done original and lasting work. He was the first to introduce a successful method of making frozen sections and his publications on [anatomical] anomalies have been recognized and quoted by anatomists in all parts of the world. Dr. Shepherd has always stood for the highest ideals in professional and scientific work and while the members of this Faculty deeply regret his decision to retire from active work in the department of anatomy, they desire to express the hope that he may enjoy a well merited rest from the arduous duties of teaching.

Towards the end of his tenure Shepherd maintained that the professor of anatomy should be a full-time position, and the incumbent should not have other major interests and appointments. Perhaps due to his recommendation, in 1913 the McGill governors appointed Auckland Geddes as McGill's first full-time professor of anatomy. Geddes came to McGill from Edinburgh after having previously worked in Dublin. In 1912 Robert Reford, a Montreal philanthropist, donated $100,000 to the medical faculty to support the anatomy department,[13] and Geddes became the first Reford Professor of Anatomy.[14]

Shortly after he came to McGill, Geddes changed the teaching program in anatomy with reduced hours. Though Shepherd was dean of the faculty, Geddes failed to consult him; but eventually Shepherd accepted the changes.[15]

War started after Geddes had been in his post for a year, and he offered his services to the British Army in August 1914. As his acceptance was delayed, he became involved with the McGill Provisional Battalion as commanding officer with the rank of major.[16] Later that year he was ordered to England, and McGill gave him leave of absence until the end of the war. Geddes's first duties in England were as director of recruiting and other government posts. His extraordinary administrative ability impressed the British government, and he became a member of the British cabinet as president of the Board of Trade. Later in the war he was knighted the Right Honorable Sir Auckland Geddes.

In 1919 Geddes resigned as professor of anatomy. In the same year Principal Sir William Peterson retired due to poor health, and the McGill governors appointed Geddes principal and vice-chancellor of McGill. However, he requested a further year's leave of absence so that he could continue in government service. Bigger and better opportunities awaited him, and instead of returning to McGill, in 1920 he resigned as principal to accept an appointment as British ambassador to the United States.[17]

From 1914 to 1919 a sequence of assistant professors, lecturers, and demonstrators taught the anatomy course, continuing the programs started by Shepherd and modified by Geddes. As his successor, in 1919 McGill appointed Samuel Ernest Whitnall, a dedicated and less political anatomist[18] (fig. 61), the Reford Professor of Anatomy and chairman of the McGill department.

Whitnall was a "pure anatomist," a charming man and an enthusiastic and dedicated teacher but a stickler for detail. Anatomy was taught in first year; students attended three one-hour lectures a week and spent anywhere from nine to twelve hours a week in the dissection

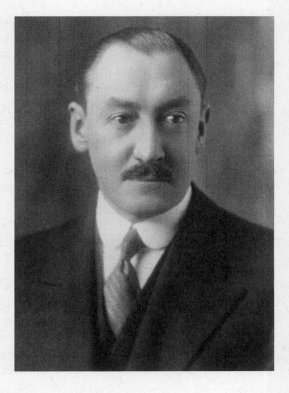

Figure 61
Samuel Ernest Whitnall,
1876–1950. Photographer
unknown

room. The class was divided into teams of four, each team assigned a
cadaver. Gross anatomy was taken in systems, as is the custom even
today. At the end of each system, such as the thorax, the abdomen, or
the nervous system, Whitnall introduced "spot examinations" for the
students. The staff placed specimens on the laboratory benches with
pins indicating certain structures and questions about them.[19] In addition there were bone identification sessions, with the students blind-
folded at times, so that they had to identify a bone by touch. Students
were graded according to their results from the these examinations, the
final written and oral examinations, and their work in the dissecting
room. Whitnall taught anatomy at McGill until 1934 when, much to
the regret of the faculty, he returned to England to accept an appointment as professor of anatomy at the University of Bristol.[20]

Whitnall left his mark at McGill in several respects. In 1922 he published a small book, *The Study of Anatomy, Written for the Medical
Student*,[21] a popular guide in the approach to the study of anatomy
and related subjects. His main research interest was the orbit. In 1921
he published *Anatomy of the Orbit*[22] and was the expert in that field.

He was also involved in the establishment of the McGill Osler Society[23] with a group of students led by C.J. Tidmarsh. The Osler Society, devoted to stoking the coals of medical history, became the most prestigious society of the medical faculty and attracted many students to its meetings and graduates to the annual banquets. As secretary of the Osler Library Reception Committee, Whitnall played an important role in the arrangements for the transfer of Osler's library to McGill.

In 1936 Cecil P. Martin came to McGill from Trinity College Dublin where he had been university anatomist from 1928 to 1936.[24] He continued as Reford Professor of Anatomy and chairman of the department until 1957.

HISTOLOGY[25]

After Osler left McGill in 1884, George Wilkins[26] carried on teaching histology, including the laboratory course. He purchased more microscopes and collected more specimens, and he also taught the histology course that Osler had started for senior students. Neal Gunn, the Holmes Medallist in 1888, assisted Wilkins for ten years. Gunn went to Johns Hopkins and earned a Ph.D. in anatomy and histology before returning to McGill. When Gunn resigned, W.M. Fisk and H. Blushing assisted Wilkins.

In 1908 J.G. Adami, professor of pathology, recommended that the teaching of histology should be a joint responsibility of the departments of anatomy, physiology, and pathology, supervised by an "advisory committee" with representatives from the three departments.[27] When Wilkins retired in 1907, C.W. Duval, a pathologist, taught the histology course that was given in the first two years. In 1910 J.C. Simpson,[28] a biologist, took over the histology and embryology courses, assisted by Fisk. With the completion of the SMB in 1910, the histology department moved to a new laboratory on the second floor of the east wing, with excellent lighting and storage facilities for students' microscopes. When Geddes became professor of anatomy in 1913, histology and embryology were made the sole responsibility of the anatomy department, and the attempted takeover by pathology was dropped.

PHYSIOLOGY[29]

In 1877 Osler travelled to Boston to visit the Harvard Medical School and the Bowdich Laboratory for Physiology. He was impressed with the facilities and convinced of the importance of laboratory experience for medical students. By 1880 he succeeded in persuading the McGill medical faculty to provide a proper physiology laboratory. His lectures and laboratory demonstrations dealt with physiological chemistry, digestion, and secretions. In 1881 the faculty appointed Thomas Wesley Mills, a promising physiologist,[30] as demonstrator to help Osler in the recently established laboratory. Mills procured apparatus for the laboratory; W.S. Morrow and A.A. Robertson assisted him.

When Osler left McGill in 1884 to go to Philadelphia, Mills was appointed lecturer and in 1886 became professor of physiology. He taught a lecture and demonstration course for first-year students and laboratory work for second-year students, using new apparatus in the physiology laboratory. By this time a great deal of basic and organ specific physiology was known. In 1628 William Harvey had demonstrated the separate arterial and venous circulations of the blood, one of medicine's great discoveries. Priestly, Lavoisier, and Haldane had isolated oxygen and carbon dioxide and determined the relationship of those gases to living cells. It was known that the stomach contained hydrochloric acid and pepsin and that the pancreas secreted digestive enzymes. After Beaumont started his work in 1833, much was understood about how food was digested. It was also known that nerves carried current that made the muscles contract and that there were afferent and efferent nerves to and from the spinal cord.

By 1890, after Mills had been professor for four years, the physiology course for first-year students consisted of lectures and laboratory demonstrations. Second-year laboratory work in physiology consisted of experiments on foodstuffs, digestion, blood, and urine. The renovations of the Medical Building in 1894 included a new physiology laboratory with proper space for a student laboratory – a large room with benches and individual sitting spaces with drawers and a small cabinet for equipment (fig. 24) – and three separate research laboratories. These facilities allowed Mills and his three assistants to gradually expand the course to include simple laboratory work in the first year and physiological chemistry. Mills wrote one of the first medical textbooks from McGill, his *Textbook of Comparative Physiology* (1890).

In 1897 the Drake Family endowed the chair of physiology in honour of Joseph Morley Drake, former professor of the institutes of medicine,[31] and Mills became the first Morley Drake Professor of Physiology. In 1903 the faculty spent $3,000 on new apparatus for the physiology laboratory. Smoked drums and spectrometers were available so that second-year students could record the results of experiments on blood pressure and respiration of animals.

In the major fire in April 1907 that destroyed about one-third of the Medical Building, the physiology laboratory was fortunately saved. By that time Mills had six assistants: W.S. Morrow, assistant professor; A.A. Robertson and A.H. Gordon, lecturers; W.B. Howell[32] and T.P. Shaw, demonstrators; and A. Gildon, assistant demonstrator. Eighty students per laboratory session worked with modern electrical (smoked drum) equipment and studied the physiological chemistry of blood, digestion, and urine. In the second semester they studied the principles of respiration and circulation of blood, and gastrointestinal, genitourinary, muscle, and nerve functions.

In 1910 when Mills retired because of ill health,[33] the faculty had considerable difficulty in finding a new chairman. In 1911 N.H. Alcock was appointed professor and chairman, but he died after two years.[34] In 1914 G.R. Mines was appointed professor of physiology, but he died one year later.[35] Because of the war it was difficult to recruit a professor of physiology from the United Kingdom. In the unsettled period from 1910 to 1920, at various times F.R. Miller and W.S. Morrow were acting chairmen, and they recruited local teachers to continue the physiology courses.[36] In 1919 while Dean Birkett was travelling in England, he sent a telegram to the medical faculty recommending John Tait, a Scottish physiologist of the classical school, for the position of Morley Drake Professor of Physiology. The faculty and the McGill board of governors concurred and offered the appointment to Tait. He accepted and arrived in Montreal in 1920.

The basic physiology course and laboratory schedule did not change over the next seven years. The advanced course in 1920 included study of physiology for three hours per week and in third year a course on mammalian physiology on cats and dogs using Sherrington's textbook *Mammalian Physiology*. In 1924 the new Biology Building (now the F. Cyril James Building) was opened, and the physiology department occupied new offices and laboratories. The frog and mammalian work continued, and hospital clinics were given with clinical/physiological correlation. Medical students formed a Physiological Society.

The physiology course still required two years, with introductory lectures and laboratory sessions in the spring term of the first year. Second year included three hours per week of lectures, frog laboratories for six hours per week in the fall term, and mammalian laboratories in the winter term.

Boris Babkin, a renowned physiologist, arrived at McGill in 1928 with appointments as research professor of physiology and professor of experimental medicine.[37] Tait had held the post of professor of experimental medicine from 1920 to 1928. Babkin introduced sophisticated research expertise to the physiology department, particularly in the function of the gastrointestinal tract. In 1928 physiology received another boost when the experimental surgery program was funded, and many of the candidates in the program worked with the physiologists.

Tait continued as Morley Drake Professor of Physiology until 1940. His main research interest was labyrinthine function, and he published numerous papers in that area with W.J. McNally from the department of otolaryngology.[38]

PHARMACOLOGY AND THERAPEUTICS (MATERIA MEDICA)

William Wright taught the course in materia medica from 1854 to 1883.[39] He did not distinguish between pure botany and the practical knowledge that students required to pass licensing examinations and to practise medicine. In a remarkable and unprecedented move, second-year students boycotted his lectures in December 1882 and petitioned for a new professor. Wright resigned in 1883 under protest because the faculty sided with the students. He was succeeded by James Stewart,[40] an internist, who was given the job by seniority. Stewart was professor of materia medica from 1883 to 1891, when he was succeeded by the remarkable Alexander Blackader.[41] One of McGill's most accomplished members of faculty, Blackader practised medicine, was head of the MGH pediatric clinic, gave a course of lectures on diseases of children with Professor J.C. Cameron, and was acting dean of medicine from 1915 to 1918 when Dean Birkett was serving with the CAMC. Editor of the CMAJ for a decade from 1919 to 1929, his strict editorial policy made it a reputable medical journal.

In 1895 the name of the course, Materia Medica, was changed to Pharmacology and Therapeutics, in keeping with the times and the developing chemical industry that had changed therapeutics. Chemical medications were displacing botanicals in the pharmacopoeia. In 1900 the course was given in the second and third years. Second year included three months of practical medicine and therapeutics, and six months of lectures and laboratory sessions on therapeutics. Blackader continued as professor, assisted by J.T. Halsey, A.A. Kerby, J. Morris, and J.W. Scane. In 1909 prescription writing was added to the laboratory course in the third year. By this time the course extended from second to the fifth year. The second and third year courses remained the same. In fourth year, a course on the action of drugs was added, and in the fifth year a course on applied therapeutics was given at the hospitals.

In 1912 the pharmacology and therapeutics course was reduced to three years, because it was taking too much time in the curriculum. In 1914 C.J. Tidmarsh was lecturer, and F.W. Nagle and W. Bourne were demonstrators.

Blackader resigned as professor of pharmacology in 1920 to make way for a new professor and chairman of the department, R.C. Stehle,[42] who modernized the course and added D.S. Lewis, S.M. Rosenthal, D.G. Campbell, and C.C. Stewart to the staff. J.C. Meakins and F.B. Gurd taught a course on immunology and infectious diseases, a new subject in the curriculum. N. Brown and F.W. Howser taught physiotherapy. The pharmacology course now started in the third year (the medical course was six years) with an introduction to pharmacology and a laboratory term to study the chemistry and action of drugs. In fourth year, lectures were given on the principles of therapeutics and the application of drugs. In the fifth year members of the department of medicine conducted ward classes at the MGH and the RVH regarding the clinical applications of drugs. After his appointment in 1924, Professor Meakins stressed bridging the gap between the science and the practical applications of pharmacology.

In the 1920s members of the departments of medicine and surgery were doing research in collaboration with the pharmacologists. By 1930 Stehle was assisted by D.S. Lewis, N.B. Drewe, and W. Bourne. The course remained unchanged in format but with the addition of information about new drugs.

CHEMISTRY[43] AND BIOCHEMISTRY

Chemistry and Materia Medica was one of four courses offered by the Montreal Medical Institution in 1828,[44] and chemistry in one form or another continued to be part of the medical school curriculum. The content of the courses depended on the instructor, the body of knowledge at the time, and the students' knowledge of chemistry prior to entering the medical faculty.

In 1879 Gilbert Prout Girdwood, a knowledgeable and practical chemist, was placed in charge of the chemistry course.[45] He lectured to the students and conducted a practical laboratory course. Robert Fulton Ruttan was appointed in 1886 to assist Girdwood in the practical chemistry course and teach chemistry to medical and undergraduate science students.[46] As most first-year medical students had very little knowledge of chemistry, the course was given at an elementary level, followed by a more advanced course in the second year. In 1888 Ruttan was placed in charge of the course in organic chemistry.[47] The construction of the new chemistry laboratories in the Medical Building in 1894 (fig. 23) was a great improvement for the practical chemistry classes.

After 1896 Girdwood became interested in the new techniques of x-rays, and gradually withdrew from teaching chemistry. Ruttan assumed more responsibility as professor of practical chemistry.[48] By the turn of the century, many first year students had already studied general chemistry in the arts faculty, so the basic course became redundant. The content was gradually altered to include physiological and biological chemistry.[49] Ruttan's appointment was changed to professor of organic and biological chemistry. He developed a particular interest and expertise in public health and water supplies.

In 1912 general chemistry was taught in three McGill faculties – medicine, arts, and applied science. The University Corporation decided that all general chemistry would be taught in the Faculty of Arts and Science using the facilities in the Chemistry Building on the east side of the campus.[50]

The separation of chemistry and biochemistry began during Ruttan's tenure as chair of the university chemistry department, which was strong and developed major interests outside of the medical field. The requirements of modern medicine for biochemistry indicated that changes were required. Consequently, with the construction of the new Biology Building in 1920, biochemistry became officially separated from the chemistry department. With the establishment of the biochemistry department in the medical faculty in 1920, professors and instructors from that department gave the lectures and supervised laboratories for the medical students. In 1923 the medical faculty made an important decision in defining the entrance requirements to include the successful completion of three years of college or university courses in general and organic chemistry, physics, and biology.[51] Thereafter only biochemistry and physiological chemistry were included in the medical school curriculum.

The first true biochemist to arrive at McGill was Archibald Byron Macallum. He gained his B.A. at the University of Toronto in 1880 and began his academic career as a schoolteacher. He completed a Ph.D. in biology at Johns Hopkins University in 1888, a medical degree at Toronto in 1889, and would later study at Harvard University and in the United Kingdom. In 1890 he was appointed lecturer in physiology at University of Toronto and professor the following year. From 1908 to 1916 he was professor and chairman of the biochemistry department. When the National Research Council was founded in Ottawa in 1917, Macallum became its first chairman. The progress and foundation of the council on sound scientific lines was in a large measure due to his far-seeing guidance. In 1920, at age sixty-two, after having spent three years in Ottawa, he accepted the position of chairman of the new biochemistry department at McGill. Under his direction the medical school curriculum for biochemistry became the full responsibility of the new department and provided a chemical basis for the practice of medicine. Macallum retired from active service at seventy in 1928 with the title of professor emeritus.

Ruttan had established a graduate program, and there were students who continued in Macallum's time, although the numbers were small. Macallum's scientific interests were wide, but his own research compared the composition of the body fluids of many organisms with that of prehistoric seawaters. Macallum was extremely well known and belonged to many professional organizations. He received numerous honours, including election as a fellow of the Royal Societies of London, Glasgow, and Canada. He had a major influence of the development of science in Canada and enhanced McGill's reputation in the scientific community.[52]

After Macallum retired in 1928, the Corporation recruited James Bertram Collip (1892–1965) to take over the chair of biochemistry.[53] At that time biochemistry was a very active field in which many fundamental discoveries were being made, none more exciting than in endocrinology. Collip was recognized as one of the world's outstanding investigators in the field of endocrinology, and his contributions to the isolation and purification of insulin had been recognized in 1921. Prior to coming to McGill, he had successfully isolated parathyroid hormone and identified its relationship to calcium metabolism. Collip received offers to accept other academic appointments, but having been a former student of Macallum, he elected to remain at McGill. He was thirty-five years old, full of energy, and an able leader and scientist. He recruited David L. Thomson from England. Hans Selye joined the biochemistry department, as did John S.L. Browne, who took a ph.d. with Collip.

In addition to medical student instruction, undergraduate programs in biochemistry (along with other basic sciences) were established during this time. Throughout Collip's tenure as chairman, there was a sense of excitement in the department. Browne isolated estriol, work proceeded on the isolation of adrenocorticotrophic hormone (ACTH), and the publication rate was extremely high. Collip was the first incumbent of the Gilman Cheney Chair of Biochemistry. In 1938 he expressed a desire to step down as chairman and devote all of his energies to research, clearly his primary interest. D.L. Thomson, who was a brilliant teacher, carried much of the instruction. However, World War II was imminent, and Collip stayed at McGill until 1941 when Thomson took over the chair of the biochemistry department.[54]

BIOLOGY – BOTANY AND ZOOLOGY

The situation for biology was similar to that of chemistry. Prior to 1900 the first-year medical students had very little knowledge of theoretical or practical biology. For many years Principal Sir John William Dawson taught botany and zoology to the medical students.[55] After he retired in 1893, P. Penhallow, F.E. Lloyd, MacBride, and Wiley taught biology for two hours per week until 1912. Those professors had joint appointments in the arts and medical faculties, and they were granted seats on the medical faculty executive.

After 1912 botany and zoology were gradually eliminated from the medical school curriculum.[56] Those subjects were taught in the arts faculty, and successful completion of a course in biology became part of the admission requirements to the medical faculty.

PATHOLOGY AND BACTERIOLOGY

The first knowledgeable pathologist at McGill, William Osler, returned from Europe in 1874 and was appointed pathologist to the Montreal General Hospital in 1877. He used his knowledge of pathology to improve student teaching. Pathology was his research interest, and he wrote many articles and books based on the 780 autopsies he did at the hospital between 1874 and 1884. The pathology in his textbook *Principles and Practice of Medicine*, published in 1892, came mainly from the Montreal General experience.

As a medical student Wyatt Johnston[57] worked with Osler in the pathology laboratory. After postgraduate study in Europe in 1886, Johnston was appointed pathologist to the Montreal General. Initially he continued teaching using the autopsy material from the hospital and published in Osler's footsteps. His quest for new frontiers gradually led him away from morphological pathology to public health and bacteriology. He realized that technological advances in handling and culturing of material from the body were needed. He published on bacteriologic technique and developed a reputation as an independent thinker.

At first the pathology laboratory was in the basement of the Montreal General Hospital. In 1895 it moved to a small building on the hospital grounds. This was enlarged, with a new Pathology Building constructed in 1909–11.

In the late 1880s the medical faculty needed a department and professor of pathology, particularly with the plans for the new Royal Victoria Hospital. On the recommendation of the faculty, the university governors appointed John George Adami professor of pathology in 1892, before the RVH was completed and an endowment had been offered.[58] The funds were forthcoming in 1893 when Lord Strathcona donated $100,000 to endow chairs in pathology and hygiene. Adami became the first Strathcona Professor of Pathology.[59]

On his arrival in Montreal, Adami settled into offices in the northeast wing of the renovated Medical Building. The Royal Victoria's postmortem facility was completed in 1894. Initially Adami was advisory pathologist to the Montreal General and the Royal Victoria. He complained about these appointments since he thought his academic reputation would suffer without the titles of pathologist to the MGH and RVH. The MGH wanted to appoint its own pathologist, so Adami continued to be advisory pathologist. However, the RVH board of governors was sympathetic to his point of view and appointed him pathologist; he was assisted by A.G. Nicholls

Adami's haven from the clinical service was his office in the Medical Building where he wrote his papers and his textbooks.[60] He became involved in many projects, studying diseases such as rheumatic fever, pneumonia, appendicitis, and typhoid fever and its complications. He published reports with members of the clinical staff on these and other subjects, including the mechanism of infection. "J. George" became involved in the medical community, reviving the Montreal Medico-Chirurgical (Med-Chi) Society by presenting new cases at each meeting and becoming an editor of the *Montreal Medical Journal*. As a community leader he helped to found the University Club.

Adami appointed Maude Abbott as curator of the Medical Museum in 1899. She made it a monument for teaching and study. The museum, an appendage to the medical school for years, was so well catalogued and developed under Abbott's leadership that it became an impetus to the founding of an International Association of Medical Museums in 1908, which Adami supported and Lord Strathcona funded. In 1907 the offices of the pathology department and the Medical Museum suffered fire damage, but that didn't stop the activities. Museum specimens that had been lost were soon replaced by generous donations from other museums. Abbott was able to save some of Osler's original specimens.

The next major figure in McGill pathology, John McCrae, arrived in Montreal in 1901 to study under Adami after a year at Johns Hopkins.

Wyatt Johnston died unexpectedly in 1901 from an infection, so Mc-
Crae went to the Montreal General to be resident pathologist under
Adami's supervision. He became a Governors' Fellow in 1902. In 1904
he moved back to the Royal Victoria to a position in pathology and
clinical medicine and started a medical practice. He was replaced as MGH
pathologist by B.D. Gillies until 1906, CW. Duval from 1906 to 1909,
and then G.B. Wolbach. Duval became professor of pathology at Tu-
lane University, and Wolbach was appointed professor of pathology at
Harvard University. D.D. MacTaggart was assistant pathologist from
1905 to 1920. In 1910 L.J. Rhea began his long and brilliant term of
service that lasted until he died in 1944.

Adami's energy and interest in infection and inflammation led him to
greater interests in public health in 1905. He also published a two-
volume *Textbook of Pathology* (fig. 7) in 1908 and 1909. McCrae by
this time had relinquished the Governors' Fellowship, which he never
properly fulfilled. Oscar Klotz, whose main research interest was arteriosclerosis, was appointed in his place. Adami's academic interest in
research led him to retire from the clinical service at the Royal Victoria
in 1909. He was replaced by Oscar Gruner, but in 1913 Gruner was retired for budgeting reasons. Adami and McCrae wrote *A Textbook of
Pathology for Students* in 1911.[61] With the opening of the Strathcona
Medical Building, Adami moved into the west wing to continue his
research and writing on inflammation, inherited diseases, and public
health issues.

McGill and the Royal Victoria then recruited Horst Oertel[62] from
Guy's Hospital in London. He came to Montreal in the fall of 1914
after the war had begun. Both Adami and McCrae enlisted with the
CAMC and went overseas in 1915, leaving Oertel as acting chairman of
the pathology department. This was an extraordinary windfall for him,
because his views about the organization and role of the department
differed from those of Adami and McCrae, and neither returned to
McGill. McCrae died overseas, and Adami remained chairman of the
pathology department until 1919. He resigned at that time from McGill,
and was vice-chancellor of the University at Liverpool until he died
1925. In 1919 Oertel was confirmed as the second Strathcona Professor
of Pathology and remained in that position until his retirement in 1938.

A bachelor, Oertel lived at the Ritz Carlton Hotel and enjoyed his
private life. Educated at Yale, trained in Berlin, he had worked in New
Haven, Connecticut, New York City, and at Guy's Hospital in London.
He was a good lecturer and was respected but allowed few friends. He
had a close association with Sir Vincent Meredith, president of the RVH

from 1912 to 1928. Meredith's autocratic, heavy-handed actions did not endear him to the hospital staff. Unfortunately, Oertel was associated with some of these actions.

Like Adami, Oertel had his office in the SMB. The Royal Victoria's autopsy room was located in what is now the outpatient department. Odours from the autopsy room and pathology laboratories began to seep through the hospital via the underground tunnels that connected the RVH buildings, including the Ross Memorial Pavilion, and the hospital administrators heard many complaints. Fortunately, while the authorities were addressing what to do with the autopsy service, Acting Principal Frank Adams helped to obtain a $1,000,000 endowment from the Rockefeller Foundation for the McGill 1921 Centennial Fund, with a promise that McGill would construct a pathology institute. Sir Arthur Currie raised the money for the construction of the Pathological Institute[63] and the renovation of the Biology Building. Fearing that the university might place the Pathological Institute blocks away from the hospital, the RVH governors, who were well-to-do businessmen, pledged $100,000 to the project. McGill contributed the land that it owned across University Street directly opposite the emergency entrance to the RVH. The McGill architect Percy Nobbs and his associates designed a building in keeping with the RVH style to house pathology, bacteriology, and jurisprudence. The autopsy rooms were now in the basement of the Pathological Institute, connected to the Royal Victoria by a tunnel. There was a large lecture room, and student and research labs, costing $460,000 in all. The Province of Quebec generously promised a million dollars for the McGill Centennial for endowment.

The official opening of the McGill Pathological Institute (fig. 66) was celebrated on Founders' Day, 6 October 1924, after the fall convocation, by an academic procession from the campus to the institute. The lieutenant governor of Quebec and A.E. Boycott, a pathologist from England, addressed the audience, praising the skill of the institute for teaching and research. Boycott was chosen to speak because he shared the opinions of Adami and Oertel that, although the clinical demands of the pathology department were a responsibility, teaching and research were of primary importance. Oertel, as chairman of the pathology department and director of the Pathological Institute, supported research but did not cooperate with anyone when his interests were not considered. He remained aloof from McGill and had a petty side that was exemplified in 1928 when W.G. Penfield, accompanied by C.F. Martin and E.W. Archibald, sought a favour from him for research space in the Pathological Institute. Remembering how Penfield had rejected his invitation to visit Montreal five years earlier, Oertel offered minimal space, and so McGill almost lost Penfield. Oertel retired in 1938 when he reached the mandatory age of sixty-five.

In 1899 the faculty introduced a compulsory course for third-year students in the spring term to teach clinical microscopy and clinical laboratory methods using techniques that could be used in a doctor's office.[64] Martin organized the course; the lecturers and demonstrators of medicine assisted him. This course continued for many years with an expanded content, and the subject became known as clinical pathology.

Before he left Montreal in 1915 Adami appointed Dr Bruère to head a small clinical bacteriology laboratory at the Royal Victoria; the lab remained independent of the pathology department until the early 1920s. When Oertel became director of the Pathological Institute, the bacteriology laboratory was moved to a few small rooms in the institute. The next important development occurred in 1930 when Everitt George Dunne Murray came to Montreal as professor and head of bacteriology and immunology and bacteriologist-in-chief at the Royal Victoria.[65]

Murray's lectures to the medical students included descriptions of bacteria of various types (identified with the light microscope), and the diseases that they caused. There was no microbiology – only descriptive biology. Students learned techniques to handle subcultures of infective material, and transferred that material to culture plates, slopes, and solutions with loops. They would culture their own material and then make smears on slides, and stain the slides with Gram and other stains to help to identify the organisms.

Within a few years Murray developed a strong department for bacteriological services, teaching medical and graduate students and carrying out research. He remained at McGill until 1955.

6 Medicine and Medical Specialties

How can we make the work of the student in the third and fourth years as practical as it is in his first and second? The answer is, take him from the lecture-room, take him from the amphitheatre – put him on the wards. It is not the systematic lecture, not the amphitheatre clinic, not even the ward class – all of which have their value – in which the reformation is needed, but in the whole relationship of the senior student to the hospital.
WILLIAM OSLER[1]

MEDICINE

By 1885 Robert Palmer Howard had been professor of medicine since 1860 and dean of the medical faculty since 1882. He lectured on the theory and practice of medicine at the Medical Building from Monday to Friday at 4:00 P.M. and gave clinical lectures and presentations at the Montreal General on Monday, Friday, and Saturday from 12:45 to 1:45 or 2:00 P.M. His academic and pathology-oriented approach to medicine made the department exciting. Most of the students read Austin Flint's (1812–86) *Principles and Practice of Medicine*, first published in 1866. It went into seven editions and was the leading textbook of medicine prior to the publication of Osler's *Principles and Practice of Medicine* in 1892. In a few years Osler's book became the most widely read textbook in medicine in the English language.

George Ross, professor of clinical medicine, made hospital ward rounds of his patients at the MGH in the morning with the house surgeons and the medical students. A house surgeon, having written a patient's medical history in a folio-sized casebook that he carried on the rounds, would read the history to the class at the bedside and then write follow-up notes in the casebook based on Ross's findings on history and physical examination. The notes might include urine output, weight, and temperature – at that time there were no laboratory tests or x-rays. The follow-up notes would be made on a weekly basis – more frequently if there were significant changes in a patient's status.

For instruction on the hospital wards, Ross would select one medical student to examine a patient in the presence of the group and test that student on his knowledge of basic sciences – anatomy, physiology, pharmacology, and pathology. After the ward round, Ross would give a lecture to the students, usually bearing on an important case they had seen that week on the ward. Students were non-participating witnesses to patient care and observers of the natural history of the disease. Although the Montreal General had the reputation of being an open hospital, essentially this meant that the door was open for students to come in and out of the hospital providing they had purchased a Hospital Card; they were forbidden to deal with the patients regarding diagnosis and treatment.[2]

When Palmer Howard died in 1889, Ross was promoted professor of medicine, and Richard MacDonnell succeeded him as professor of clinical medicine. They continued a similar teaching program. However, this arrangement was short lived – MacDonnell died in 1891 and Ross in 1892.[3] The deaths of three senior members of the teaching staff within three years created a problem for Dean Craik. He promoted James Stewart, professor of materia medica and attending physician at the Montreal General, to succeed Ross as professor of medicine.

When the Royal Victoria opened in 1894,[4] one professor of clinical medicine could no longer supervise the practical teaching at both hospitals, and so the position of professor of clinical medicine was abolished. Stewart was professor of medicine and clinical medicine and taught the lecture course in medicine. He moved to the Royal Victoria where he admitted his private patients and consulted as chief of medicine. C.F. Martin and W.F. Hamilton assisted him with the clinical teaching there.

After Stewart's departure, William Alexander Molson became the senior physician at the Montreal General.[5] Although he had a busy medical practice, particularly amongst poor patients, he was not interested in teaching medical students on his own patients and did his own round unaccompanied. To continue the teaching program at the MGH, in 1894 Dean Craik appointed two young physicians, F.G. Finley (fig. 62) and H.A. Lafleur (fig. 63),[6] as lecturers of medicine and clinical medicine. They were each in charge of a medical service at the Montreal General, and they continued as senior attending physicians until they retired in 1924.

In 1894 there were forty-eight members of the medical faculty; twenty-two were professors. By 1900 the faculty had expanded to sixty-seven, including eight teachers in the department of medicine. These eight were: James Stewart, professor of medicine and clinical medicine

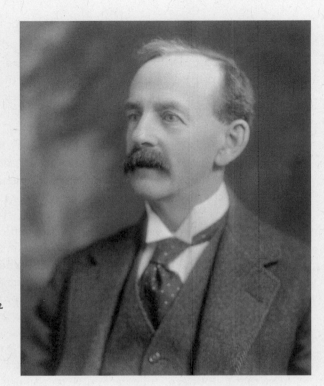

Figure 62
Frederick Gault Finley,
1861–1940. Photo by
William Notman, 1922

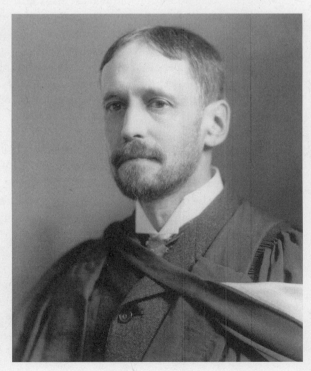

Figure 63
Henri Amédée Lafleur,
1862–1939. Photo by
William Notman, 1903

(RVH); Alexander D. Blackader, professor of pharmacology and therapeutics (MGH); Frederick G. Finley, associate professor of medicine and
clinical medicine (MGH); Henri A. Lafleur, associate professor of medicine and clinical medicine (MGH); Charles F. Martin, assistant professor of medicine and clinical medicine (RVH); G. Gordon Campbell,
lecturer in clinical medicine (MGH); William F. Hamilton, lecturer in
clinical medicine (RVH); and S. Ridley MacKenzie, demonstrator of
medicine. He did not have a hospital appointment.[7]

With an enlarged Medical Building for the pre-clinical departments,
and with the clinical facilities at both hospitals, the class size gradually
increased so that by 1900 there were more than one hundred students
in each class.[8] The teaching program consisted of sessions for the whole
class and other sessions for small groups. The whole class attended lectures on the theory and practice of medicine in the Medical Building
and amphitheatre clinics at the hospitals. The previous practice of the
professor of medicine giving all the lectures was abandoned. The professor, associate, and assistant professors gave the lectures and the amphitheatre clinics in rotation, according to their particular interests and
expertise. For the practical teaching, the class was divided into groups
of twelve to fourteen students who were assigned to either of the hospitals. For instruction on the wards, each group was divided into sub-
groups of six or seven,[9] with a junior member of the teaching staff in
charge of each subgroup. This arrangement required the appointment
of numerous physicians who had appointments as demonstrators or assistant demonstrators and often were assistant physicians in the outpatient clinics.[10] Generally they taught for a term of twelve weeks each
year. They were practising physicians in the community, and they made
major contributions to the teaching program.

Student teaching in medicine was conducted in a similar manner at
both hospitals. Some students requested that all their clinical training
be at either the Montreal General or the Royal Victoria. After some debate the faculty executive decided that students would rotate between
hospitals in the senior years. All students had to report cases assigned
to them in specific beds. The final-year students attended outpatient
clinics every week. The nagging deficiency in the clinical teaching persisted – that is, a lack of any involvement by students in the care of the
patients. When the number of house surgeons increased at the hospitals, they assisted in teaching students, but their teaching was limited
because they had many duties and responsibilities.

After 1904, Stewart stopped attending meetings of the faculty executive because of the onset of illness, and Martin took over his hospital

and teaching duties. When Stewart died in 1906, Martin, Lafleur, and Finley were promoted to professors of medicine.

Prior to 1924 all McGill clinical teachers were part time, and their incomes came from their medical practices. Their private offices were outside the hospitals, and they were relatively isolated from the medical school. (J.C. Meakins was the first full-time clinical appointment in 1924.) The full-time pre-clinical professors received salaries and had their offices in the Medical Building.[11] The primary goal of the McGill teaching hospitals was to treat patients. Research was not done in the hospitals because there were no facilities and no time for the busy physicians to be involved in research. The exceptions were Edward Archibald and Francis Scrimger in the department of surgery – they worked together on experimental surgical projects before World War I.

During World War I many members of the medical faculty served overseas with the CAMC. The doctors who remained in Montreal had a double load – increased teaching responsibilities and more patients. They carried on as best they could but, as discussed in chapters 3 and 4, major changes in the faculty had to wait until after the Armistice in 1918. At that time, with skilful negotiations C.F. Martin was able to start the reorganization of medical services at McGill.

The Royal Victoria staff supported the idea of a university clinic and a full-time professor, but such was not the case at the Montreal General. In 1924 when Finley and Lafleur retired, Dean Martin appointed Campbell Howard as professor of medicine and encouraged him to organize a McGill-MGH University Clinic similar to the McGill-RVH University Clinic. Martin hoped that Howard as MGH physician-in-chief would have a full-time role, similar to Meakins's appointment at the Royal Victoria. However, there was a power struggle at the Montreal General. The old guard, headed by A.H. Gordon, insisted on maintaining the two medical services system, with Howard the head of one service and Gordon the head of the second. Howard also wanted a private practice, and this made it impossible for him to establish himself as the Montreal General's full-time physician-in-chief.[12] Both physicians had their offices outside the hospital where they conducted their private practices – Howard on Mackay Street and Gordon in the Drummond Medical Building where he shared an office with A.T. Bazin for many years.

Howard met resistance, indifference, and silence when he attempted to get the MGH medical board to agree to establish a research clinic. Nevertheless, with his colleagues he completed clinical projects and reported them at national meetings of the American College of Physicians and the Association of American Physicians.[13] His struggle to reorganize the medical department lasted until 1936 when he died suddenly while on a lecture tour in California. Gordon and his followers wanted to maintain their power and the traditions of the Montreal General and seriously set back progress in research at the hospital until after World War II. In surgery a similar oligarchy existed with A.T. Bazin, E.M. Eberts, and F.S. Patch.

After the turn of the century there had been many advances in the practice of medicine – in radiology, clinical chemistry, electrocardiography and other diagnostic techniques such as measuring basal metabolic rate. New therapies were developed, including insulin for diabetes mellitus after its discovery in 1921. At the Royal Victoria, E.H. Mason developed a diabetic clinic within the University Clinic and on Ward K. At the Montreal General, I.M. Rabinowitch developed clinical chemistry and founded the Department of Metabolism, which later became the Department of Metabolism and Toxicology. He started a diabetic clinic in that department rather than in the department of medicine, and it became one of the largest diabetic clinics in Canada.

Most of the attending physicians at the two hospitals were general internists but some developed special interests. At the Montreal General, C.C. Birchard and N. Feeney had special interests in diseases of the heart and circulation and developed electrocardiography. At the Royal Victoria C.F. Martin, J.C. Meakins, C.F. Moffatt, and G.R. Brow had similar interests. By 1936 anesthesia, dermatology, neurology, and radiology were the recognized medical specialties. Specific divisions for other medical specialties in the departments of medicine were developed after World War II.

In 1936 Meakins published his textbook *The Practice of Medicine*, with chapters on endocrinology and metabolism by E.H. Mason, neurological diseases by J.M. Peterson, and diseases of the urinary tract by W. de M. Scriver. Meakins's book documented recent progress in diagnosis and treatment of medical diseases.[14] The first edition was written before the antibiotic era, and Meakins described the serum treatment of pneumonia. By 1936 the antibiotic era had started with the use of sulphapyridine.

PEDIATRICS

McGill was slow to recognize the need for a department and specialty in pediatrics, even though Johns Hopkins formed a department in 1913. Considerable resistance from internists and obstetricians was mounted at the suggestion, because they would lose their pediatric office patients and consultations in the hospitals. Despite opposition, A.D. Blackader had developed the first pediatric service in 1874 as an outpatient clinic at the Montreal General. The obstetricians continued to provide all in-patient pediatric care. Blackader had a major interest in childcare and had special training in London, but he was never able to make a living from the practice of pediatrics. From 1886 to 1912, Blackader and J.C. Cameron, professor of obstetrics, gave a lecture course to the students on diseases of children.

At the turn of the century, pediatric surgical problems and children's crippling orthopedic diseases were neglected. Fortunately there was enough public support to establish a hospital for the treatment of those problems. In 1902, led by an orthopedic surgeon, Alexander MacKenzie Forbes, a group of concerned citizens formed a committee of organization. They announced plans to form a children's hospital, and by 1903 rented a large home at 500 Guy Street for $20 per month. Renovations totalled $298, and the estimated monthly operation costs were approximately $300.

The founders decided to dedicate the hospital to Queen Victoria. After royal assent was obtained, they named it the Children's Memorial Hospital (CMH) as a memorial to the queen. Blackader was the first physician-in-chief from 1904 to 1905, and Harold B. Cushing succeeded him until 1938. The hospital was initially an orthopedic hospital with pediatric consultants. The main thrust was the correction of some crippling orthopedic diseases.

MacKenzie Forbes was the first surgeon-in-chief and served until 1929. Sir Melbourne Tate was president of the hospital from 1902 to 1907. The medical and nursing staff worked in the cramped Guy Street quarters, drawing support from both the anglophone and francophone communities. The Carsley family,[15] wealthy neighbours across the street, had sympathy for the patients and staff in the crowded house, and in the summer they permitted the erection of a tent hospital on their property to get the children outside, particularly those who were staying in the hospital for a long time. This was a great success and emphasized the need for a larger facility.

A suitable site for a new building was located and purchased on Cedar Avenue, across the street and up the mountain from the present Montreal General Hospital, a splendid location on the south-west side of Mount Royal where there was a view of the St Lawrence River and the Eastern Townships. The property cost $29,000 and the hospital building an estimated $55,000. The patients and the staff moved from Guy Street to the new CMH building (fig. 64) on 6 April 1909. For many years it remained mostly a surgical institute, with some medical pediatric patients cared for by Harold Cushing. Chief of pediatric medicine at the hospital from 1904 until 1938, Cushing was reticent and seldom made himself known within the McGill community, let alone outside it. Blackader had many other responsibilities and he did not want to compete with Cushing for his position at the hospital.

The location of the CMH was ideal for inpatients, but it was almost an impossible and inaccessible site for outpatients and visitors. Uphill from Cedar Avenue, it required a steep walk from the nearest streetcar stop on Côte des Neiges. Outpatients were seen in a large ground floor room that soon became overcrowded. As the outpatient population increased, there was a pressing need for a more accessible facility. After many delays because of financial problems, the outpatient building on Cedar Avenue was constructed and opened in 1920.

Initially the nurses, in addition to all their other duties, taught the children with prolonged hospital stays as best they could. Subsequently the Protestant Board of School Commissioners appointed a teacher whose full-time duty was at the hospital. Children with physical disabilities presented another problem, as most were confined to their homes with no educational possibilities. The construction of a special building was started in 1914, and the School for Crippled Children opened in 1916 near the corner of Pine and Cedar Avenues. Initially there were seven pupils, but by the end of one year ninety-seven pupils had enrolled. They were carried to and from their homes to the school on special buses.

The CMH and the nearby school had a good working relationship. By 1920 the hospital was flourishing with new outpatient and x-ray facilities. In the same year McGill finally decided to include the CMH in its circle of teaching hospitals. This meant that the medical students could have official rotations at the CMH and McGill had some control over the teaching schedule. McGill established a pediatrics department in 1937 and appointed Cushing (fig. 65) as its professor and chairman. When he retired in 1938 at the mandatory retirement age of sixty-five, R.R. Struthers succeeded him and served until 1948.

The CMH Nursing School opened in 1907. Ruth Harrington R.N., at Forbes's request, designed the magnificent Nursing Pin with a circle of maple leaves around a brilliant Geneva Red Cross, with the letters "CMH" clearly imprinted on the cross. It was Forbes's idea to put large letters on the pin so that it would be easy to see where the graduates had trained. In the 1920s virtually all the sub-specialties were also available at the Children's Memorial Hospital. In addition to the pedi-

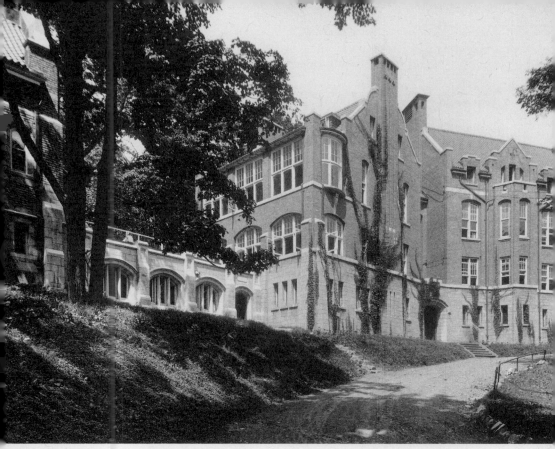

Figure 64
Children's Memorial Hospital, Cedar Avenue, Montreal, 1909–56.
Photo by William Notman, 1909

atric, medical, surgical, orthopedic, ear nose and throat, and genito-urinary clinics, there was a dental clinic.

Pediatric medicine was expanded with the addition to the staff of a
brilliant young pediatrician, Alton Goldbloom (1890–1968), who
became one of the first Jewish doctors to make it through the McGill
clinical system. In 1948 he succeeded Struthers as professor and chairman of the department of pediatrics, and physician-in-chief at the
CMH. Edward Archibald succeeded MacKenzie Forbes as chief of surgery at the hospital and served until 1933.

ANESTHESIA

In 1885 two anesthetics were available: ether and chloroform, both
highly volatile liquids, the fumes of which were potent anesthetics. Each
had different properties. At times chloroform produced serious cardiac

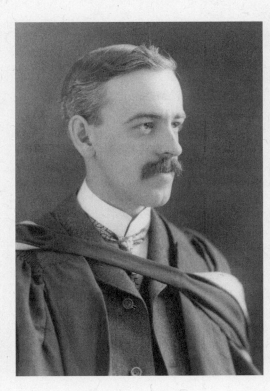

Figure 65
Harold Beveridge Cushing,
1873–1947. Photo by
William Notman, 1920

problems, and its use was gradually phased out by 1920.[16] Inducing anesthesia with ether was difficult because the patient frequently had to be tied down. House surgeons and/or medical students were given the job of administering anesthesia in the operating room supervised by the surgeon, neither having detailed knowledge about the highly toxic substances that were being used. They were literally learning while doing, which was the only guide for their use at the time.[17]

Ether or chloroform was administered by the "open drop" method, in which a cone with gauze stretched over a metal frame was held over the patient's nose and mouth, and drops of the fluids were put on the gauze. The patient inhaled the fumes while also breathing room air and gradually became anesthetized. Once induction was accomplished, the patient went into the deeper stages of anesthesia, and maintaining the anesthetized state was fairly routine.

Prior to 1892 house surgeons performed anesthesia at the Montreal General on rotation. In 1892 because of the increase in surgical procedures and the beginning of some surgical specialties at the hospital, H.P. Carmichael, one of the house surgeons, decided to spend a year learning the practical use of anesthesia and was appointed anesthetist. Thereafter one house surgeon was appointed on an annual basis to give the anesthetics – usually a surgeon-in-training who wanted to increase his knowledge and skills in anesthesia. By 1913 the practice was sophisticated enough to attract a full-time physician, W.B. Howell, whose job it was to provide anesthesia for all the surgeons at the hospital on an outpatient and inpatient basis. Howell started to develop a department of anesthesia at the Montreal General, but his work was interrupted in 1915 when he went overseas with No. 3 Canadian General Hospital (McGill). W.G. Hepburn became the anesthetist at the General from 1917 until 1926. C.C. Stewart followed him and developed the modern General department of anesthesia.[18]

In 1911 George Armstrong introduced endotracheal anesthesia at the hospital. It was successful, and he reported fifty cases in one year.[19] The development of the first anesthetic gas – nitrous oxide and the apparatus to administer it – was an important step, because nitrous oxide had to be mixed with oxygen to prevent the patient from becoming anoxic. Nitrous oxide could only be used for short procedures such as removing sutures, cleaning wounds, or dental procedures, because the patient stopped breathing and became anoxic. Anesthesia could not be maintained with nitrous oxide alone.

During World War I, morphine plus nitrous oxide and oxygen were used extensively for minor procedures such as changing dressings, repairing superficial wounds, making incisions and draining abscesses. Ether anesthesia was used for major surgical procedures. Chloroform was rarely used because of its toxic effects. Other developments during and after the war were the introduction of rectal and spinal anesthesia and special anesthetic techniques for chest, neurological, abdominal, and pelvic surgery.

At the Royal Victoria, anesthetists were appointed annually from its opening in 1894 until 1908. As a McGill medical student, Francis Willard Nagle developed an interest in anesthesia. When he graduated M.D., C.M. with honours in 1908, he was appointed house anesthetist at the Royal Victoria. From 1910 to 1912 he took postgraduate training in anesthesia, probably at the suggestion of Edward Archibald, who was also interested in gas-oxygen mixture anesthesia.[20] When Nagle returned to Montreal, he was appointed the RVH's chief anesthetist. He introduced endotracheal anesthesia using a laryngoscope for insertion of the endotracheal tube, and gas-oxygen mixtures that required special apparatus with valves to mix the gases and pipes running from the tanks to the anesthetic mask. In 1918 he died tragically at age thirty-eight from accidental carbon monoxide poisoning, one of the first known cases of fatal inhalation of car exhaust fumes. W.B. Howell, who had extensive experience in anesthesia during the World War I with No. 9 Field Ambulance and No. 3 Canadian General Hospital, replaced Nagle as chief anesthetist at the RVH and served in that capacity until he retired in 1937. John W. Alex Armstrong assisted him.[21]

Wesley Bourne (1886–1965) graduated M.D., C.M. from McGill in 1911. He was one of the first to apply the study of basic sciences to anesthesia with physiological and pharmacological research on the effects of anesthesia on the human body. His work on respiratory, cardiac, hepatic, renal, and central nervous functions as well as on electrolytes, hormone levels, hemoglobin, and hematocrit during anesthesia formed the scientific basis for the specialty of anesthesia.

Bourne was offered a full-time position in anesthesia at the Royal Victoria, but he refused the salaried appointment. He preferred to continue his established private anesthetic practice at St Mary's Western, and Montreal Maternity hospitals, and later at the Royal Edward Hospital, the Grace Dart Home and in private dental practice. He had an extraordinary ability to get things done and worked regularly at the McGill physiology and pharmacology laboratories in addition to practising anesthesia. Bourne made anesthesia a scientific specialty and became one of McGill's most famous anesthetists.

Bourne remained in private practice from 1922 until 1945 with a McGill appointment as lecturer in pharmacology. He could do his research unencumbered by administrative and major teaching duties. In 1945 he was appointed chairman of a new McGill department of anesthesia with the rank of assistant professor – probably the only assistant professor to head a McGill department. He resigned his McGill positions in 1950 when he reached age sixty-five. During his career he published 137 papers and a book.[22]

Harold Randall Griffith (1884–1951)[23] graduated M.D., C.M. from McGill in 1922. His medical studies had been interrupted during the war with service in the CAMC and the Royal Navy. Before he enlisted, he was a student-intern at the Montreal Homeopathic Hospital and worked with his father, Dr A. Griffith, who was a general practitioner-surgeon and medical superintendent of the hospital. While a medical student, Harold Griffith learned to "drop ether," and he had further experience with anesthesia in the armed services. By the time he graduated in 1922 he had given four hundred anesthetics. He started a general medical practice with his father and his brother, and soon was giving most of the anesthetics at the Homeopathic Hospital.[24] Though offered a position as staff anesthetist, like Bourne he preferred to be in private practice and work at several hospitals.

Griffith was an innovative anesthetist, and in his career his many contributions to the practical applications of anesthesia earned him a worldwide reputation. One of his first innovations was the use of ethylene in 1923 to replace nitrous oxide. On 30 October 1933 he administered cyclopropane for a surgical procedure for the first time in Canada. Cyclopropane, a potent anesthetic agent, was used in a 15 per cent concentration with an 85 per cent concentration of oxygen – conditions approaching the ideal. Patients were routinely intubated for cyclopropane anesthesia because the gas was highly flammable, and a closed circuit was essential to prevent an explosion in the operating room. By 1937 Griffith reported three thousand cases of the use of cyclopropane in anesthesia and by 1945, ten thousand cases. Much of his work was done at the Homeopathic Hospital. By 1933 he had practically abandoned general practice in favour of anesthesia and hospital administration.

Griffith's greatest contribution to anesthesia was to develop curare as a useful muscle relaxant. This enabled the anesthetist to use lighter anesthesia, which reduced the toxic side effects. He administered the first dose of curare in 1942 at the Homeopathic Hospital and published the first paper on the surgical use of curare in anesthesia in the same year. Also in 1943 he established the first post-operative recovery room.

Griffith succeeded Bourne as chairman of the McGill department of anesthesia in 1950 and served until 1957. His exceptional work on curare, cyclopropane, and the recovery-room concept was widely recognized. He was president of every major anesthesia organization and was decorated and honoured by many organizations in World War II. He received the Order of Canada in 1974. When he died in 1985 he was emeritus professor of anesthesia at McGill.

From 1885 to 1936 there was no course in anesthesia in the medical school curriculum. Medical students learned the principles of anesthesia in the physiology and pharmacology courses, and the practical aspects during the surgical rotations.

NEUROLOGY

Development of a special interest in diseases of the nervous system at McGill began with the autopsy reports of William Osler between 1874 and 1884 when he was performing post-mortems at the Montreal General.[25] He was a remarkable observer of pathological changes. During his McGill years he published thirty-five pathology reports on diseases of the nervous system including congenital abnormalities, tumours, infections, aneurysms, and strokes. He also published clinical reports on epilepsy, brain tumours in children, concussion, and the localization of diseases of the nervous system, chronic dementia, tabes dorsalis, and Parkinson's disease. This remarkable production of papers went without recognition at the time because there was little interest or understanding at McGill in neurology and neuropathology.[26]

When Osler moved to Philadelphia in 1884, James Stewart, a practising physician and professor of materia medica at McGill, developed an interest in neurological diseases. In 1893 when he became physician-in-chief at the Royal Victoria and professor of medicine at McGill, he was considered the leading consultant on neurological diseases.

McGill's first official appointment in neurology was in 1904 when David A. Shirras was appointed as a lecturer. He was also professor of neurology at the University of Vermont and went there on a regular basis to teach. He taught and practised at McGill from 1904 to 1920 and published numerous clinical and neuropathological reports. When he retired in 1920, Fred H. McKay (1884–1947) succeeded him. McKay had trained at Queen Square in London after World War I for one year before returning to Montreal. Like all neurologists, he diagnosed and treated both neurological and psychiatric diseases.[27]

After Stewart died in 1906, Colin Russel (1877–1956) was the prominent consultant in neurology at the Royal Victoria. When he returned after three years of postgraduate training at Johns Hopkins and Queen Square,[28] he assumed the informal role of consultant for neurology. He was appointed neurologist at the Royal Victoria in 1910, lecturer at McGill in 1913, and clinical professor in 1922.[29] Russel's publications, although mostly on neurological subjects, also touched on psychiatry. During the war he went overseas as neurological consultant for the British Army and returned to Montreal in 1918 to resume his practice at the RVH. He developed a strong division of neurology within the department of medicine. Arthur Young joined him in 1923 and Norman Peterson a little later. Russel at the RVH and Shirras at the MGH practised both neurology and psychiatry because there was no organized psychiatry service at either of the two hospitals until 1930 and no department of psychiatry at McGill until 1943.[30]

Before the war little or no therapy could be given for neurological disease except bromides for seizures. There were no antibiotics, anticonvulsants, or antidepressants. Neurological diagnosis was based on exquisite clinical examination. Except for x-rays, there were no tests to localize and identify intracranial and intraspinal diseases until 1918 when Walter Dandy reported the use of the ventriculogram with air in the ventricles as a way of indirectly demonstrating space-occupying intracranial lesions. This was followed in 1919 by the pneumoencephalogram with air injected into the lumbar subarchnoid space and rising to the head. These were followed by a series of new investigations for the central nervous system. Myelography with contrast dye was reported in 1922. Moniz developed angiography using a radioactive gamma emitter – thorium dioxide – but this was a tragic event. Thorium was not excreted from the body, and it eventually killed every patient to whom it had been administered by causing radioactive-induced liver and spleen failure.

Russel, Mackay, Young, and Peterson established neurology at McGill and formed a strong base at the RVH and the MGH. Wilder Penfield appointed them to the Montreal Neurological Institute staff when it opened in 1934.

DERMATOLOGY

In 1879 T.G. Roddick started a weekly clinic for skin diseases at the Montreal Dispensary on St Antoine Street. He published one paper, "A Remarkable Case of Favus," from his experiences there.[31] After 1880 F.J. Shepherd continued the clinic for skin diseases – seeing on average fifty patients in about an hour! In 1883 he transferred the clinic to the Montreal General, and continued it until he retired in 1914. Final-year medical students attended the clinics, and for many years that was their only teaching in dermatology.

Shepherd's interest in skin diseases began during his postgraduate study in Europe from 1873 to 1875. While in London he attended the clinics of Jonathan Hutchinson at the Stamford Street Skin Hospital. In his memoirs Shepherd recalled, "Few students attended this clinic and we had excellent opportunities to see skin diseases of all kinds under the instruction of a very able man. I owe much of my knowledge of skin diseases to my regular attendance at those wonderful clinics." Shepherd read Hutchinson's books *Rare Skin Diseases*, *Atlas of Illustrations in Clinical Surgery*, and *Skin Diseases*. He continued his interest by attending Kaposi's and Herb's clinics in Vienna in 1874, as well as a course by Hebra and Neumann.[32]

Recognition of dermatology as a specialty by the medical faculty and the teaching hospitals was a slow process. At a faculty meeting in 1901, Shepherd called attention to the absence of dermatology from

the curriculum, whereas it was a part of the curriculum in many leading American and European medical schools. No decision was taken at
that meeting, and there was no follow-up for several years.[33] Dermatology was first listed as one of the subjects on the curriculum in the
medical faculty calendar for the 1905–06 session: "The course will be
given by Professor F.J. Shepherd and Dr G.G. Campbell (fee $5.00)
and will consist of instruction at outdoor clinics. It will also include a
lantern demonstration of skin diseases by Professor Shepherd."[34]

The 1906–07 calendar included the following: "Dermatology –
Professor F.J. Shepherd; G.G. Campbell (Montreal General) lecturer;
W.P. Burnett (Royal Victoria) demonstrator. The course is entirely clinical – a weekly theatre clinic at the General by Professor Shepherd on
specially selected cases, and outdoor clinics by Campbell at the MGH
and Burnett at the RVH throughout the session." Starting in 1909–10
there was a clinical examination in dermatology for the fifth (final)
year students.[35]

Campbell, J.J. McGovern, and A.O. Freedman assisted Shepherd at
the General's dermatology clinic for more than twenty years. Campbell
replaced Shepherd when he was not available. For several years after
his graduation from medical school, Campbell was interested in pediatrics; later in his career he specialized in dermatology.

Although Shepherd said he was not a "pure dermatologist" and considered dermatology "an entertaining hobby and sideline," in 1886 he
was elected the second Canadian member of the American Dermatological Association.[36] There were forty members – Shepherd was the only
non-specialist, all other members being full-time dermatologists. In 1901
he was president of the American Dermatological Association; his pres-
idential address was published in the Montreal Medical Journal. In 1928
he was honorary president of the Canadian Branch of the British Dermatology Association (the forerunner of the Canadian Dermatological
Association). He accepted the honour and wrote a thank-you note but did
not attend the meeting. Thirteen of his 123 publications were on dermatological subjects.[37] When he retired in 1914, Campbell was placed
in charge of the MGH dermatology clinic and in 1920 published the first
Canadian textbook on dermatology.[38]

Prior to 1900 dermatology was considered a surgical specialty because it mainly involved removal of polyps and other skin lesions. With
the development of effective medical treatments, particularly for syphilis
with its many skin manifestations and for other venereal diseases,
dermatology became a medical specialty. It was often referred to as

"dermatology and syphilology." Syphilis treatment included the use of arsphenamines, bismuth, and mercury.

In 1921 the Montreal General's board of management established the department of dermatology. Campbell was head of the department from 1921 to 1928 and clinical professor of dermatology from 1924 to 1928. J.F. Burgess followed him from 1928 to 1950.

A dermatology clinic was established at the Royal Victoria in 1906 with Burnett being in charge until 1940. Drs Bruère, Ereaux, Joyce, and Mason assisted him. After 1920 they held three to five dermatology clinics each week. Most of their work was in the outpatient department. Occasionally they admitted patients with skin diseases to the medical wards.[39]

In the 1920s few doctors confined their practices to dermatology. In 1921 Dr Cleveland asked Shepherd for a letter of reference to support his application for a dermatology post. Shepherd said: 'I do not think there is much of a future in dermatology in Montreal." Dr Barney Usher called on Shepherd when starting his dermatology practice in Montreal. Shepherd's opinion was that he would starve. Usher said Shepherd was partially correct; after starting his practice, it took him years to pay off his accumulated debts.[40]

From a slow start, by 1936 dermatology was well established as a medical specialty in the community, the medical school, and the teaching hospitals. Some doctors devoted their whole practice to dermatology. There were local and national specialty societies and professional publications.

PSYCHIATRY

In the late 1800s mental disease was treated poorly around the western world. Patients with psychiatric diseases were referred to neurologists, all of whom had some psychiatric training. Patients with serious mental disease such as general paresis of the insane (GPI) needed custodial care. Neither the Montreal General nor the Royal Victoria had proper facilities for such patients. Custodial care otherwise was given in large state-constructed institutions where patients were committed and disappeared from their communities. The Quebec government, bowing to pressures from society, built a large institution for the mental patients in Verdun – the Verdun Protestant Hospital (VPH).[41] Incorporated in 1881, it opened in 1890 with a large campus and accommodation for hundreds of patients. William Douglas, M.D., was a member of the first board of governors. William Burgess was a major figure in the development of the VPH, the first medical chief and a member of the board of directors. In 1895 he became the first teacher of mental diseases on the McGill faculty and arranged demonstrations at the VPH by 1903. He was professor of mental diseases (1898–1920), and professor of psychiatry (1920–23). After 1916 C.A. Porteus, with the rank of lecturer, assisted Burgess.

By 1923 the psychiatric service (not a department) expanded dramatically because of the great need. Burgess retired in 1923 and Porteus succeeded him as professor, with W.D. Tarte as assistant professor, G. Mundie as lecturer, and H.A. Sims and A.G. Murphy as demonstrators. The course on mental disease by that time was taught in the fourth and fifth years at the medical school and at the VPH. It consisted of discussion of the main psychiatric diseases and the limited treatment that was available – sedation with barbiturates, arsenicals for syphilis, and custodial care for the remainder of the patients.

By 1936 the knowledge base in psychiatry was expanding and the staff increased, but psychiatry was not granted department status in the medical faculty until 1943.

RADIOLOGY

Wilhelm Conrad Röntgen discovered x-rays on 8 November 1895 and published his results on 25 December 1895, for which he received a Nobel Prize.[42] Many physicists around the world repeated his experiments. At McGill John Cox (1851–1923), Macdonald Professor of Physics, developed an x-ray machine in his department by early 1896 which caused great excitement as word spread around the Montreal medical community.

In February 1896 Robert C. Kirkpatrick, a thirty-four-year-old surgeon at the General, had a patient with a bullet in his lower leg. He wanted to locate the bullet prior to surgery and went to the McGill physics department to talk with Professor Cox about his x-ray machine. Cox, along with H.L. Calender, H. Barnes, and F. Pitcher, took the first x-rays at McGill of Kirkpatrick's patient on 7 February 1896. The bullet was found after prolonged exposure to x-rays (nearly forty-five minutes). The picture of the leg together with an x-ray of a normal hand were presented the next evening at a meeting of the Med Chi. Kirkpatrick removed the bullet. Cox and Kirkpatrick thought that they had performed the first clinical use of x-ray in Canada and published an article in the *Montreal Medical Journal* – "The new photography with a report of a case in which a bullet was photographed in a leg."[43] For years this article was considered to be the first clinical use of x-ray published in Canada. (However, in 1962 Charles Roland found prior articles.[44])

In 1896 Gilbert Girdwood, professor of chemistry, developed an x-ray apparatus in his laboratory on University Street and proceeded to do x-ray examinations for the General and Royal Vic. The Vic records reveal ten patients sent to Girdwood in 1897 and more the following year, but no written reports of the x-rays exist.

In 1901 the Royal Victoria appointed Girdwood as director of the Medical Electrical Department, and he went to England to purchase new equipment. For the next seven years he did x-ray work for the RVH until he retired in 1908 at age seventy-six. The hospital appointed R.H. Pirie, a well-trained radiologist from Scotland, to succeed Girdwood. With new techniques and equipment, the department expanded rapidly, and the name was changed to "diagnostic radiology." In 1925 Pirie was appointed radiologist-in-chief; E.C. Brooks and J.C. Lanthier assisted him. Brooks was radiologist-in-chief from 1935 to 1938.[45] At the Montreal General, radiology developed at a similar pace. W. Wilkins was radiologist from 1908 until 1925 and L. Ritchie from 1925 to 1947.[46]

Within months of Röntgen's discovery, Henri Becquerel discovered radioactivity and also later received a Nobel Prize. Techniques were developed for the use of radioactive substances – chiefly radium – for the treatment of a variety of diseases. In 1909 George E. Armstrong went to the Radium Institute in Paris to study the use of radium in the treatment of patients with cancer. On his return to Montreal he began to use radium at the Montreal General and continued after he moved to the Royal Victoria in 1911. In 1922 the Quebec government appropriated $100,000 for the purchase of radium to found the Institut du Radium at the Université de Montréal with Joseph-Ernest Gendreau, M.D. PH.D., as director. The Institut functioned until 1947.[47] For several years the Royal Victoria and Montreal General obtained some of their supplies of radium from the Institut. In 1926 Mrs W.W. Chipman donated 100 milligrams of radium for use in the newly opened RVH Women's Pavilion.[48] At the General, J.C. Newman donated $50,000 to purchase a supply of radium.[49] Eleanor Percival from the department of obstetrics and gynecology took special training and used the radium for the treatment of cancer of the cervix. It was several years before departments of radiation therapy were established at the two hospitals. C.B. Pearce was appointed radiologist-in-chief in 1938 at Royal Victoria and director of therapeutic radiology. Later the name of the specialty was changed to radiation oncology.

In 1911 the medical faculty announced a summer course for "Teaching in Radiography and Radioscopy," open to medical graduates and optional for undergraduates. In 1922 the medical faculty offered a diploma in radiology. However, prior to 1936, medical graduates who wanted to specialize in radiology usually went to Europe or the United States for training. McGill developed residency programs in diagnostic radiology and radiation oncology after World War II. Medical students had some instruction in the use of x-rays in their clinical rotations, but there was no formal instruction in diagnostic and therapeutic radiology.

7 Surgery and Surgical Specialties

The surgeon [has] the obligation to know thoroughly the
scientific principles on which his art is based, to be master
in the technique of his handicraft, ever studying, modifying,
improving ...
WILLIAM OSLER[1]

SURGERY

Prior to 1882 the attending doctors at the Montreal General were generalists. If one of their patients required an operation, they did the operation. If the patient died, they might do a post-mortem examination.
The first separation of medicine and surgery occurred in 1882 when
Thomas Roddick limited his practice to surgery and George Ross specialized in medicine. Some of the hospital's attending staff continued to
practise medicine and surgery, but with the development of antisepsis,
better anesthesia, and new surgical procedures, the generalists who
practised general medicine and performed surgery disappeared from
the McGill teaching hospitals by the end of the World War I.

In the 1880s Roddick demonstrated to the doctors at the Montreal
General the use of antiseptic techniques, and as operating room standards were established, the control of operating room protocol and
procedures was gradually taken out of the individual surgeon's hands.
Surgical procedures began to extend into the abdomen, pelvis, chest,
neck, and finally the head. In 1885 Fenwick, Roddick, Shepherd, and
Bell were the attending surgeons at the MGH.[2] Shepherd was the most
innovative, and in 1884 he performed his first successful thyroid
operation. In 1885 he was the first surgeon in Canada to successfully
remove a kidney. On 14 September 1889 he performed the second pre-
diagnosed appendectomy at the hospital (Bell performed the first on
5 May 1889).[3] Shepherd contributed many specimens to the McGill
Medical Museum, some of which were lost in the fire in 1907.[4]

Fenwick retired in 1890, and Roddick became senior surgeon at the MGH and professor of surgery. George Armstrong (fig. 53) was appointed as the fourth attending surgeon on the indoor service.[5] He introduced endotracheal anesthesia, known as "endotracheal insufflation."[6] Entries in the MGH Operations Book showed that in the 1880s more and a greater variety of operations were done each year.[7] The big boost for surgery at the hospital occurred when the Greenshields and Campbell surgical wings were constructed from 1890 to 1892, including a new operating room suite. This provided the surgical services with four wards, and separated the surgical from the medical wards. Previously this had been a problem because many infectious-disease patients were admitted to the hospital wards.

In 1885 the course in surgery for students consisted of two components: a lecture course at the Medical Building by Fenwick, professor of surgery, on the principles and practice of surgery, and classes and demonstrations at the General by Roddick, professor of clinical surgery. His classes were usually held in the operating room because it was the only room large enough to accommodate the students. When Roddick became professor of surgery in 1890, he gave the surgical lectures at the Medical Building and continued to do so until 1907, long after he retired from active surgery in 1894. His work as a member of parliament promoting the Roddick Bill, and with the Dominion Medical Council, took him out of Montreal a great deal. His lectures had become out of date by 1900, and he had no real interest in promoting or discussing surgical research.

When Roddick and Bell (fig. 17)[8] moved to the Royal Victoria in 1894, Shepherd was the senior attending surgeon at the Montreal General.[9] As professor of anatomy he was not available to teach surgery to the medical students during the October to March academic term. He took the surgical ward duty from April to September. His title was lecturer in operative surgery, relating to his activities with the summer postgraduate courses.

After the Royal Victoria Hospital opened for patients in 1894, the class gradually increased to more than one hundred students. Ward classes in surgery were conducted in small groups at the both hospitals, and most of the senior and junior surgeons assisted in the surgical teaching program. Student training in surgery was poor. It was bad enough to have the students as non-participating witnesses watching the experts perform on the hospital wards and in the operating rooms, but there was a lack of practical experience for the students and little or no involvement with the care of patients.

When Roddick retired in 1907, Bell and Armstrong were appointed professors of surgery. The custom of one professor of surgery giving all the lectures at the Medical Building was stopped. The professors and the junior staff gave the surgical lectures according to their special interests and expertise. This was an important change in policy in order to keep the teaching current. There was not a director of the McGill surgical department until 1923, when Edward Archibald was appointed. Thereafter he organized the teaching program in surgery.

At the Royal Victoria, James Bell succeeded Roddick as chief surgeon in 1895. Bell had worked closely with Roddick for ten years. Highly disciplined and a stickler for details, he demanded sacrifices from his house surgeons. He took advantage of his position to establish a training program in surgery at the Royal Victoria – not seen before at McGill. He supervised the house surgeons' training for three or four years and insisted on proof of competency. His house surgeons had to be available day and night. A house surgeon spent the first year studying surgical pathology, then two years as an intern on the surgical service, and the fourth and final year as surgical resident and Bell's assistant.[10] In 1905 Bell's associates were E.W. Archibald (fig. 54),[11] A.E. Garrow, and W.B. Keenan. This team constituted the RVH department of surgery and worked with Bell to run the surgical service and train the house surgeons.

In 1911 after seventeen years as the RVH's chief surgeon, Bell died from an acute abdominal illness, the diagnosis of which was not obvious at the time. At autopsy, the pathologist found a ruptured appendix and peritonitis. F.A.C. Scrimger, one of the junior staff surgeons at the time, confided later that he had mentioned that a diagnosis of appendicitis was a possibility, but because of the atypical symptoms and signs, it was not considered.[12]

After Bell's sudden and unexpected death, the Royal Victoria needed a new chief surgeon whose patients would fill the surgical beds to keep the hospital's income stable.[13] Garrow was forty-nine, Keenan forty-four, Archibald thirty-nine, and all were possible candidates. Garrow, the 1889 Holmes Medallist, was popular, had a large surgical practice, and was clinical assistant professor of surgery. However, he was not a good teacher, and it was doubtful that McGill would promote him to full professor. Keenan also had a large surgical practice but was not interested in research, so neither Garrow nor Keenan was considered for appointment as chief surgeon. Archibald was known for his experimental work in pancreatitis. Together with his interests in neurological and pulmonary surgery, he was also an excellent teacher. He was interested in a position that would combine practice and research but not in full-time private practice. However, he was frequently late for appointments (including his own operations), he was partially deaf, he had had pulmonary tuberculosis, and he operated on animals in the laboratory. All of this worried the RVH board of governors, and Archibald was not appointed chief surgeon.[14]

At a critical meeting of the RVH medical board, Garrow realized that he was not going to get the job and recommended George Eli Armstrong, the senior MGH surgeon, as Bell's successor. The medical board approved the suggestion. The RVH governors offered Armstrong the position, and he accepted. He was a forceful, somewhat bombastic, but energetic and innovative general surgeon who could fill the surgical beds and continue where Bell had left off. Armstrong brought his experience with endotracheal anesthesia to the RVH, but this did not become standard procedure for anesthesia for almost two decades.

Armstrong's associates – Garrow, Keenan, and Archibald – were not a cohesive group. Garrow was busy with his large surgical practice. Archibald and Keenan, as Bell trainees, carried on his traditions. Armstrong never really generated personal support and had no close friends in the department. He didn't need them because he was the favourite of Sir Vincent Meredith (fig. 52), president of the Royal Victoria's board of governors, who essentially ran the hospital in a dictatorial manner after he took office in 1912. Meredith wanted the surgical wards and the Ross Pavilion[15] full of patients to keep the hospital solvent, since the hospital lost so much money with the teaching programs. Armstrong was able to do this.

In 1923 after twelve years as RVH chief surgeon, Armstrong wanted to retire. This threw Meredith into a panic – he had to find a surgeon who would keep the Ross Pavilion full of paying patients. In a desperate move, at Armstrong's suggestion Meredith chose Sir Henry Gray as chief surgeon – an untried, questionably competent Scottish surgeon who had not impressed his peers, although he had received a knighthood for his service in the South African War and World War I.[16] Sir Henry was chief surgeon at the Royal Victoria from 1923 until he resigned in 1925.

From 1925 to 1928 Archibald acted as the RVH chief surgeon. His appointment was confirmed in 1928, and he served until December 1935.[17] From his appointment to the hospital's surgical staff in 1902, he had been involved in surgical research, often in collaboration with his junior associates. He reported his work on pulmonary surgery, the gastro-intestinal system, and the treatment of pancreatitis, and developed a wide reputation as an experimental surgeon. However, a pro-

gram for basic research in surgery and the effects of surgery on body
functions was lacking until the hospital formed a centre for experimental surgery in 1929. Thereafter academic general surgeons were trained
at that centre in the basic sciences of anatomy, physiology, chemistry,
and pharmacology. F.A.C. Scrimger succeeded Archibald in 1936 but
died in 1937.

After 1894 when Roddick and Bell went to the Royal Victoria,
Shepherd, Armstrong, Kirkpatrick, and Hutchison were the attending
surgeons at the Montreal General. Shepherd applied his knowledge of
anatomy to his surgical practice and reported cases of fractures, nephrectomy, appendectomy, inguinal hernia, bowel obstruction, breast cancer,
excision of the tongue for cancer, and gall-bladder surgery. He had performed the first thyroid operation in 1884 and the second in 1889,
using antiseptic techniques. He became famous for the surgical treatment of goitre. By 1906 he had performed one hundred thyroidecto-
mies, by far the largest series in Canada.[18]

When Shepherd retired from the surgical staff in 1912, Hutchison
was the senior surgeon and professor of surgery at McGill from 1913
to 1923.[19] Elder, Bazin, and Eberts had waited for years for senior MGH
and McGill appointments and were fully qualified academic general
surgeons. Eberts was experienced in operating on pulmonary diseases
such as tumours, abscesses of the lung, and tuberculosis. Archibald had
similar experience at the RVH. In 1923 when Elder retired, the MGH department of surgery gradually expanded to include associate, assistant,
and junior surgeons. The junior surgeons worked in the surgical clinics
and assisted with the ward classes for the medical students. Surgery at
the MGH was controlled by strong personalities who worked hard at
their practices, their academic responsibilities, and their professional
and community activities.

SURGICAL SPECIALTIES

Obstetrics and gynecology were the first surgical specialties to be recognized at McGill, followed by ophthalmology and otolaryngology.
After 1908 urology and orthopedic surgery developed as surgical specialties, followed by neurosurgery in the 1920s. Departments for other
specialties such as plastic, vascular, and cardiac surgery were developed
after World War II.

Obstetrics and Gynecology
In 1841 William MacNider introduced the concept to Montreal of a

lying-in hospital where women would be confined before and after delivery. He established the Montreal Lying-In Hospital on St James Street (then Bonaventure) near what is now Victoria Square. MacNider was one of a group of anti-McGill physicians, and he made it clear that he would not allow McGill students in the door of the hospital. This sentiment against the McGill medical faculty was shared by a number of MacNider's associates and led to the opening of a rival medical school in 1843, the Montreal School of Medicine and Surgery (L'École de Médecine et Chirurgerie de Montréal).[20]

Not to be outdone by the upstart MacNider, the McGill medical faculty, with the help of a committee of capable women, opened its own University Lying-In Hospital on the main street of the St Lawrence District (St Lawrence Boulevard) in 1843. The hospital's patients were indigent pregnant women who needed care when giving birth. Midwives performed the main work, delivering the babies and teaching the nurses and students. The first chief, Michael McCulloch (1795–1854),[21] visited the hospital regularly and was called in cases of difficult deliveries or complications. MacNider's hospital failed and closed in 1848, but the McGill obstetrical facility thrived and moved to larger quarters in 1847. In 1852 it moved again to a building on St Urbain Street, where it remained until 1906. A "Ladies' Committee" (later the medical board) ran the hospital with representation from the McGill faculty. As the hospital became established, the committee changed the name in 1884 to the University Maternity Hospital and in 1887 to the Montreal Maternity Hospital.

Michael McCulloch died unexpectedly in 1854, and the talented Archibald Hall (1813–1868)[22] was appointed chief. Duncan MacCallum (1824–1904)[23] succeeded him from 1868 to 1883 and was the last chief of both obstetrics and gynecology until Chipman's appointment in 1912. In 1883 William Gardner (1842–1926)[24] was appointed McGill professor of gynecology. He had had no surgical training and consequently went to England in 1885 to spend six months with Lawson Tait, one of Britain's renowned gynecologists.

In 1883 Arthur Browne[25] was appointed professor of obstetrics and diseases of infants, and chief at the Lying-in Hospital. This split in the specialties of women's diseases was in line with the faculty's promotion of new specialties. Browne had a large private practice and resigned his professorship in 1886 because he was too busy to teach at McGill. James Chalmers Cameron, professor of obstetrics at Bishop's Medical College, came to McGill to replace him.[26] Cameron was born in Ontario in 1852 and graduated from Upper Canada College as head boy, and was first in the final examinations at the McGill medical faculty in 1874. This earned him an appointment as a house surgeon at the Montreal General where he remained until 1877. He then went to Dublin, obtained his MRCP in 1879, and travelled in Europe, where he learned new developments in obstetrics as well as surgical antisepsis for gynecology. On his return to Montreal he was appointed professor of obstetrics at Bishop's Medical College, where he would have remained had it not been for Browne's resignation. Cameron was the first obstetrician at McGill with extensive training in the specialty. He was influential at McGill and internationally, and introduced modern techniques at the Montreal Maternity Hospital that brought its standards up to date and helped to establish obstetrics and gynecology as academic specialties at McGill.

In February 1886 the medical faculty appointed a committee to "investigate the professional management of the Montreal Maternity Hospital and to suggest such amendments as they deem proper." The members of the committee were F.J. Shepherd, W. Gardner, and A.A. Browne. This was the beginning of Shepherd's interest in the affairs of the Montreal Maternity, an interest he maintained until he died in 1929. For many years he was a member of its medical board, and for a period its chairman. The committee reported in March 1887 and recommended, among other things, "that a resident accoucheur be appointed from among the member of the graduating class if possible, who shall board and lodge within the Maternity Hospital. He shall keep the roll of students in attendance, shall cause to be called to each case never more than six men [medical students] and shall see that none are present who are not called. He shall be responsible for the quiet behaviour of the students while in hospital. He shall also be responsible for the proper reporting of all cases admitted. By the creation of such an appointment the necessity for a matron and a midwife would be obviated and the professional work of the institution greatly facilitated."[27] In 1887 the medical faculty appointed J.H.Y. Grant as the first resident at the hospital. Later Grant went on to practise in Buffalo. David J. Evans followed him as resident, and in 1892 he was promoted assistant professor of obstetrics at McGill. He published a student textbook that was used for years.

In 1893 the Royal Victoria established a department of gynecology with William Gardner, professor of gynecology at McGill, as its head. T.J. Alloway became chief of gynecology at the MGH until 1898 and then A.L. Lockhart succeeded him until 1925. In 1897 J. Clarence Webster, who had graduated from Edinburgh M.B. in 1888 and M.D. in

1890, was invited to come to Montreal to be Gardner's assistant at the RVH. Webster resigned three years later, and Walter William Chipman (fig. 66)[28] succeeded him as assistant gynecologist at the RVH and demonstrator of gynecology at McGill. The Royal Victoria had no obstetrics department and only a small gynecology service – all obstetrical patients went to the Montreal Maternity Hospital. There was a similar arrangement at the Montreal General where there was a gynecological service but not public obstetrical service.

By the turn of the century the Montreal Maternity Hospital began to change from a purely obstetrical hospital to one where both obstetrical and gynecological patients were treated. By 1910 additional room for gynecological patients was created in the hospital by moving the nurses to adjacent housing and taking over the nurses' residence. In 1912, 230 gynecological patients were admitted, in addition to the obstetrical cases.

From 1900 to 1910 McGill's medical faculty had considered forming a single obstetrics/gynecology department, but this could not be accomplished until Cameron resigned. Chipman was appointed professor of gynecology in 1910 when Gardner retired; however, it appeared that Cameron was going to go on for years. When he died unexpectedly in 1912, the medical faculty was able to re-establish a department of obstetrics and gynecology to be headed by Chipman as professor and chairman.

The war suspended many activities at McGill and indirectly began to affect the admissions to the Montreal Maternity Hospital. Most of the attending doctors had been admitting patients to the small gynecological services at the MGH and the RVH. The general lack of trained aides at those hospitals because of the war made the Maternity Hospital more appealing to the staff for their private patients. This led to the need for more space at the hospital than was available. In 1920, 503 private gynecological patients were admitted to the Maternity Hospital, pressing the fifteen-year-old facility to its limits. Because of its lack of facilities for gynecological surgery, financial deficits began to accumulate. Rising costs led to a deficit in 1921 of $25,000, which was paid by the Hospital Emergency Fund of Quebec in 1922.

In 1922 the Royal Victoria expanded its gynecological service. Chipman was appointed gynecologist-in-chief, with J.R. Fraser and H.C. Burgess as assistants and W.A.C. Bauld and G.C. Melhado as clinical assistants.

The financial problems of the Maternity Hospital persisted, so in January 1923 the Royal Victoria's board of governors (undoubtedly influenced by Chipman) offered an amalgamation proposal to the board

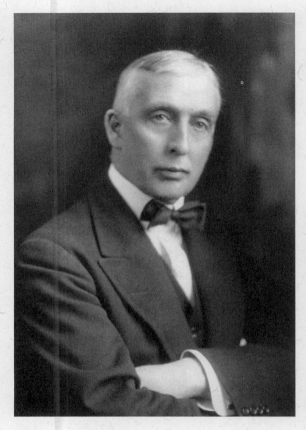

Figure 66
Walter William
Chipman, 1866–1950.
Photo by William
Notman, 1922

of management of the Montreal Maternity. The RVH proposed the construction of a large separate building for obstetrical and gynecological medicine and surgery on the grounds of the RVH to the east of the Ross Pavilion. In addition to improved facilities for treating patients, there would be facilities for teaching residents, students and nurses. F.J. Shepherd, chairman of the medical board of the Maternity Hospital, and Mrs Miller, chairman of the board of management, met with the RVH governors. The plan to amalgamate was accepted in August and signed in December 1923. The Montreal Maternity Hospital would be sold with all its assets to help meet the cost of the new building, to be constructed at the top of University Street. The new building (soon known as the "Mat") was built on the mountainside, but the main entrance (fig. 67) was on its north side, necessitating a circuitous road from Pine Avenue to the back of the Ross Pavilion. An entrance to the outpatient clinics was built on the south side of the hospital at the top of University Street.

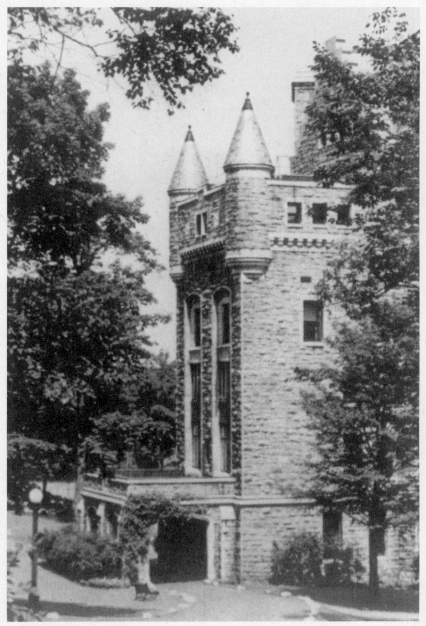

Figure 67
Main entrance of RVH Montreal Maternity Hospital on the north side of the hospital. Photographer unknown

A francophone group purchased the former Montreal Maternity Hospital building in 1924 and changed the name to Hôpital Ste Jeanne d'Arc. The sale of the hospital and its assets brought in $400,000. The Province of Quebec donated $200,000, and private donations raised $150,000, for a total of $750,000 – less than half the final cost of $1,750,000 of the new building. The imposing nine-storey building contained 213 beds and 100 cribs for public and private patients, case rooms, operating rooms, laboratories, offices, quarters for nurses and students, and teaching rooms. On 1 June 1926 the nurses, support staff, and patients moved from the Maternity Hospital to the new building.

Chipman was then at the peak of his career, professor and chairman of the McGill department of obstetrics and gynecology with ten associates and assistants and a new hospital building. His remarkable teaching skills and organizational strengths were known outside McGill. He was president of the American College of Surgeons in 1925 and a member of many professional organizations. Although the specialties of obstetrics and gynecology were recognized from the opening of the Montreal Medical Institution, it was Cameron and then Chipman who established the specialty of obstetrics and gynecology. With the opening of the "Mat," the department of obstetrics and gynecology had finally taken its place in the McGill Medical School along with medicine and surgery. Pediatrics remained the only other major area that was undeveloped at McGill, mainly because the obstetricians, who traditionally treated infants and children, did not want to see a new specialty created to take away their practices. Due to the influence of powerful figures such as Cameron and Chipman at the Royal Victoria and Lockhart at the Montreal General, a department of pediatrics was not established at McGill until 1937, when Harold Cushing was appointed the first chairman.

OPHTHALMOLOGY

Ophthalmology as a specialty did not exist at McGill or at the Montreal General until after Frank Buller (1844–1905)[29] arrived in Montreal in 1876 trained in ophthalmology, otology, and laryngology. The following year he was appointed lecturer on diseases of the eye and ear at McGill without salary. He lived in a three-storey house at 1351 St Catherine Street West and for a while shared it with William Osler. At the time it was the custom to train in Europe, and Buller selected celebrated ophthalmologists and scientists to study under in Germany –

Von Graefe, Virchow, and Helmholtz. From the latter he learned to use the ophthalmoscope. In 1872 he imparted this knowledge to his colleagues at Moorfields (the common name for the Royal London Ophthalmic Hospital founded in 1805), where he was junior and then senior house surgeon. He was attracted to Moorfields because of its staff, traditions and ophthalmological training. He worked with Bowman, Critchett, Hutchison, Nettleship, and Marcus Gunn – the senior staff. While at Moorfields he developed the "Buller eye shield" used in the prevention of gonorrhoeal conjunctivitis.

Buller was the first to practise ophthalmology in Montreal and brought with him from Germany and England the ophthalmoscope, the perimeter, accurate refraction technique, knowledge of ocular muscle defects, ocular pathology, and a modern scientific approach. The first ophthalmic clinic was established at the Montreal General in 1876, and all clinical teaching in ophthalmology became Buller's responsibility. He delivered lectures on eye and ear diseases to the medical students and operated at the MGH. Consequently, McGill appointed him the first chairman of ophthalmology and otology in 1883, and he held that position until 1905. At first, senior MGH physicians were unwilling to give up their ophthalmic patients, but as Buller's training and knowledge became generally accepted, all such patients were assigned to his care. His competence convinced his colleagues that specialization was essential in the medical and surgical care of diseases of the eye. Treatments consisted of solutions for eye infections (gonococcus or syphilis), refraction for glasses, removal of cataracts, other surgery including plastic and lachrymal procedures, operations for glaucoma, repair of trauma, and removal of foreign bodies in the eye. The retina was examined with the ophthalmoscope, but little could be done for diseases of the retina at that time.

With the department developing at the Montreal General in 1895, Buller resigned to take charge of ophthalmology at the newly opened Royal Victoria Hospital. The department grew, and he brought in younger ophthalmologists. Despite a large practice and a department to run, he was able to author seventy-six publications. He died of pernicious anemia in 1905. While his scientific contributions were important, his greatest achievement probably lay in the high standards he set and maintained. He played a major role in the early development of academic ophthalmology in Canada and in establishing the requirements for ophthalmology training in North America. He saw the creation of departments of ophthalmology at the MGH and RVH, both of which grew and developed successfully over the years.

John Stirling (1859–1923) succeeded Buller as head of the department at the Royal Victoria and McGill professor and chairman in 1906. He had graduated in medicine at the University of Edinburgh in 1884 and went on to become house surgeon in the Royal Infirmary under Argyll Robertson. He then spent two years in eye clinics in Vienna, Heidelberg, and Berlin, and later became assistant to Marcus Gunn at Moorfields. Moving to Montreal in 1887, he was appointed professor of ophthalmology at Bishop's Medical School. In 1895 he resigned to become assistant oculist and aurist to J.J. Gardner, who succeeded Buller as chief of the MGH eye department from 1895 to 1905.

The ophthalmology department at the Royal Vic grew rapidly after 1895. F.T. Tooke took charge of pathology, becoming second assistant ophthalmologist alongside W.G. Byers in 1910. In 1920 A.G. MacAuley and J. MacMillan became associate ophthalmologists. Stirling became a member of the consulting staff in 1922, and he was noted for his humanitarian, friendly attitude and his loyalty. His publications dealt with a variety of subjects and were well received. He presided over a period of consolidation in the McGill department when clinical excellence was emphasized at both the General and Royal Victoria.

By 1910 the student course in ophthalmology consisted of ten lectures for students in fourth and fifth years, delivered by the chairman, and biweekly clinics at the two hospitals.

G.W. Mathewson was appointed ophthalmologist-in-chief at the Montreal General in 1905 and associate professor of ophthalmology at McGill. He advanced to clinical professor of ophthalmology in 1923 and remained in those positions until his retirement in 1931. He had graduated in medicine at McGill in 1894 and worked as a clinical assistant with Buller for four years before pursuing further training in Europe. During his tenure as chief, the volume of patients at the Montreal General increased greatly, and additional ophthalmologists joined the department – S.H. McKee, A. Bramley-Moore, L.G. Pearie, and W.G. Richer. In 1922 S.O. McMurtry and G.S. Ramsey were added to the staff. This was a period characterized by clinical excellence and growth at both hospitals.

S. Hanford McKee (1875–1943), one of Montreal's most distinguished ophthalmologists, succeeded Mathewson as ophthalmologist-in-chief at the MGH in 1931 and carried on in this position until his retirement in 1941. He graduated M.D., C.M. from McGill in 1900 and for several years was a house surgeon under Buller at the Royal Victoria, following which he studied in Germany. In 1906 he was appointed assistant oculist and aurist at the Montreal General and assistant oculist and assistant demonstrator of ophthalmology at McGill. He was the official ocular pathologist in the department and contributed significantly in this field over the years. In World War I he was given command of the Canadian Eye Hospital at Shorncliffe, England, where he was awarded the Companion of the Order of St Michael and St George (CMG). He was McGill professor of ophthalmology from 1931 to 1941. The Montreal General annual reports from 1928 to 1930 record that McKee had taken an active interest in the laboratory aspects of his specialty. In 1931 he was elected president of the American Academy of Ophthalmology and Otolaryngology.

W.G. Byers (1872–1955) was appointed ophthalmologist-in-chief at the Royal Victoria in 1921 and in 1923 became professor and chairman of the McGill department to succeed J.W. Stirling. He had a special interest in ocular pathology and was an excellent surgeon, a perfectionist, and a superb teacher in the operating room. After studies abroad he worked with Buller from 1899 to 1905. He developed an interest in research, and in 1909 McGill conferred on him the degree of Doctor of Science.

Byers was an important leader in ophthalmology. In 1920 he founded the Montreal Ophthalmology Society and later established the pathological laboratory of the ophthalmology department. Over the years he advanced the medical and surgical therapy in his specialty and was widely known and respected in ophthalmological circles in Canada, the United States, and Europe. In 1906 he became president of the American Ophthalmological Society and was the driving force in founding the Canadian Ophthalmological Society. In 1937 he convened fifty ophthalmologists from across Canada for this purpose and became the first president of the Canadian society. His many interests included the medical library, and he played an important role in persuading Casey Wood to leave his outstanding ophthalmological library to McGill. His greatest contribution was the organization of ophthalmology in Canada. It is fair to say he was Canada's most noted ophthalmologist of his time. In 1934, he resigned as ophthalmologist-in-chief of the Royal Victoria and chairman of the McGill department, and F.T. Tooke succeeded him as professor and chairman.

From 1885 to 1936 ophthalmology grew from a one-man service under Frank Buller to a strong, well-established department at McGill and the teaching hospitals. Buller, Byers, and McKee had international reputations.

OTOLARYNGOLOGY

In 1885 the designation "specialist" appeared for the first time in the sixty-third annual report of the MGH: Frank Buller was listed as "oculist and aurist."

George Major (1851–1923), a laryngologist, was appointed to the medical faculty and the MGH in 1887 and kept his McGill positions until 1893. His expertise was in treating diseases of the nose, throat, and windpipe.[30] In 1894 H.S. Birkett was appointed to the General as a laryngologist. He resigned his position there in 1898 to pursue his career at the Royal Victoria.

In 1895 H.D. Hamilton was appointed as a laryngologist at the Montreal General. He was laryngologist-in-charge from 1898 to 1919 and then otolaryngologist-in-chief from 1919 to 1928. During his thirty-year tenure, otolaryngology achieved departmental status at the Montreal General and the Western General hospitals.[31]

Following the emergence of specialization at the MGH in the late nineteenth century, separate reports appeared from the department of ophthalmology and otology, and from the department of laryngology in the annual hospital reports. This continued until 1919 when in the MGH's ninety-eighth annual report, separate reports appeared from the department of ophthalmology and from the department of otolaryngology.

During Hamilton's tenure, fourteen part-time specialists who had private offices outside the Montreal General assisted him in otolaryngology. Hamilton retired as otolaryngologist-in-chief in 1928 and had consulting status until he died. G.E. Hodge was the MGH's otolaryngologist-in-chief from 1928 to 1948. During his tenure, the clinical service was enhanced, and audiology, speech therapy, and research were established. Under his leadership the Montreal General became a pioneer in audiologic development and research in Canada.

When the Royal Victoria opened for patients in 1894, there were four clinical departments: medicine, surgery, diseases of women, and ophthalmology and otolaryngology. The medical staff was largely recruited from the Montreal General. Buller was in charge of the RVH's ophthalmic clinic. Birkett was the laryngologist and professor of laryngology at McGill. He was associated in practice with Buller, who according to the customs of the time practised otology as well as ophthalmology. At the onset Birkett assisted Buller with procedures such as refractions, but after a time Buller practised ophthalmology more exclusively and Birkett otolaryngology. In 1905 after Buller's untimely death, the governors of the Royal Victoria and McGill decided to associate otology with laryngology at both the hospital and in the medical faculty.

Birkett organized the department of otolaryngology at the Royal Victoria and at McGill in its present departmental form. McGill's first professor and chairman of otolaryngology, he introduced to Canada bronchoscopy, submucous resection of the nasal septum, the Killian radical operation on the frontal sinus, radiography of the mastoid and of the nasal accessory sinuses, audiometric examination of hearing, and modern dissection methods of tonsillectomy. In 1893 he was the first in Canada to perform a thyrotomy for malignant disease of the larynx.

In the early 1920s Birkett collaborated with John Tait, professor of physiology and experimental medicine, in setting up a research laboratory to study vestibular physiology. W.J. McNally worked with Tait, and they established for the first time the mechanism of labyrinthine stimulation. In 1930 Birkett retired as otolaryngologist-in-chief but continued in private practice. He became emeritus professor at McGill and consultant at the RVH, positions he held until his death on 19 July 1942. In the course of his term of office he was assisted by eight part-time otolaryngologists with private offices outside the hospital. At that time the otolaryngologists developed bronchoscopy and bronchograms for investigation and treatment of pulmonary diseases.

D.R. Brown was the first laryngologist and D.A. Kerry was the oculist and aurist appointed at the Montreal Children's Hospital (originally the Children's Memorial Hospital). Later, associate specialists and consultants were appointed to cope with the increased outpatient services and the specialty clinics. For years the most frequent operation performed was tonsillectomy-adenoidectomy, which was done on an outpatient basis. In the hospital's 1935 annual report, the first in which a separate report from the division of otolaryngology appeared, it is recorded that the waiting time for this procedure was at least nine months. The directors of otolaryngology, a division of the department of surgery at the Montreal Children's Hospital, were D.R. Brown, 1909–14; H.S. Muckleston, 1914–18; and R.R. Wright, 1919–39.

With the establishment of the faculty department of otolaryngology in 1906, undergraduate teaching consisted of a series of six to eight lectures encompassing the breadth of the specialty presented in the pre-clinical period to second-year medical students. In the early clinical period there was small group instruction at the two teaching hospitals on physical examination in otolaryngology, arranged by the chairmen of the department of otolaryngology, H.S. Birkett, 1905–30; E.H. White, 1930–33; and D.H. Ballon, 1933–50.[32]

UROLOGY

Prior to 1900, general surgeons performed operations on the genito-urinary tract – dilation for urethral stricture, prostatectomy, cystosto-my, and circumcision. Shepherd, a general surgeon, performed the first nephrectomy in 1884. After 1900, with the development of x-rays, radio-opaque dyes, and improved instruments such as cystoscopes (1909), detailed investigation of the urinary tract was possible.

In the early 1900s Roland Campbell and Frank Patch at the General began to take a special interest in diseases of the urinary tract. The General and the Royal Vic established outpatient clinics for treatment of genito-urinary diseases – at first, mostly for venereal diseases. In 1911 Campbell was appointed chief of a new Montreal General department for genito-urinary diseases, or urology, as it came to be called. A similar department was established in 1914 at the Royal Victoria with J.W. Hutchinson as the first chief of urology. He had postgraduate training in urology in Germany in 1908. For the 1914–15 session at McGill, Campbell, and Hutchinson were lecturers for genito-urinary surgery, and F.S. Patch was demonstrator.

In 1914 Campbell joined the CAMC and was commanding officer of No. 5 Field Ambulance. After he was killed in action at Courcelette in France in 1916, Patch succeeded him as chief of the Montreal General's urology department. He had graduated from McGill Medical School in 1903, interned at the General from 1903 to 1905, and went to Europe for the next two years for postgraduate study in Bonn, Vienna, and London. On his return to Montreal in 1907, he was appointed medical superintendent at the General, assistant demonstrator of surgery at McGill, and assistant surgeon (outpatient) at the General. He lectured to the senior medical students on diseases of the genito-urinary tract.

Hutchinson went overseas with the CAMC during World War I and was given a leave of absence from the Royal Victoria. David W. MacKenzie, a native of Prince Edward Island who had trained in urology in New York City, came to the hospital in 1916 as joint head of the department of urology with Hutchinson. Hutchinson returned from overseas in 1919 but, after a short period as joint chief of urology with MacKen-zie, did not like the arrangement. He resigned from the Royal Vic in

March 1919 and went to the Ottawa Civic Hospital as chief of urology from 1919 to 1938.

After the war there was increased recognition of urology as a speciality at the medical faculty and the two teaching hospitals. The faculty formed a department of urology with Patch and MacKenzie as clinical professors. At the General, Patch was the senior urologist, assisted by R.E. Powell. At the Vic, MacKenzie was head of the department from 1920 to 1938, assisted by M. Seng.

MacKenzie developed Ward L at the Royal Victoria into "a hospital within a hospital," with cystoscopy and operating rooms and other special facilities. He established a three-year training program for urologists – senior intern, assistant resident and resident. There were many successful graduates of the Vic training program in urology.[33] The General did not have similar facilities or training program.

In the 1920s there was a course of fifteen lectures on diseases of the genito-urinary system for the fourth-year medical students, and they attended fifteen outpatient clinics at the hospitals. For fifth-year students, group instruction included case presentations stressing differential diagnosis and methods of treatment. Students followed the progress of patients on the wards. Patch and Mackenzie continued as clinical professors, Powell was promoted to lecturer, and Seng continued as a demonstrator in urology.

The period from 1885 to 1936 saw constant improvements in techniques for diagnosis and additional treatments for diseases of the genito-urinary tract. By 1936 urology was a well-established surgical specialty in the medical faculty and the teaching hospitals, and there were numerous professional societies and associations.[34]

ORTHOPEDIC SURGERY

Alexander MacKenzie Forbes (fig. 68), an 1898 McGill medical graduate,[35] started orthopedic surgery practice in Montreal in 1903 by founding a small children's hospital for orthopedic surgery not associated with McGill – the Children's Memorial Hospital (later renamed the Montreal Children's Hospital). Forbes was the first surgeon-in-chief.

Forbes's first appointment at McGill in 1903 was as assistant demonstrator of anatomy. He advanced with appointments in clinical surgery in 1907, assistant demonstrator of orthopedic surgery in 1908, demonstrator of orthopedic surgery in 1909, lecturer in 1912, and clinical professor in 1920. At the Montreal General his first appointment

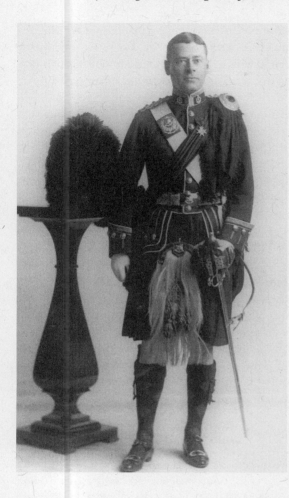

Figure 68
Alexander MacKenzie
Torrance Forbes,
1874–1929. Photo by
William Notman, 1920

was in 1906 as a surgeon in the outpatient department without operating privileges

At the turn of the century, general surgeons treated fractures and
musculo-skeletal injuries. This continued to be a significant part of their
practices at the MGH and the RVH through the 1930s. Numerous musculo-skeletal problems required special attention, many of them in children: club feet, scoliosis and tuberculosis of the spine, spina bifida with
its associated complications, spastic diplegia, deformities of the spine
and joints from poliomyelitis, birth defects of arms and legs, torticollis,
and dislocations. In 1907 clinics for those problems were started, with
Forbes in charge at the Montreal General and W.G. Turner at the Royal

Vic. At first they were confined to manipulative treatments, and the general surgeons continued to operate when necessary. As orthopedic surgery became better recognized, orthopedic surgeons began to operate under the auspices of a division of the department of surgery at both hospitals.

Turner had appointments similar to Forbes at McGill, including that of clinical professor of orthopedic surgery from 1920. J.A. Nutter and W.J. Patterson assisted as demonstrators in orthopedic surgery. The course in orthopedic surgery for the medical students consisted of introductory lectures on diseases of bones and joints. Demonstrations were arranged in the outpatient clinics at the two hospitals.

In 1925 Forbes had such a reputation for orthopedics that the Shriners organization began to consider building a hospital in Montreal. The Montreal Shriners Hospital opened in 1925, located on Cedar Avenue near the Children's Memorial Hospital; Forbes was its first chief of orthopedics. Turner succeeded him in the position in 1929.

N.T. Williamson was appointed assistant demonstrator of orthopedic surgery in 1927. By 1929, when he died suddenly of mycardiopathy, Forbes controlled orthopedics at the teaching hospitals. Orthopedic surgery continued with Turner as clinical professor of orthopedic surgery at the Royal Victoria and Nutter at the General. By 1935 Turner and Nutter were clinical professors of orthopedic surgery, Patterson was lecturer, and Williamson demonstrator.[36]

NEUROSURGERY

The development of neurosurgery at McGill from 1893 to 1936 is described in chapter 4. Bell did some neurosurgical procedures from 1893 to 1911, but neurosurgery at McGill really started when W.G. Penfield and W.V. Cone came to Montreal in 1928 and the Montreal Neurological Institute opened in 1934. At first the MNI had forty-seven beds, and bed and board cost $3 per day. The staff included Penfield and Cone as neurosurgeons and C. Russel and J.M. Peterson as neurologists. The house officers were Theodore Erickson, John Kershman, E. Baldrey, Francis McNaughton, William Gibson, and Webb Haymaker, all of whom became prominent neurologists or neurosurgeons. The dynamic Eileen Flanagan was the institute's director of nursing from 1934 until she retired in 1961. Her experiences convinced her that special skills were required in neuroscience nursing, leading her to establish a twenty-two week neuroscience nursing program that attracted students from around the world.

8 Other Subjects

From 1871 the medical school curriculum included a course on hygiene that dealt with community rather than individual health. George Ross, a junior member of the medical faculty, was the first professor of hygiene. It was a lecture course, and the appointment as professor of hygiene was considered "entry level," since it was more poorly paid and had less prestige than one of the major courses in the medical school curriculum.[1] The first few professors of hygiene had no particular training or interest in the subject and lectured using one of the standard textbooks.

Gradually, the hygiene course increased in scope, importance, and prestige as the population increased, urban centres grew, and governments assumed more responsibility for public health problems. Over the years different titles were used for the course – hygiene, public health, preventive medicine. In addition to the basic course content there were add-ons such as industrial medicine, forensic medicine, and mental health. By the early 1900s the professors and teachers were qualified and interested in their subjects.

In 1885 Richard L. MacDonnell, a brilliant young internist whose father had been on the McGill staff in the 1840s, started to give the hygiene lectures. The content of his course included discussion of public water supplies, conditions of soil and water that affected community health, drainage and sewer systems, the atmosphere (including heating and ventilation), industrial hygiene regarding food and drink, physical exercise and bathing, and public health facilities in Montreal and the Province of Quebec.

In 1889 Robert Craik[2] succeeded Howard as dean of the medical faculty and MacDonnell as professor of hygiene. In 1893 Sir Donald Smith donated $50,000 to endow the chair, and Craik became the first Strathcona Professor of Hygiene. Craik's course consisted of two lectures per week for the entire third year. In 1896 the department was renamed "public health and preventive medicine," and that title was used for the next decade.[3]

New subjects were added to the course: bacteriology, infectious diseases, and serum therapy. A museum directed by R.F. Ruttan, professor of chemistry, was equipped to demonstrate public health systems. By 1900 the Public Health Museum had models illustrating the principles of sterilization, disinfection, filtration, and ventilation. A number of private companies contributed to the museum. A laboratory course was held for three months. Craik and Ruttan taught chemistry and physics, J.G. Adami bacteriology, and Wyatt Johnston[4] preventive medicine. As public health issues became greater, H.B. Yates was added to the staff in 1897 and A.J. Williams in 1898, and Craik was able to devote more time to the deanship. In 1900 the faculty offered a one-year postgraduate course leading to a McGill Diploma in Public Health – an indication of the increased interest in public health problems in the community.[5]

Craik retired as dean and professor in 1902, and Wyatt Johnston was appointed Strathcona Professor of Hygiene. The department now occupied the north end of the Medical Building on the mezzanine floor, and included a sixty by fifty foot laboratory, a thirteen by fifteen foot balance room, and a forty-five by thirty foot model systems room. When Wyatt Johnston died unexpectedly from pulmonary embolism in 1902, as his replacement the faculty appointed T.A. Starkey as Strathcona Professor of Hygiene and Bacteriology; he would continue in that post until 1935.[6] He gave compulsory lectures three times per week in the third year covering all aspects of public health in detail, and the broader aspects of the influence of air, water, heating, plumbing, climate, housing, and lighting on community health, and of public facilities for disposal of waste, drainage, burial of the dead, and hospital sanitation. He also discussed epidemics and infectious diseases. After 1900 the population of Montreal had increased rapidly, and so did the number of public health problems.[7] In 1907 the faculty appointed three staff members who held diplomas in public health (DPH) – B. Jones, F.C. Douglas, and J.A. Lundie.

By 1914 the general focus of the public health course changed to include discussion of the causes of disease, channels of communication, and modern prevention measures. One lecture and demonstration were given per week for one year. The students continued to use the Public Health Museum.

After 1920 T.A. Starkey, F.B. Jones, and R. St John MacDonald taught the course and gradually introduced changes. In 1928 hygiene was introduced into the first-year curriculum. Groups of students were taken to industrial sites, schools, and public works to see how public health was monitored. In 1926 Starkey stepped down as director of the department, though he remained Strathcona Professor until 1935. In 1927 A.G. Fleming was appointed professor and director, and the department was renamed Public Health and Preventive Medicine. Experts in mental hygiene (Mitchell) and industrial hygiene (F. Pedley) assisted Fleming. In 1927 the faculty formed a subdepartment of industrial medicine. The Metropolitan Life Insurance Company supported an industrial medicine clinic at the Montreal General with a grant of $25,000. This was the start of a specialty that became known as "occupational medicine."

By 1930 Fleming directed a department of eight physicians, including professors, lecturers, and demonstrators – three of them in mental hygiene. Short introductory courses were given in first and second years. The major course was given in the third year, followed by a course on communicable diseases in the fourth. The mental hygiene course was concerned with measures to prevent nervous and mental disease, delinquency, crime, and social failure in home, school, and work environments. Its objective was to teach students the principles of social behaviour. In 1936 McGill probably offered the best public health course in the Province of Quebec.

MEDICAL JURISPRUDENCE

The chair of medical jurisprudence was founded in 1845. The average physician needed knowledge of the subject matter of this course to pass the provincial licensing examinations and for medical practice. For the next few decades the professor of medical jurisprudence was an "entry-level" appointment filled by a series of young physicians with academic aspirations,[8] often without any special knowledge or interest in the subject. Senior physicians were not interested in medical jurisprudence because it was not considered to be real medicine.

Medical jurisprudence was a lecture course, and the professors used standard textbooks by Husban, Gay, and Ferrier that were often out of date. The subjects covered in the course included the medical and legal aspects of insanity; attention to blood stains (blood typing was not done yet); recent research in the differences between animal and human blood cells; the names and classification of poisons; the most common food poisons; the post-mortem appearances and tests demonstrating the presence of poisoning.

In 1883 George Wilkins[9] started to teach the course and continued to lecture until he retired in 1911. In 1895 medical jurisprudence was one of thirteen subjects in the medical school curriculum. T.W. Burgess lectured on the medico-legal aspects of mental disease. Wyatt Johnston lectured on forensic pathology, illustrating his lectures with specimens from the coroner's court; he attempted to demonstrate the pathological conditions seen in violent or sudden death that raised suspicion of homicide.

In 1901 Johnston offered an optional course in legal medicine (forensic medicine) at the Montreal General. A certificate was presented to students passing the examination.[10] In 1903 D.D. MacTaggart, a forensic pathologist, was appointed lecturer in medical jurisprudence. Wilkins and MacTaggart continued teaching the course until Wilkins retired in 1911; then MacTaggart was appointed professor. He remained in that post until 1929 when the course was discontinued and the material was incorporated into other courses. I.M. Rabinowitch, director of the department of metabolism and toxicology at the General and a recognized expert in medical jurisprudence, gave interesting lectures to the third-year students as part of the public health course.

MEDICAL HISTORY

In 1907 the medical faculty appointed Andrew Macphail (1864–1938) professor of the history of medicine. A friend of John McCrae and Stephen Leacock, he was considered to be one of the great Canadian men of letters before and after World War I. From 1903 he was editor of the privately owned *Montreal Medical Journal*. In 1911 he became the founding editor of the *Canadian Medical Association Journal* when the decision was taken to convert the *Montreal Medical Journal* into the official organ of the CMA. He continued editing the CMAJ and teaching the history of medicine at McGill until the outbreak of war in 1914, when he and his assistant, W.W. Francis, went overseas on active service with the CAMC. Macphail was knighted for his literary work during the war.[11]

Macphail taught an optional course of twelve lectures on medical history that was available to all medical undergraduates. Except for the war years, he continued to give those lectures until 1937. In spite of two events that might have given a major boost to interest in medical history – the founding of the Osler Society in 1921 by C.J. Tidmarsh and the arrival of the Osler Library at McGill in 1929 – few students attended Macphail's lectures towards the end of his term. The appointment of Francis, now the Osler Librarian, to succeed Macphail as professor of the history of medicine and his continuation of the lecture series did little to stimulate the interest of the students. The Osler Society, however, kept the subject of medical history alive amongst the students and the annual Osler Banquet amongst the graduates.

9 Governance of the Medical Faculty, 1885–1936

The evolution of the Faculty of Medicine from 1885 to 1936 required close cooperation between the faculty, the university, and the teaching hospitals. In 1885 these included the Montreal General and the Montreal Maternity Hospital; by 1936 the Royal Victoria, the Children's Memorial Hospital (later the Montreal Children's Hospital), the Verdun Protestant Hospital for the Insane, and the Alexandra Hospital for Infectious Diseases had been added. Although the hospitals were independent bodies with separate governing boards and at times with interests that conflicted with those of the McGill medical faculty, for the most part the university and the hospitals cooperated with the faculty to enhance the quality and scope of its teaching and its reputation.

In 1885 there were eighteen members of the teaching staff – fourteen professors, one lecturer, and three demonstrators. Their incomes were from their medical practices, with some additional income from student fees. Palmer Howard was a part-time professor of medicine and received some remuneration for his additional responsibilities as dean. James Stewart, a practising physician, was professor of materia medica and the part-time registrar (1884–93.) In the 1880s an average of thirty-five students graduated from the McGill medical faculty each year.

On the evening of 16 April 1885 Dean Howard held a faculty meeting at his home at 47 Union Avenue. Ten of the eighteen members of the teaching staff attended. The minutes of the meeting recorded discussions about the curriculum, the Medical Library, the Medical Museum, and the proposed enlargement of the Medical Building. The business of the meeting was settled by consensus. When the teaching staff increased, this informal "family" type of governance did not continue, and there were major changes in the next fifty years.[1] By 1936 there were more than one hundred members of the teaching staff – a few full time with salaries and most part time with an annual honorarium. Since 1923 C.F. Martin had been the first full-time dean. J.C. Simpson, histologist and embryologist, was part-time secretary of the faculty with an annual honorarium. In the 1930s more than one hundred students graduated from the medical faculty each year.

In May 1893 the faculty made an important decision regarding the curriculum, a change in policy that had been discussed informally for several years. In keeping with educational trends in North America, the faculty decided that there should be more practical instruction with less reliance on lectures.[2] By 1900 the faculty had appointed assistant professors, lecturers, demonstrators, and assistant demonstrators for most of the departments and subjects in the curriculum, and the teaching staff increased from eighteen to one hundred. There were four salaried professors: T.W. Mills in physiology, J.G. Adami in pathology, R.F. Ruttan in chemistry, and R. Craik in hygiene.[3] The assistant professors and lecturers received an annual honorarium; demonstrators received $100 and assistant demonstrators $50 per annum.

In 1893 the committee structure of the faculty was formalized by the appointment of five standing committees: education, finance, house, museum, and library. Each committee had a convenor and four or five members.[4] Only the professors were members of the standing committees, and some professors served on more than one committee. Although all members of the teaching staff were entitled to attend the monthly faculty meetings at the Medical Building, generally only the professors attended.

The question was raised: Who was empowered to make decisions on behalf of the faculty regarding curriculum, finances, promotions, and other important items? When J.G. Adami joined the faculty in 1892 as professor of pathology, he recommended that a small group, or an executive, of the teaching staff should be appointed to run the business of the faculty. After several years of discussion at faculty meetings, on 11 April 1896 the faculty adopted its first constitution[5] defining the Faculty of Medicine as "all members of the teaching staff appointed by the University Board of Governors." The constitution named a faculty executive consisting of the principal, the dean, the registrar, the titular professors in thirteen subjects,[6] the professors of clinical medicine, and the professors of clinical surgery at the two teaching hospitals.[7] The faculty executive was empowered to direct and control the affairs of the faculty. The remaining members of the teaching staff – the junior faculty – would elect one representative to sit on the executive. The appointment of this executive made governance efficient but also more autocratic; the inclusion of a representative of the junior faculty was an attempt to make governance somewhat democratic and representative. Wyatt Johnston was the first elected representative of the junior faculty, and for several years he attended most meetings. Principal Peterson chaired the monthly meetings from September to June,[8] and the dean presided in his absence.

In 1899 the faculty executive adopted formal guidelines for the five standing committees.[9] At the annual April meeting, the executive appointed the convenors and members of the standing committees for the following academic year. Every committee was required to give an annual report to the executive, preferably written. The executive referred important business and controversial items to these committees for study and by and large accepted the recommendations.[10]

In 1907 the university governors appointed Andrew Macphail as professor of the history of medicine. Since medical history was not a major subject in the curriculum, a new category was created – a professor without a seat on the faculty executive. Professors from the Faculty of Arts who taught in the medical school, for example, P. Penhallow, professor of biology, had a seat on the faculty executive.

After these arrangements had been in place for more than a decade, the junior faculty wanted to have more input into the business of the faculty. Wesley Mills, professor of physiology, was sympathetic to this position and suggested that the junior faculty should hold regular meetings, formulate views, and report to the executive.[11] In 1920 the "junior faculty" was renamed the "associate faculty" – comprised of all members of the teaching staff not on the faculty executive, including demonstrators but not assistant demonstrators.[12]

The relations of the associate faculty with the faculty executive were defined in a revised constitution. The associate faculty would elect a president, a secretary, and two representatives to sit on the executive. For the 1910–11 session, J.M. Elder was president, and F.T. Tooke secretary of the associate faculty, while W.F. Hamilton and J. McCrae were the representatives on the executive.[13] After 1912 the associate faculty also had one representative on the Education Committee.[14]

In the following months the associate faculty began to have an expanded role in faculty affairs and in April 1912 proposed that botany should be eliminated from the medical school curriculum and taught in the arts faculty. It would be replaced by a course on infections and immunity. The executive adopted that proposal and appointed J.C. Meakins and F.B. Gurd to give the course. The associate faculty also recommended that A.D. Blackader be appointed professor of pediatrics without a seat on the executive, since pediatrics was a sub-department of medicine. Blackader had been professor of therapeutics and pharmacology since 1890 but up to then had little recognition of his role as a pediatrician.[15] In 1914 the faculty executive also revised the constitution so that the associate faculty would have better communication with the dean.[16]

After World War I there were lengthy discussions about the future organization of the faculty. H.S. Birkett had been dean since 1914 and was anxious to retire. The question was raised of who would succeed him as dean and with what terms of reference. Birkett, as a part-time dean, and J.W. Scane, as part-time registrar, were having difficulty handling the increasing administration. Two options were proposed: first, that the dean would be an honorary part-time position that would be rotated amongst the department heads while a full-time assistant dean would be the faculty's administrative officer; and second, that a full-time salaried dean would be the faculty's administrative officer assisted by a part-time secretary of the faculty.

In 1918 the Education Committee recommended the second option, and the following year the university governors agreed.[17] However, arrangements for appointment of a full-time dean could not be completed at that time, and the first option for the role of the dean was adopted. F.G. Finley was dean in 1921–22 to succeed Birkett, and G.E. Armstrong was dean in 1922–23, both on a part-time basis. Scane, who had been part-time registrar from 1903 to 1921, was appointed assistant dean on a full-time basis. He would have been the faculty's administrative officer, but unfortunately his health declined and he was on sick leave from 1921 until he died in 1924. J.C. Simpson was appointed part-time secretary of the faculty in his place. This arrangement was not satisfactory, and in 1923 the university governors announced the appointment of C.F. Martin as the first full-time dean of the faculty "on a somewhat more permanent basis."[18]

In 1921 the faculty approved a revised and more elaborate constitution. All members of the teaching staff were invited to attend the faculty meetings, which were held quarterly. A council consisting of all the professors would monitor decisions taken at the meetings. An executive committee of the council would run the day-to-day business of the faculty.[19] This new model of governance was an attempt to be democratic by including all members of the teaching staff, and at the same time to have the efficiency of a small executive committee.

After his appointment in 1923, however, Dean Martin instituted a new organization of the faculty that was more autocratic and less representative. In his opinion small groups were more efficient at decision-making than large groups, and the members of the teaching staff were spending too much time attending meetings. He suggested that there should be meetings of departments, for example, medicine, surgery, obstetrics, and gynecology. He disbanded the five previous standing committees (education, finance, house, museum, and library) and replaced them with one standing committee comprised of the dean, secretary, and three members of the teaching staff: a physician, a surgeon, and a representative of the pre-clinical departments, each of whom would serve for one year. Thereafter three new members were appointed each year with rotation amongst the departments and hospitals.[20] From time to time Martin appointed special committees to address specific problems and report to the standing committee.[21] The quarterly faculty meetings of all teaching staff continued.

As outlined in chapters 3 and 4, with this organization Martin was able to introduce major changes to the faculty. In 1930 the teaching staff wanted to have more input into running faculty affairs. Martin agreed to this, and in the last six years of his deanship he made the governance of the faculty more democratic by appointing additional members to the standing committee. These would now include the dean, the secretary, two representatives from medicine, two from surgery, and one representative from each of obstetrics/gynecology, public health, pathology, pharmacology, physiology, biochemistry, and anatomy. After 1936 the dean's office accepted more responsibilities for postgraduate medical education, research and community medicine, and at various times vice-deans and associate and assistant deans were appointed.

Epilogue

As the 1930s drew to a close, McGill's Faculty of Medicine found itself in a world still mired in the Depression and on the brink of a second catastrophic world war. While war activities would put the North American economy on a stronger footing, they clearly would place most development activities within medical schools on hold.

Referring to Ludmerer's monumental history of medical education[1] in the United States and Bonner's[2] examination of activities in that country as well as in Europe, one can state with confidence that McGill was not just a Canadian medical school. It was completely integrated into the fabric of North American medicine, while maintaining the strong links that had always been present with the United Kingdom. The developments that had occurred during the previous seventy-five years had closely paralleled those in the United States. Thus, when medical faculties were becoming integral parts of universities, the same process was happening at McGill. The development of student laboratories, reflecting an emphasis on science, likewise closely paralleled those activities in the better American schools. In the 1880s when President Charles William Eliot was chairing faculty meetings at the Harvard Medical School, Principal William Dawson was exerting a similar influence at McGill. It must be remembered that these events took place before the Flexner Report of 1910 and indeed were the reasons why Flexner rated McGill so highly.[3]

Trends in the United States were also present at McGill following the Flexner Report. The development of full-time clinical faculty was encouraged by Rockefeller Foundation grants to McGill, as was true of so many medical schools around the world, and further development of the scientific underpinnings of medical education took place. The development of facilities for both science and clinical teaching occurred on both sides of the border. The expansion of the old Medical Building, the new Strathcona Medical Building, the development of the Montreal General, the building of the Royal Victoria and the Royal Victoria's Women's Pavilion (the Mat), the addition of the Montreal Neurological Institute and the Pathological Institute all created the foundation of what would subsequently become an academic health-science centre in Montreal.

Finally, the composition of the student body also reflected a North American rather than solely a Canadian character in McGill's medical school. The first medical graduate in 1833, William Logie, pursued his career in the United States. American students have always studied at McGill's many faculties in great numbers, thus making it somewhat different from other universities in Canada, whose student bodies have been more regional in composition.

World War II represented an interlude when development largely stopped as McGill University and the medical faculty coped with obligations imposed by the war. Many doctors and nurses served overseas in the armed forces, adding to the burdens in patient care and education of those left behind. The curriculum was accelerated to produce more physicians, and graduating physicians and nurses went overseas to join their more senior colleagues. When World War II ended, those individuals often returned to the faculty with immense experience and a tangible sense of camaraderie.

While the facilities available to the medical faculty had been adequate in the 1930s, after World War II medicine was changing rapidly, and new facilities and equipment were required. The major trends that emerged were certainly global with, as always, some local shifts in emphasis. The most dominant trend, of course, was the enormous expansion in biomedical science and technology that rapidly made existing clinical and research facilities obsolete. A second trend was the emergence of a feeling in Canada that health care was a right, not a privilege. This resulted in the gradual remodelling of Canada's national health policy, beginning with federal underwriting of hospitalization in 1958 and ending with the arrival of payment for physicians' services in the country in general and in Quebec in 1970. Most of the activities taking place within the medical faculty and its associated teaching hospitals from 1945 until the present have constituted efforts to adjust to the reality imposed upon it by these two trends.

The medical faculty and all of McGill's major institutions embarked upon building programs to meet the new demands. The Royal Victoria opened a new surgical wing in 1956, and a new medical wing followed in 1958. The Montreal Children's Hospital moved from its cottage-style buildings on the side of Mount Royal to a building on Tupper Street that had previously housed the Western Division of the Montreal General. This was renovated and occupied in 1957. An expanded research base was present in all buildings, often using what had previously been occupied by clinical activities. The Jewish General Hospital, which was a large community hospital, changed its focus in the 1980s and 1990s; it expanded, built extensive research facilities, and became more academic in its orientation. Other community institutions, such as the Queen Elizabeth and Saint Mary's hospitals, also became involved in teaching and provided outstanding clinical rotations. The Verdun Protestant Hospital (subsequently known as the Douglas Hospital) and the Shriners Hospital expanded their facilities and became important for both teaching and research. Finally, in order to draw closer to the community and to provide community-based teaching opportunities, the Faculty of Medicine used Quebec's community health network and established several rural rotations.

The medical school also required a great expansion in facilities. Class size had increased to 160 in response to a shortage of physicians in the country, and space for instruction was lacking. The requirements of modern science could not be met in the existing facilities. Consequently, the McIntyre Medical Sciences Building and the Stewart Biology Building opened in 1965, offering modern laboratories for the departments of pharmacology, biochemistry, and physiology and for the newly developed Aerospace Medicine Unit. Anatomy and histology remained in the Strathcona Medical Building along with an expanded dental faculty. Pathology had expanded facilities in both hospitals with its headquarters remaining at the Pathological Institute (subsequently renamed the Lyman Duff Medical Sciences Building), sharing the facilities with microbiology and immunology. Activities that did not require laboratories occupied several houses on Pine Avenue close to the McIntyre Building. Thus, epidemiology and biostatistics, occupational health, and the Centre for Medical Education all moved into these areas and freed up central space that could be devoted to basic science laboratories.

As the physical facilities expanded, so did the medical faculty. The postwar period saw a great increase in funding of education in Canada, and all medical faculties benefited. The number of full-time faculty members, particularly in clinical departments, increased tremendously. Partly this increase was in order to free faculty time for research. The great expansion in subspecialty medicine also played a major role. The number of generalists diminished significantly, and as specialties proliferated, all required their full-time staff. Fortunately, resources were available from provincial funding, private sources, and research grants to support these changes. In addition, clinical earnings were on the rise, and major departments in the larger teaching hospitals pooled these resources utilizing a portion for academic advancement. Once more, these trends mirrored those seen south of the border.

The development of Canada's national health plan had a major impact on the medical faculty. Medicare, as it was known, was viewed with suspicion by a substantial number of physicians, and the faculty lost important members as a result of its imposition. However, this occurred when McGill had enlarged training programs, and the deficits were rapidly made up with young individuals who had not worked in the previous system and were not as hostile to Medicare. A reorganization of teaching programs resulted because all patients were now "fee-capable," there thus being no more "ward patients." A policy decision was made to include as many patients as possible in teaching programs, and this met with general acceptance from the patients. Finally, physicians' incomes actually went up during the first decade after the institution of Medicare, facilitating the maintenance of a full-time system while adequately supporting clinicians who, as had always been true, gave freely of their time to teach.

The great increase in health-care expectations and the recession of the 1980s changed this relatively optimistic picture. University and health-care funding was cut dramatically, making it more difficult to maintain faculty support. At the same time, fee schedules from Medicare did not increase consonant with the cost of living. Thus pooled income from clinical earnings was down, and, more seriously, physicians had to work harder, processing more patients than before in order to maintain clinical earnings, leaving less time for academic activities including teaching. Once again, this situation was similar to that found in the United States.[4] There it was managed care that was interfering with teaching time, whereas in Canada it was the national health plan itself.

Thus as the millennium drew to a close, all medical schools in Canada, including McGill, were struggling with Canadian problems that found parallels to those in the United States, and indeed throughout the world. The faculty actually appeared to be weathering difficult times reasonably well, in large part because of the great dedication of the McGill teachers. Throughout its history, McGill has provided an intellectual milieu that its members cherish and wish to foster. Faculty members have given freely of their time and have never been remunerated for everything that they did. This atmosphere and these attitudes persisted, and at the start of a new century indications are that the public is demanding higher levels of funding for health care, which should alleviate some of the difficulties.

Beginning in the 1990s, a plan was developed to merge McGill's traditional teaching institutions. The Montreal General, Royal Victoria, Montreal Neurological Institute, and the Montreal Children's Hospital legally merged and embarked upon planning to build a new McGill University Hospital Centre (MUHC). Once more the global trend towards concentration at major teaching institutions is found at McGill. As medical problems, illnesses, and procedures become more complex in the major teaching hospitals, community teaching sites become even more important, and the Faculty of Medicine has moved to actively maintain existing sites and expand into new ones.

As Canada's oldest medical faculty moves into the twenty-first century, it remains what it has always been – a highly respected academic institution whose graduates are first of all skilled clinicians, respected by their patients and their peers. McGill medical graduates occupy important positions in their communities as well as in academic institutions throughout the world. The outlook of the faculty and the university is broad and inclusive, the student body and the faculty extremely diverse, reflecting as they always have the reality of Canadian society.

Appendices

Appendix One

Index of Biographical Sketches

McGill Medicine, Volume 1

Name	Dates	Page
Sir William Osler	1849–1919	179
William Robertson	1784–1844	144
Sir Thomas George Roddick	1846–1923	172
George Ross	1845–1892	171
William E. Scott	1823–1883	161
Francis (Frank) John Shepherd	1851–1929	183
John Stephenson	1794–1842	145
William Sutherland	1815–1875	157
William Wright	1827–1908	165

McGill Medicine, Volume 2

Name	Dates	Page
Maude Elizabeth Seymour Abbott	1869–1940	212
John George Adami	1862–1926	213
Edward William Archibald	1872–1945	214
George Eli Armstrong	1855–1933	216
Alfred Turner Bazin	1872–1958	217
James Bell	1852–1911	218
Herbert Stanley Birkett	1864–1942	219
Arthur Annesley Browne	1848–1910	220
James Chalmers Cameron	1852–1912	220
Walter William Chipman	1866–1950	221
James Bertram Collip	1892–1965	222
William Vernon Cone	1897–1959	223
Frederick Gault Finley	1861–1940	225
Alexander MacKenzie Torrance Forbes	1874–1929	226
Alva H. Gordon	1876–1953	227
Sir Henry McIlree Williamson Gray	1870–1938	227
Campbell Palmer Howard	1877–1936	228
Robert Jared Bliss Howard	1859–1921	229
Henri Amédée Lafleur	1862–1939	230
Charles Ferdinand Martin	1868–1953	231
John McCrae	1878–1918	232
Robert Tait McKenzie	1867–1938	233

Biographical Sketches

MAUDE ELIZABETH SEYMOUR ABBOTT
(1869–1940)

As the first woman appointed to the McGill Faculty of Medicine in 1910, Maude Abbott epitomized the work ethic of the Victorian era. Initially barred from the men's world at McGill, she thrived by relying on her astonishing industry and genius. She became a pathologist, author, historian, and woman's advocate, and she excelled at each endeavour.

Born Maude Babin at St Andrew's East, Quebec, in 1869, she was orphaned at seven months. Her father had abandoned the family after being involved in a murder trial, and her mother died of tuberculosis. Her sixty-two-year-old grandmother, Mrs William Abbott, adopted Maude and her sister, Alice, and changed their surname to Abbott. After schooling the children at home, Grandmother Abbott sent Maude to a private girl's school in Montreal for one year; she then entered McGill University in 1886 on a Donald Smith grant. The students on this grant were known as "Donaldas," after their benefactor. She graduated B.A. from McGill in 1890 with a gold medal for general proficiency. Denied admission to McGill's medical faculty, she graduated M.D., C.M. with honours from Bishop's Medical Faculty in 1894.

After studying for two years in Europe she started a medical practice in Montreal. A chance meeting with C.F. Martin on the McGill lower campus changed her life forever. She had done work on hemosiderosis in Europe and wanted to work with Martin. He introduced her to J.G. Adami, professor of pathology, who was also interested in blood diseases. Adami hired her as assistant curator of the Medical Museum in 1898 and promoted her to curator one year later, a position she held until 1932. She was established in a screened-off corner of the Medical Museum and began to publish an extraordinary number of papers with expertise and depth on the history of medicine and nursing, McGill University, cardiology, and congenital heart disease. She classified the hundreds of specimens in the Medical Museum using a modified Dewey Decimal library system. In 1904 she published an in-depth history of the medical faculty. At the request of William Osler, she wrote a chapter on congenital heart disease for his multi-volume text *System of Medicine*. Osler said that her chapter was the best description of congenital heart-disease conditions ever written.

In 1910 McGill awarded her M.D., C.M. *honoris causa*. Her greatest contribution to medicine was the classification of cyanotic and acyanotic congenital heart disease. After classifying and recording one thousand cases, she published the definitive *Atlas of Congenital Cardiac Disease* in 1936. Inspired by Osler, a personal friend for many years, she wrote much about him, nursing, and Florence Nightingale. She was the first woman member of the Med-Chi, assistant editor of the *CMAJ*, a charter fellow of the RCPSC in 1931, and received an LL.D. from McGill in 1936. She was acting chairman of pathology at the Woman's College of Pennsylvania from 1923 to 1925, and compiled the first comprehensive bibliography of the writings of Sir William Osler.

Maude Abbott became a famous McGill character and renown for her knowledge and description of congenital cardiac disease, her love of and frequent articles about Osler, and the first definite history of the McGill medical faculty. Although she was initially excluded from the man's world of McGill, there was not a man in the university who did not respect her.

References: H.E. MacDermot, *Maude Abbott – A Memoir* (Toronto: Macmillan, 1941); D. Waugh, *Maudie of McGill: Dr. Maude Abbott and the Foundations of Heart Surgery* (Toronto: Hannah, 1992).

JOHN GEORGE ADAMI (1862–1926)

After Osler left Montreal to go to Philadelphia in 1884, Wyatt Johnston taught the course in pathology, but by the late 1880s he became more interested in bacteriology and public health. With the enlarging classes, McGill needed a professor of pathology. The faculty executive compiled a list of twelve possible candidates. When these were approached, only Adami, a fellow at Christ's College, Cambridge, was interested in applying for the post.

Adami's early education was at Owens College, Manchester, and from there he continued his studies at Christ's College, Cambridge, graduating M.B. in 1889 and M.D. in 1892. Most of his postgraduate work was in experimental physiology, but he had enough confidence to accept an appointment as McGill's first professor of pathology in 1892. In 1893 Lord Strathcona endowed the chair, and Adami became the first Strathcona Professor of Pathology.

Adami arrived in Montreal in the autumn of 1892 and set up his department of pathology in an extension to the Medical Building that had been made possible by a generous grant from J.H.R. Molson. After 1894 suitable accommodation was available at the Royal Victoria for Adami's work. In 1910 he moved his department to the newly opened Strathcona Medical Building.

Adami had great energy, and soon became an academic pathologist and a prominent member of the medical faculty executive. An enthusiastic public speaker, he was frequently asked to address audiences in Montreal and elsewhere. He was an inspiring teacher and a prolific writer and enjoyed working with the clinical staff. In 1908 he published his magnum opus, the two-volume textbook *The Principles of Pathology*, and in 1912 with John McCrae, *A Textbook of Pathology for Medical Students*.

In August 1914 Adami enlisted in the CAMC and went to England and France as one of the officers attached to No. 3 Canadian General Hospital (McGill). After the war, instead of returning to McGill, he accepted an appointment as vice-chancellor at the University of Liverpool. During his time at McGill he built up a strong department of pathology and his successors, Horst Oertel and Lyman Duff, continued the good work that he had started.

Reference: M.J. Adami, *J. George Adami: A Memoir* (London: Constable, 1930).

EDWARD WILLIAM ARCHIBALD (1872–1945)

Archibald was a sophisticated Victorian gentleman who was ahead of his time in interests and ability. He was a research-oriented surgeon whose primary interest was not private practice. The surgical department he built at the Royal Victoria Hospital became recognized internationally. His great achievement was to establish a Surgical Research Centre at McGill and the RVH in 1929, funded by the Rockefeller Foundation. In addition, he helped to persuade Wilder Penfield to come to McGill to develop a program in neurosurgery.

Archibald was born in Montreal in 1872, twenty-one years after Francis Shepherd and twenty-three years after William Osler. His parents educated three sons in English and French at home and in Grenoble, France. He went from the High School of Montreal to McGill in 1888, graduating with a gold medal in modern languages in 1892; he then entered the medical faculty, graduating M.D., C.M. in 1896. After three years as a surgical house officer at the RVH under James Bell, he went to Europe for further training in pathology and general surgery. Returning to Montreal in 1900, he was appointed to the surgical departments at the RVH and McGill.

In 1901 Archibald contracted pulmonary tuberculosis and spent a year at the Trudeau Sanatorium in Saranac Lake in upper New York State. On his return to McGill he began a remarkable career of surgical research, publishing on many subjects. Because he was doing neurosurgery with James Bell, in 1906 he went to get training with Sir Victor Horsley, the British neurosurgeon at Queen Square, London. In 1908 Archibald published an eight-hundred-page monograph on neurosurgery. However, after Bell died in 1911, Archibald did little brain surgery. He published books on diseases of the pancreas in 1927 and 1936, and monographs on surgical treatment of tuberculosis, writing on neurosurgical procedures, gastric surgery, and surgery for pancreatitis, and publising twenty-nine articles on pulmonary tuberculosis between 1913 and 1936.

Archibald rose in academic rank to professor and chairman of surgery at McGill in 1923 but was not appointed surgeon-in-chief at the RVH until 1928. Although he was a general surgeon, he was most widely known for his work in the surgery for pulmonary tuberculosis, a field in which he is regarded as an outstanding pioneer. In H. Rocke Robertson's opinion, Archibald was the father of thoracic surgery in North America. He retired in December 1935.

References: W.G. Penfield, "Edward Archibald: 1872–1945." *Canad J Surg* 1 (1958): 167–74 (includes a complete bibliography); H.R. Robertson, "Dedication of the Archibald Amphitheatre." *Canad J Surg* 24 (1981): 447–8. 1981. Obituary and appreciations: *CMAJ* 54 (1946):

194–7. M.E. Entin, "Edward Archibald, Surgeon of the Royal Vic," McGill University Libraries, Montreal 2004.

GEORGE ELI ARMSTRONG (1855–1933)

Born in Leeds, Quebec, a railway junction in the upper Ottawa River Valley near the Ontario border, Armstrong graduated M.D., C.M. from McGill in 1877, in the same class as James Bell. After postgraduate training, partly in Europe, he was appointed attending surgeon at the Montreal General in 1890 and McGill professor of surgery in 1907 when Roddick retired.

He was a skilled and innovative surgeon and a dedicated teacher. E.W. Archibald said that McGill medical graduates always remembered Armstrong's clinics, which were assiduously prepared and presented. He was one of the first to use endotracheal anesthesia, by 1920 reporting experience with fifty patients. He also introduced the use of radium in medicine in Canada, which he had learned at the Radium Institute in Paris in 1909.

When Bell died in 1911, the Royal Victoria's governors wanted to appoint a chief surgeon who would keep the private beds occupied so that the RVH could operate in the black. They offered the appointment to Armstrong, and he accepted. He was chief surgeon at the hospital from 1911 to 1923 and developed an extensive private practice in addition to his teaching duties as professor of surgery. However, he did not establish the same loyalty his associates had had for James Bell. When he decided to retire in 1923, he threw the RVH administration into a panic because he did not recommend one of his associates as his successor. In a desperate move he suggested a Scottish surgeon, Sir Henry Gray, who could operate but had no academic, teaching, or administrative ability. Gray was RVH surgeon-in-chief from 1923 until he resigned in 1925. This episode raised serious questions about Armstrong's judgment.

Armstrong served with the CAMC in 1916–17 and was discharged with the rank of colonel. He was dean of the medical faculty in 1922–23, received many honours, and held prominent positions in numerous medical associations, including president of the CMA, the American College of Surgeons and the American Surgical Association. He died on 25 May 1933 in Montreal, at age seventy-eight. E.W. Archibald said that Armstrong was remembered for many years for his well-prepared surgical clinics at the RVH.

Reference: Obituary and appreciations, *CMAJ* (1933) 29: 103–4.

ALFRED TURNER BAZIN (1872–1958)

Bazin was born in Montreal on 31 December 1872. After attending the High School of Montreal, he graduated M.D., C.M. from McGill in 1894. For the next four years he was a member of the MGH house staff, rising to the post of medical superintendent. In 1912 he was appointed attending surgeon at the Montreal General and was secretary of the hospital's medical board and then chairman from 1923 to 1930.

His first appointment to the McGill medical faculty was as demonstrator of anatomy. He continued with that appointment through the 1907–08 session and resigned when he was appointed demonstrator of clinical surgery for the 1908–09 session. He rose to become professor of surgery at McGill in 1924 and chairman of the McGill department of surgery in 1937–38, succeeding F.A.C. Scrimger. On his retirement from teaching in 1939, he was appointed emeritus professor of surgery.

Bazin went overseas in 1915 with the CAMC. One of his early assignments was as commander of No. 9 Canadian Field Ambulance. Later he was officer-in-charge of surgery at No. 3 Canadian General Hospital (McGill) in Boulogne with the rank of lieutenant colonel. He was commanding officer of that hospital for the month of July 1918. He was awarded the Distinguished Service Order and was twice mentioned in dispatches.

He took an active part in the reorganization of the CMA in the 1920s as a member of general council and the executive committee. He was managing editor of the *CMAJ*, honorary treasurer of the CMA (1923–27), and president (1929–30). He continued as chairman of the CMA executive committee and general council (1930–34), and then became honorary life president. While he was president of the CMA in 1929, the Royal College of Physicians and Surgeons of Canada (RCPSC) was incorporated. He was a member of the first RCPSC Council from 1929 to 1931. He retired from council in 1939, having served for ten eventful years, including a term as RCPSC president from 1935 to 1937.

Bazin also belonged to and held senior executive positions in other medical organizations. For years he was a devoted supporter of the Canadian Red Cross Society. A man of immense energy, he was an excellent teacher and an able organizer. In 1951 he was awarded the Starr Memorial Medal, the CMA's most prestigious honour. He received honorary degrees from Bishop's University in 1945 and McGill in 1956. He died in Montreal on 3 September 1958 at the age of eighty-five.

Reference: H.E. MacDermot, "Dr. Alfred Turner Bazin: An Appreciation." *CMAJ* 79 (1958): 600–1.

JAMES BELL (1852–1911)

Bell enrolled in the McGill Faculty of Medicine after high school, graduating in 1877 with the Holmes Gold Medal. He was appointed to the Montreal General as a house surgeon and then as medical superintendent until 1885, when he advanced to attending surgeon. In 1885, when Roddick was appointed deputy surgeon general of the Medical Services for the Canadian Militia during the Riel Rebellion in Western Canada, Bell was appointed surgeon in Field Hospital No. 1. His performance was so good that on returning to Montreal in July 1885, with Roddick's help he rapidly developed a private practice in surgery. He was a strong advocate of Lister's antisepsis in the operating room and had a very good surgical record. At the MGH he was the first surgeon to make a preoperative diagnosis of appendicitis and perform a successful appendectomy on 5 May 1889.

When the RVH opened in 1893, Roddick was appointed chief surgeon. He took Bell with him, with the intention of having him assume the chief surgeon's position after one year when Roddick intended to retire from active surgery. Bell was appointed professor of clinical surgery at McGill in 1891, and in 1907 professor of surgery and clinical surgery.

Bell instituted a training program for surgeons at the RVH, one of the first in Canada. House surgeons started the program with a year in pathology, then internship on the surgical service, and finished the program as Bell's surgical resident. He attracted outstanding house surgeons who were willing to make considerable sacrifices to be trained by him. The program produced many competent surgeons, including Archibald, Scrimger, Garrow, and Keenan.

Bell died at the peak of his career on 11 April 1911 of acute appendicitis, which his associates failed to diagnose. Scrimger later admitted that he had proposed a diagnosis of appendicitis, but because he was the junior man on the team, no one took him seriously.

E.W. Archibald described Bell as "indefatigable as a worker, conscientious, accurate and thorough in everything he undertook. He was a most helpful and valued counsellor in all matters pertaining to medical education."

References: Obituary, *CMAJ* 1 (1911): 453–4; D.A. Murphy, "James Bell's Appendicitis." *Canad J Surg* 15 (1972): 335–8.

HERBERT STANLEY BIRKETT (1864–1942)

Birkett was the first chief of the department of otolaryngology at McGill in 1906 and raised the standards for ear, nose, and throat treatment. He was a natural medical leader of immense ability, an historian, and an administrator. He celebrated his golden jubilee in otolaryngology while he was still in active and vigorous practice.

Born in 1864 in Hamilton, Ontario, he received his early education at Forest House School, Chester, England. He entered medicine at McGill at age eighteen and graduated with the Holmes Gold Medal in 1886. Howard, Ross, Roddick, Buller, Osler, and Shepherd taught him. He was a house surgeon at the Montreal General for one year. After some months in general practice in Montreal, he went to Europe to study ear, nose, throat, and eye diseases with professors in Austria, Berlin, Paris, and London. On his return to McGill in 1889, he rose rapidly in academic rank and was chief of laryngology at the MGH after three years and chief of laryngology at McGill University after five years. In 1898 he was invited to start departments of laryngology at McGill and the Royal Victoria Hospital.

When he started his practice, Birkett shared an office with Frank Buller, but they soon divided their practices, Buller specializing in ophthalmology and Birkett in laryngology. After Buller died in 1905, McGill formed a department of otolaryngology, and Birkett was appointed professor of otolaryngology at McGill and chief of otolaryngology at the RVH. In 1906 he introduced bronchoscopy to Canada. He pioneered new surgical techniques, radiography of the mastoid bone, and numerous innovations in his specialty.

Birkett's most notable contribution to McGill and to Canada was the founding of No. 3 Canadian General Hospital (McGill) in the fall of 1914 at the request of the federal government. As commanding officer he organized the hospital and directed the transfer of the McGill Unit to Dannes-Camiers in France in 1915. He was awarded Companion of the Order of the Bath and was promoted to the rank of brigadier general in 1918.

President or vice-president of every Canadian, American, and British otolaryngology society that he joined during his career, in his later years Birkett developed an interest in medical writing and published *The Early History of Medicine in the Province of Quebec*.

Reference: W.J. McNally, "Herbert Stanley Birkett." *CMAJ* 47 (1942): 280–3.

ARTHUR ANNESLEY BROWNE (1848–1910)

Born in Quebec's Eastern Townships, Browne graduated B.A. from McGill in 1866 and worked as a bank clerk for two years before entering the McGill Faculty of Medicine in 1868. He graduated M.D., C.M. in 1872 in the same class as his friend William Osler and spent the next year in London with Osler. On his return to Montreal, Browne specialized in obstetrics and gynecology. He succeeded Duncan Mac-Callum as professor of midwifery and diseases of women and children at McGill 1883 to 1886 and chief obstetrician at the Montreal Maternity Hospital.

Browne was a kind, devoted, and busy practitioner. After three years as professor, he was tired of teaching at McGill and resigned his academic position. For the remainder of his life he continued with private practice in general medicine. He maintained close relationships with his friends at McGill, and his company was sought at most university social occasions. He died in 1910 at the age of sixty-two. In 1911 his friends raised $10,000 dollars for the Arthur A. Browne Memorial Fund for Research.

Reference: Obituary, *Montreal Medical Journal*, 1910.

JAMES CHALMERS CAMERON (1852–1912)

Cameron was born in Aultsville, Ontario. He was destined to make a major contribution to obstetrics and gynecology at McGill. He was head boy at Upper Canada College in 1870 and, as was typical of the time, went directly from high school into McGill's medical faculty, graduating in 1874 with the prize for the final examination. He was a house surgeon at the Montreal General from 1874 to 1877. He went to Dublin to train in obstetrics and gynecology at the Rotunda Hospital, and then to Berlin, Paris, and Vienna for further training, returning to Montreal with up-to-date experience and academic training. At the time there was no position at McGill for him because Arthur Browne was professor of obstetrics, so Cameron went to Bishop's medical college as the chairman of obstetrics.

When Browne resigned in 1886, Cameron was offered the professorship of obstetrics and diseases of children at McGill. He accepted, bringing a modern approach to obstetrics and greatly improving the standards and procedures at the Montreal Maternity Hospital.

Cameron wrote many articles updating obstetrics and obstetrical procedures. He was a fellow of the American Gynecological Society, a member of the Royal College of Physicians of Ireland, and president of the section on pediatrics for the Pan-American Obstetrical Congress in Mexico in 1896. When he died on 16 March 1912, Walter Chipman succeeded him, and obstetrics and gynecology were recombined in one department at McGill.

A colleague wrote, "He was an ardent lover of music and an excellent German scholar. He wrote in an admirable style and his pen was always at the disposal of the profession."

Reference: Obituary, CMAJ 2 (1912): 329–31.

WALTER WILLIAM CHIPMAN (1866–1950)

Chipman was one of McGill's remarkable academic physicians as chief of obstetrics and gynecology. He was an able administrator to the end of his life, and like Alexander Blackader, was blessed with multiple talents and used them in many ways.

Born in 1866 in Wolfville, Nova Scotia, near the Bay of Fundy, after graduation from Acadia University in 1890 he went to Edinburgh University and obtained his M.B. in 1895, winning a gold medal. After additional study he was awarded M.D. in 1898. Following two more years of training in Europe in obstetrics and gynecology (part of it with Alexander Simpson, the nephew of Sir James Simpson, the first to use chloroform as an anesthetic), he returned to Montreal in 1900. When Webster resigned, Chipman was invited to be an assistant gynecologist at the Royal Victoria and demonstrator of gynecology at McGill. From the beginning of his career at McGill he showed above-average organizational and teaching ability. This resulted in his appointment as professor of gynecology in 1910 on Gardner's resignation, and as professor of obstetrics and gynecology in 1912 when J.C. Cameron died. In the same year Chipman was also appointed professor and chairman of the newly created McGill department of obstetrics and gynecology.

He made a major contribution to McGill by convincing the financially distressed Montreal Maternity Hospital to move to the grounds of the RVH. His careful negotiations resulted in the willingness of its board of governors to move the institution and to sell its building to help to pay for a new one. The new building at the RVH, known as the Women's Pavilion or the Royal Victoria Montreal Maternity Hospital (and generally referred to as the "Mat"), was opened in 1926. Three obstetricians (particularly Chipman) and the architects suggested the design, with little consultation with the dean's office or the university principal because they were interested in other projects at the time. With Chipman as chief, the Mat was a clinical teaching and research centre and a great addition to McGill.

Chipman's administrative ability led to his second career. In 1929 he retired as chairman of obstetrics and gynecology. He became a member of the RVH board of governors from 1933 to 1947, president of the RVH from 1943 to 1947, and a McGill governor from 1932 to 1947. He was president (1925) and governor (1938–41) of the American College of Surgeons. He was also one of the founders and honorary fellow of the Royal College of Obstetricians and Gynecologists.

Men like Chipman with international reputations who took responsibility for international organizations helped to keep McGill's reputation in clinical medicine at a high level.

Reference: Obituary and appreciation by N.W. Philpott, CMAJ 62 (1950): 519–20.

JAMES BERTRAM COLLIP (1892–1965)

Collip was one of the most productive scientists on the McGill staff from 1928 to 1947, pioneering in endocrine research and publishing many scientific papers. His first graduate degree was PH.D. in 1916 from the University of Toronto. He was appointed assistant professor at the University of Alberta in Edmonton and full professor in 1920. With a Rockefeller Traveling Scholarship in 1920 he worked at the University of Toronto with J.J.R. Macleod in the physiology department and A.B. Macallum in the Biochemistry Department. At that time Banting and Best began to work on the relation of the pancreas to diabetes mellitus. After preparing a crude extract from the pancreas that lowered the blood sugar, Banting asked Macleod to arrange Collip's help to purify the hormone insulin. Collip found the key to purification of insulin in 80–90 per cent alcohol and produced a relatively pure hormone in absolute alcohol. The fundamental and productive work by Collip with Banting and Best led to the famous paper "Pancreatic Extracts in the Treatment of Diabetes Mellitus" in the 22 March 1922 issue of the CMAJ by Banting, Best, Collip, et al. This brought hope to the world that there would be an effective treatment of diabetes. The work from the University of Toronto stimulated research in the field of endocrinology and resulted in a Nobel Prize awarded to Banting and Macleod, which they shared with Best and Collip.

Collip returned to the University of Alberta in 1922 as professor of biochemistry where he perfected a method to estimate blood calcium levels, isolated parathyroid hormone that regulated calcium metabolism, and revolutionized protein extraction techniques. In addition he graduated M.D. in 1926.

In 1928 at age thirty-five Collip was appointed professor and chairman of biochemistry at McGill. David L. Thomson and Hans Selye joined the department, and their collaborative research resulted in two hundred papers in the next ten years. Collip became interested in female sex hormones which eventually led to research on emmenin, a hormone with estrogenic activity that became known as Premarin from the work at the pharmaceutical firm of Ayerst, McKenna and Harrison. The group studied pituitary hormones, including gonadotrophic and adrenocorticotrophic hormones. By 1936 the laboratory team began to disband. Thomson became dean of graduate studies at McGill. Selye developed a major interest in the alarm reaction and stress, transfering from the department of biochemistry to McGill's department of anatomy, and later to the Université de Montréal.

In 1941 Collip turned the biochemistry department over to David Thomson and became director of a newly established Institute for Endocrinology in the Strathcona Medical Building and Gilman Cheny Professor of Endocrinology. He became involved in war research sponsored by a committee for medical research of the National Research Council, chaired by Frederick Banting. When Banting died in 1941, Collip became chairman of the committee. He continued with war-related research into subjects such as motion sickness, traumatic shock, blood preservation, chemical lung irritants, and the value of exercise.

After the war Collip became chairman of the Division of Medical Research for the National Research Council. He developed a master plan in 1946 to establish an endocrine laboratory at Macdonald College, but in 1947 he accepted appointment as dean of medicine at the University of Western Ontario. He retired from that position in 1961 and died in 1965.

Reference: R.L. Noble, "Memories of James Bertram Collip," CMAJ 93 (1965): 1356–64.

WILLIAM VERNON CONE (1897–1959)

Wilder Penfield said that Cone's tireless care of patients at the Montreal Neurological Institute allowed him – Penfield – to promote epilepsy surgery and to write and travel, thereby making the MNI world famous.

Cone was born in 1897 in Conesville, Iowa – a town named after his family. He attended the State University of Iowa undergraduate college and medical school, graduating in 1922. After studying neuropathology in Iowa, in 1924 he went to study with Fred Tilney, professor of neurology at Columbia University and a famous research neurologist and neuroanatomist. Cone developed a prime interest in surgery and trained under Allan Whipple, chief of surgery at the Presbyterian Hospital and Columbia University, while continuing his interest in neuropathology. When Penfield returned to New York City after working in Spain with Ramón y Cajál (1906 Nobel Prize winner for physiology and medicine), Cone became his assistant, and they established a laboratory for neuropathology. The pair quickly became responsible for the neurosurgical service under Whipple. Cone began to show his greater interest in neurosurgery and patient care than in research and scientific writing.

In 1928 Penfield and Cone accepted positions at McGill University and started a neurosurgical service at the RVH. Cone's first McGill appointment was as lecturer in neurosurgery. In 1929 he was promoted to assistant professor, and later in his career to professor of surgery.

Penfield planned a separate and independent neurosurgical institute funded by the Rockefeller Foundation and local donors. The Montreal Neurological Institute opened in 1934 with Cone as director of neurosurgery and neuropathology; later he became neurosurgeon-in-chief. For twenty-five years he established the standards for operative neurosurgery and nursing care at the institute. He was an indefatigable perfectionist, up day and night, and spent literally all his time at the institute. He would do midnight rounds on patients to be operated on the following day to check their scalps for infection. He developed many surgical instruments and devices including head tongs, rongeurs, air drills, under-the-mask air conditioning, and suturing equipment. He developed a special bed on which to rotate injured patients and also techniques in shunting, spine surgery, and biopsy as well as many nursing techniques and procedures.

During World War II Cone served overseas with the CMAC with the rank of lieutenant colonel. Together with Col. Colin K. Russel, he organized No. 1 Neurological Hospital.

As time progressed, Penfield's and Cone's paths diverged. Penfield, the neurological politician and creative author, was becoming more famous. Cone was spending more time directing surgery at the institute. Cone's lack of interest in research and scientific writing was a problem. He became progressively depressed, frequently walking with his head down and talking to himself. When it became apparent that the MNI was going to be directed by someone else after Penfield's retirement because he did not have the academic interests, Cone ended his own life in 1959. Despite his despondent end, Cone had made an enormous contribution to neurological surgery in terms of procedures and techniques, even though he rarely published.

References: Obituary, *CMAJ* 80; (1959): 1921; M. Entin, "Dr. William Vernon Cone: An Appreciation," *McGill Medical Journal* 29 (1960): 63–9.

FREDRICK GAULT FINLEY (1861–1940)

Finley was born in Melbourne, Australia, on 31 October 1861. In 1865 his family moved to Montreal. He attended the High School of Montreal and afterwards graduated M.B. at the University of London and M.D., C.M. at McGill in 1885. After graduation he was an intern at the MGH and later was assistant physician, physician, and consulting physician. In all he was connected with the MGH for fifty-seven years.

His first appointment at McGill was in the department of anatomy. He then joined the department of medicine and was lecturer in 1893, assistant professor in 1894, associate professor in 1896, professor in 1907, chair of the McGill department of medicine in 1920, and dean of medicine 1921–22.

In 1914 he joined the CAMC and was medical director of the No. 1 Canadian General Hospital in France from 1915 to 1918 and later a consultant to the Canadian Hospitals in England and France, with the rank of colonel. He was made a Commander of the British Empire for his service.

The team of Finley and Lafleur was for many years a tower of strength at the MGH and the McGill medical faculty. Due to the work of Finley, H.A. Lafleur, and A.H. Gordon, medicine at the MGH dominated the medical faculty from 1907 to 1924. Finley was an enthusiastic and dedicated teacher, known for the breadth of his knowledge and the soundness of his judgments. A quiet unassuming man, he influenced students and staff for years with his clear thinking.

Finley retired from the active staff at McGill and the MGH in 1924. For the next sixteen years he maintained his interests in medical and community affairs. He helped to found the Jewish General Hospital of Montreal and served as chairman of its medical board.

Reference: Obituary and appreciations, *CMAJ* 43 (1940): 192–3.

ALEXANDER MACKENZIE TORRANCE FORBES
(1874–1929)

Forbes, a pioneer in orthopedic and pediatric surgery, founded the Children's Memorial Hospital of Montreal and the Montreal School for Crippled Children. He was the first orthopedic surgeon at the MGH and chief surgeon and the first orthopedic surgeon at the Montreal Shriners Hospital.

Born in Montreal in 1874, he attended the High School of Montreal and then graduated B.A. at McGill in 1894 and M.D., C.M. with honours in 1898. He developed an interest in children's orthopedic problems and was an intern at the Hospital for Ruptured and Crippled in New York City. In 1902 he started his career at McGill as an assistant demonstrator of anatomy with an appointment to the MGH surgical outpatient clinic with no operating privileges. To have facilities for operating, in 1904 he organized the small Children's Memorial Hospital (CMH) for orthopedic problems – a memorial to Queen Victoria. This enterprise thrived, and in 1906 a new building was constructed for the CMH on the southwest side of Mount Royal, opening in 1909. At that time Forbes was a demonstrator of anatomy and assistant demonstrator of orthopedic surgery. He proceeded to repair a wide variety of orthopedic problems – congenital and acquired – at the CMH and later at the Shriners Hospital.

Volunteering to serve in World War I with No. 1 Canadian General Hospital, Forbes went to France in 1915. In 1916 he returned to Montreal because he was needed at the CMH. He instituted a teaching program for young patients requiring prolonged hospitalizations after orthopedic procedures. Eventually he founded the Montreal School for Crippled Children for those children who could not leave their homes to attend regular schools without being helped. Forbes's work attracted the National Shriners Organization to Montreal to build the tenth hospital in the Shriners series, on Cedar Avenue between the CMH and the School for Crippled Children.

Forbes was not an academic and published very little; his reputation was for action and organization. Despite founding the CMH and the School for Crippled Children, and being the first orthopedic surgeon at the MGH and the Montreal Shriners Hospital, he was slow to be promoted at McGill. He was finally appointed clinical professor of orthopedics at McGill in 1920. He died of a myocardiopathy in 1929.

References: H.B. Cushing, "Dr. A. MacKenzie Forbes," CMAJ 21

(1929): 109; H.E. MacDermot, "Dr. MacKenzie Forbes and His Hospital," *McGill News*, 37 (1956): 35, 62.

ALVA H. GORDON (1876–1953)

Gordon was born in 1876 on Prince Edward Island. While he was working at a local drugstore, a physician friend of the family urged him to study medicine. He enrolled at McGill in 1895 and graduated M.D., C.M. in 1899 with the Holmes Gold Medal. He was an intern at the MGH for one year, then worked as a paid assistant to a doctor in British Columbia for a year before returning to Montreal to open a medical practice. His McGill career started with an appointment as demonstrator of physiology at the university and a junior staff appointment in medicine at the MGH.

Gordon went on to become a senior physician at the MGH, chief of one of the two medical services, assistant professor of medicine from 1924 to 1936, and professor from 1936 to 1939. He was recognized as an outstanding physician and teacher. He was president of the Association of American Physicians and was granted LL.D. by McGill and McMaster and D.C.O. from Acadia University during the course of his career.

Reference: Obituary and appreciation, CMAJ 68 (1953): 300.

SIR HENRY MCILREE WILLIAMSON GRAY (1870–1938)

The controversial appointment of Gray was the centre of a power struggle between McGill, the academic institution, and the Royal Victoria's president (1912–28) Sir Vincent Meredith. The controversy, created by Meredith, boiled down to what was more important: the proper committee evaluation of a senior McGill academic appointment, or the privilege of the RVH to appoint a surgeon whose patients would fill surgical beds and keep the institution in the black.

Gray was born 14 March 1870 in Aberdeen, Scotland. After education at Aberdeen University, graduation from the medical school, and postgraduate study in Europe, he had a private practice of surgery in Aberdeen from 1896 to 1903. He was a surgeon in the Boer War but was invalided home with the rank of major. As a colonel in World War I, he served in France, and despite his abrasive personality, apparently performed well as a surgeon and was awarded CB (1916) and CMG (1918).

He was knighted in 1919 and after the war returned to Aberdeen.

In May 1923 at Meredith's insistence, the Royal Victoria's medical board and board of governors appointed Gray as RVH surgeon-in-chief. Principal Currie, who had been slighted by Meredith, refused to offer Gray a senior academic position at McGill. Gray was a poor teacher, refused to wear surgical gloves in the operating room, and was insensitive, crass, and unpopular. He had few friends, and even Meredith in the end admitted that it had been a terrible mistake to appoint him. In the two years Gray was at the RVH he generated bad publicity for McGill. The RVH governors and Principal Currie requested his resignation, which he submitted on 29 September 1925. He elected not to return home to Scotland and remained in practice in Montreal, opening a small private hospital in the Medical Arts Building on Sherbrooke Street. He died in 1938.

Reference: Obituary, *CMAJ* 39 (1938): 612.

CAMPBELL PALMER HOWARD (1877–1936)

Campbell Howard, the youngest son of Robert Palmer Howard, continued the family tradition of scholarship and excellence in medicine. Born in Montreal in 1877, he attended the High School of Montreal and graduated B.A. from McGill in 1897 and M.D., C.M. in 1901. He was a house officer at the Montreal General for four years and then at Johns Hopkins with William Osler for another four years. In 1909 he went to London, Paris, and Munich for further postgraduate study. On his return to Montreal, he received appointments as physician to the MGH outpatient department and demonstrator of clinical medicine and clinical chemistry at McGill. In 1910 he resigned those appointments to accept an appointment as professor and chairman of the department of medicine at University of Iowa. His tenure there from 1910 to 1924 was interrupted by service with the CAMC during World War I as assistant physician at No. 3 Canadian General Hospital with the rank of major. After the war he reorganized the department at Iowa, and with his leadership it was recognized as one of the leading departments of medicine in America.

Campbell Howard returned to Montreal in 1924 with appointments as professor of medicine and physician-in-chief at the MGH. F.G. Finley and H.A. Lafleur had established the two medical services at the MGH, and this arrangement continued after they retired in 1924. Although Campbell Howard was physician-in-chief, in reality he was in charge of one of the medical services and A.H. Gordon was in charge of the second. Both had private offices outside of the hospital, Howard at 1487 Mackay Street and Gordon in the Drummond Medical Building where he shared an office with A.T. Bazin. Although chief of medicine, he didn't have an office in the hospital, which put him at a major disadvantage when it came down to who was in charge.

During his postgraduate training and his years at the University of Iowa and the Montreal General, Campbell Howard was active in clinical investigation in a variety of subjects, with particular emphasis on cirrhosis of the liver and the relationship of liver function to various types of anemia. He reported his findings in numerous articles in the medical literature and at medical meetings. He was president of the Med-Chi, the Society for Clinical Investigation, and the Association of American Physicians.

In May 1936 he developed phlebitis that was responding to treatment, but he insisted on meeting a commitment for a lecture tour in California. He had started his lectures when there was an exacerbation of the phlebitis and he died suddenly of a pulmonary embolus on 3 June 1936 in his sixtieth year.

In an appreciation Dean C.F. Martin wrote that Campbell Howard was remembered by his colleagues and students not only because of his teaching ability and his skill in practice but as a leading consultant and the highest type of professional gentleman.

Reference: Appreciations, CMAJ 35 (1936): 78 and 104.

ROBERT JARED BLISS HOWARD (1859–1921)

Jared Howard, the eldest son of Robert Palmer Howard, was born in Montreal in 1859. His mother died in 1872. He enrolled at McGill College and graduated B.A. with first-class honours in natural sciences in 1879. His brilliant academic career continued in the medical faculty. He won Osler's prize for excellence in the primary examination in 1881 and graduated with the Holmes Gold Medal in 1882. After graduation he went to London to train at the London Hospital and was one of the first Canadians to pass the coveted Fellowship Examination of the Royal College of Surgeons of England.

In 1884 he studied in Berlin, Vienna, and Leipzig, often travelling with William Osler. He returned to Montreal with outstanding credentials to appointments as assistant pathologist and assistant surgeon at the Montreal General and demonstrator of anatomy and surgery at McGill.

In 1888 he married Margaret Charlotte Smith, the only child of Sir Donald Smith (later Lord Strathcona). After a few more years in Montreal, the couple moved to London, where Howard practised medicine for several years. His father-in-law was raised to the peerage as Lord Strathcona in 1897. Soon after, Howard gave up practice and moved to an English country estate. During World War I he organized the Mount Royal Hospital and worked at the third London General Hospital, receiving an OBE for his services. His wife, Margaret, by special provision, succeeded her father after his death in 1914 as Baroness Strathcona, and Howard became the Honorable R.J.B. Howard. During the war his brother Robert, Palmer Howard's second son, was killed in action in 1915. Another brother, Arthur, was severely wounded but survived. Jared Howard died in England on 9 January 1921. His wife died in 1926.

Reference: Obituary: *CMAJ* 11 (1921): 279–80.

HENRI AMÉDÉE LAFLEUR (1862–1939)

Lafleur was born in Longueil, Quebec, into a family of academic achievers. A distinguished scholar from his early days, he won the Outstanding Graduate Award for his High School of Montreal class, the Gold Medal in Science at McGill in 1882, and was an exceptional student in the medical class of 1886. His ability was recognized in an appointment as a house officer at the Montreal General.

In 1889 Osler invited him to come to Johns Hopkins Hospital in Baltimore as his first resident physician, a prestigious position. Lafleur did research with W.T. Councilman on amoebic dysentery, and they published a monograph on the subject in 1891. Returning to the General and McGill, Lafleur was appointed lecturer in 1894 in the department of medicine, assistant professor in 1895, associate professor in 1897, and professor in 1907. He and Finley were senior physicians at the General for many years, each directing a medical service. Lafleur retired in 1924 and was appointed emeritus professor.

A brilliant physician and a Victorian autocrat who totally dominated his hospital rounds, Lafleur required perfection in history-taking and physical examination. McGill and Queen's University awarded him LL.D. for being a brilliant teacher. He was vice-president of the Quebec College of Physicians and Surgeons for years. The General staff honoured him in 1925 by establishing the Lafleur Reporting Society. So respected was he by his associates and students that A.H. Gordon wrote,

"Those of my generation who knew Lafleur cannot in reason expect to see his like again."

References: Obituary, CMAJ 41 (1939): 96. C.A. Peters, "Henri Amédée Lafleur," CMAJ 62 (1950): 607–8.

CHARLES FERDINAND MARTIN (1868–1953)

Martin was born in Montreal on 14 April 1868 to an Alsatian merchant family that had emigrated from Europe in 1866. An honours graduate at the High School of Montreal, he entered McGill in 1884, graduating B.A. with honours and M.D., C.M. in 1892. He was an intern at the Montreal General for one year and then went to Europe to study pathology and general medicine. After he had been in Europe for a few months, J.G. Adami offered him a faculty position in the department of pathology, and in 1893 Martin was McGill's youngest appointee. While doing autopsies at the General, he found that he preferred clinical medicine and so sought and obtained a junior staff position in the department of medicine when the Royal Victoria opened for patients in 1894. Bright, energetic, and a born leader, over the next decade he established a reputation as a clinical diagnostician. He so impressed the medical faculty that he was appointed assistant professor of medicine in 1899 and professor in 1907. Unmarried at that time, he was devoted to his career. His travels in Europe helped to develop his political skills and brought him in contact with world medical leaders including William Osler. At the Royal Vic, Martin had his own clinical research projects and published enough that in 1907 Osler asked him to write a chapter on organic diseases of the stomach for his seven-volume series *Modern Medicine*. As a result Martin's name became widely known.

In 1912 he married Margaret Angus, daughter of Richard B. Angus, a major financier of the Canadian Pacific Railroad, president of the Bank of Montreal, and chairman of the RVH board of governors from 1893 to 1910. Angus gave the newlywed couple a dowry of $1 million. Martin's marriage brought him under the influence of his father-in-law, an astute man from whom he learned about dealing with organizations such as McGill University. Angus shared with Martin observations about the members of the Royal Vic's board of governors and the general comportment of various committees and groups of individuals. He told Martin that committees do not like to make sudden changes and prefer not to make irreversible decisions, but they could be persuaded to accept provisional action about a distant event. Furthermore, committees would often make commitments about important issues when they were told that another organization had already agreed to do the same. Angus thus provided Martin with information and insight regarding the inner workings of the RVH that he used in his reform efforts a decade later.

As chairman of the faculty Education Committee, in 1916 Martin began to assume responsibility for improving the McGill medical clinical services, teaching, and research which Harry Goldblatt had criticized in his valedictory address at the medical convocation ceremony of 1916. Martin's role in the appointments of J.C. Meakins and C.P. Howard as professors of medicine is detailed in chapter 3.

Appointed the first full-time dean of medicine in 1923, Martin played a prominent role in the major events during his deanship: the opening of the McGill-RVH University Medical Clinic, the Pathological Institute, the Biology Building, the RVH's Surgical Research Centre, and the MNI.

As well as his work at the hospital and McGill, Martin was president of several medical organizations including the Med-Chi, the CMA, and the American College of Physicians. He was a member of the CMA committee that led to the founding of the RCPSC. Retiring from McGill in 1936 having passed the mandatory retirement age of sixty-five, he became president of the Montreal Art Association and helped to improve its financial management.

References: W.B. Spaulding, "Charles F. Martin (1868–1953): A Notable Dean of McGill University," *Annals* RCPSC 24 (1991): 29–31; obituary and appreciations: *CMAJ* 70 (1954): 95–7.

JOHN MCCRAE (1878–1918)

McCrae was born in a small stone cottage in Guelph, Ontario, into a family of Scottish Presbyterians who revered the military. A biology major at the University of Toronto from 1888 to 1894, he then went to medical school in Toronto from 1894 to 1898, graduating with a gold medal and a scholarship. He started an internship in Toronto and then transferred to Johns Hopkins Hospital in Baltimore to work under William Osler; his brother, Thomas McCrae, had been there since 1895. In the fall of 1899 John McCrae went to McGill as a fellow to study pathology under J.G. Adami.

McCrae was a staunch and vocal imperialist, and after a short time in Montreal he joined the Canadian Contingent to the Boer War in

South Africa and served as lieutenant in an artillery brigade from 1899 to 1900. The misery, waste, widespread infectious diseases, and deaths unrelated to military action eventually made him hate war.

He returned to the Montreal General in 1901 where he was a governors' fellow and assistant pathologist under Adami and assumed the position of pathologist to the General in 1902. In 1905 he transferred to the McGill department of pathology and also had a staff position in the Royal Vic's department of medicine and began a medical practice. He continued teaching pathology at McGill and also at the University of Vermont from 1903 to 1911. In 1912 he co-authored with Adami *A Textbook of Pathology for Students of Medicine* and published several medical papers.

From 1908 to 1914, he lived on the top floor of Edward Archibald's house. As a bachelor and a great storyteller, he had an active social life and was on the guest list for many dinner parties. He began writing poetry as well as clinical articles, and he found that he was more interested in medical practice than in research. His imperialistic political leaning made him friends with Andrew Macphail, Stephen Leacock, and John McNaughton.

At the outset of World War I, McCrae joined the CAMC as a medical officer. From June 1915 he was chief of the medical service at No. 3 Canadian General Hospital and went to France with the unit. In the following months one of his best friends, Alex Helmer, was killed in action. McCrae became depressed and shortly after wrote his famous poem "In Flanders Fields," published in December 1915 by *Punch* magazine. He never recovered from Helmer's death. He died of pneumonia, meningitis, and septicemia on 28 January 1918 and was buried in Wimereaux, France.

Reference: D. Graves, *A Crown of Life: The World of John McCrae* (St Catharines, Ont.: Verwell Publishing, 1997); J.F. Prescott, *In Flanders Fields: The Story of John McCrae* (Erin, Ont.: Boston Mills, 1985).

ROBERT TAIT MCKENZIE (1867–1938)

McKenzie was born in 1867 in Almonte, west of Ottawa. He developed a great interest in athletics and physical training, and as a McGill undergraduate he thrived on athletic competition and was the all-around gymnastic champion. He set a Canadian inter-collegiate high jumping record, ran the hurdles, boxed, and played on the varsity football team. His interest in physical education was so great that while a medical student he went to Boston in 1891 to attend Dr Dudley Sargent's summer course in physical education at Harvard.

McKenzie graduated M.D., C.M. from McGill in 1892, interned at the Montreal General, and then spent a year as a ship's surgeon. He returned to McGill in 1894 as instructor in physical culture and assistant demonstrator of anatomy. He had an abiding interest in promoting athletics and later was appointed medical director of physical training, but found the athletic facilities at McGill seriously lacking. One of his first publications in 1894 was *Therapeutic Uses of Exercise in Education.*

McKenzie's artistic talents were stimulated in 1897 when he went to Paris and met the renowned sculptors Auguste Rodin and Paul Bartlett. He began to be interested in sculpting athletes. His first efforts in 1899 were the facial masks of athletes showing four expressions "Violent Effort," "Breathlessness," "Fatigue," and "Exhaustion." These four small masks, casts of which are in the Montreal General library, were based on photographs of athletes in competition. He worked on them for three years before having them cast in bronze.

In 1904 McKenzie accepted an appointment as director of the physical education department at the University of Pennsylvania in Philadelphia, an institution with advanced athletic facilities. He remained there for twenty-six years, developing an international reputation for his sculpting of athletic and military figures, now on public display in London, Greenwich, Ottawa, Calgary, McGill, University of Pennsylvania, Edinburgh, and Balmoral Castle in Scotland.

During World War I he developed a third career in rehabilitation medicine and wrote two books on the subject. A founding member of the American Academy of Physical Education in 1926, he was its president for eight years. He received many awards and honorary degrees and was inducted into the McGill Athletic Hall of Fame. His retirement home from 1930 to 1938 was the "Mill of Kintail," near Almonte, now a nature conservatory centre and museum that displays many of his sculptures.

Among his many achievements, McKenzie introduced the idea of exercise as important to improve health and prolong life. He was an athletic director at a major university, was one of the first to recognize the need for a specialty in rehabilitation medicine, and became an acclaimed sculptor of athletic and military figures.

Reference: J. McGill, *The Joy of Effort: A Biography of R. Tait McKenzie* (Bewdley, Ont.: Clay Publishing, 1980).

JONATHAN CAMPBELL MEAKINS
(1882–1959)

Jonathan Meakins was born in Hamilton in 1882, one of six children of Charles William Meakins and Elizabeth Campbell. After attending the Hamilton Collegiate Institute he graduated M.D., C.M. from McGill in 1904. He spent the next two years as C.F. Martin's intern at the Royal Vic, and then continued his postgraduate training in the United States – the first year as assistant resident in medicine at the Johns Hopkins Hospital and the next three years as resident pathologist at the Presbyterian Hospital in New York City.

He returned to McGill in 1910 as demonstrator of medicine and bacteriology. In 1912 he was appointed assistant physician at the RVH, lecturer in medicine and pathology, and director of experimental medicine at McGill. He was also Martin's assistant in private practice. Together they introduced electrocardiography at the Royal Vic. In 1913 he was granted a leave of absence from the hospital and McGill and went to London, England, to study cardiology with Sir James McKenzie and Sir Thomas Lewis. He also visited several European medical centres including Paris and Munich, returning to Montreal in 1914.

During World War I Meakins served with the CAMC from 1915 until 1918, initially in France as registrar and chief of medicine of No. 3 Canadian General Hospital with the rank of major. After a year in France, he was transferred to England to join the British Research Council for research on soldiers' hearts and the effects of war gases. During that period he worked with Haldane, the eminent British physiologist, as well as with Sir Henry Dale, Cushny, and Lewis. During the last stages of the war, he was officer-in-charge of medicine at Connaught Red Cross Hospital, Taplow, England.

He returned to Canada in late 1918 and was discharged from CAMC with the rank of lieutenant colonel. Martin urged him to rejoin the Royal Vic staff; however, on 14 July 1919 Meakins accepted an appointment as full-time Christison Professor of Therapeutics and Clinical Medicine at the University of Edinburgh and physician to the Royal Infirmary with a five-year contract.

In 1923 Martin obtained funding, including some from the Rockefeller Foundation, for a full-time professor of medicine at McGill. In 1924 at the completion of his five-year contract at Edinburgh, Meakins returned to Montreal with appointments as physician-in-chief at the Royal Vic, chairman of the McGill department of medicine, and director of the

McGill University Clinic. He continued with those appointments until his retirement in 1947. He also served as dean of the medical faculty from 1941 to 1947 and in 1942 was acting principal of McGill. In 1947 he was appointed emeritus professor of medicine.

At the McGill-RVH University Clinic, Meakins was a pioneer in applying scientific methods to the study of disease. His clinic developed a series of young men and women who later occupied prominent positions in research and teaching in North America and Great Britain. A prolific writer, he published articles covering a wide field in internal medicine, ranging from a study of bowel perforation in typhoid fever in 1905 through studies of immunity and vaccine treatment to articles on many aspects of cardiovascular disease, pulmonary disease, and diabetes. His best-known work was his textbook *The Practice of Medicine*, first published in 1936. Three of his colleagues, E.H. Mason, J.M. Peterson, and W. de M. Scriver, contributed chapters. The sixth edition was published in 1956, with Meakins as editor and a list of eighty-seven contributors from Canada, United States, and Britain.

Meakins was elected president of the RCPSC at the first meeting of the council in Ottawa on 20 November 1929. He remained on the RCPSC Council until 1935. He returned to military service in 1942 as deputy director of Canadian Medical Services with the rank of brigadier.

In 1934–35 Meakins was president of the American College of Physicians, and in 1935–36 president of the CMA. He also served as president of the Mental Hygiene Institute and the Canadian Cancer Society from 1949 to 1951. After his retirement from McGill he was editor of the *American Heart Journal* from 1950 to 1958.

Meakins received many honours: OBE (Commander of the Order of the British Empire) for war services; LL.D. Edinburgh; honorary M.D., University of Sidney, Australia; FRCP (Edinburgh, London and Canada); honorary FRCS (Edinburgh); FRS (Canada and Edinburgh); Master of the American College of Physicians, 1949; senior member of the CMA, 1957. He died in Montreal on 12 October 1959 at the age of seventy-seven. In 1972 the Meakins-Christie Laboratories, a research centre for pulmonary pathophysiology, was opened at the Royal Vic.

Reference: Obituary and appreciations: CMAJ 81 (1959): 857, 956.

WILLIAM ALEXANDER MOLSON
(1852–1920)

William Molson was born 27 August 1852 in Montreal to one of the most prestigious families in Canada, the son of John Molson III and

Anne Molson, who were cousins. He was educated at Bishop's College, Lennoxville, Quebec, and at the High School of Montreal. At McGill he graduated M.D., C.M. in 1874 at the age of twenty-two. Following graduation he went to London where he spent a year studying at the Royal College of Surgeons and as a house officer at St Thomas's Hospital. He passed the examination for LRCP, continued his studies in Vienna and Edinburgh, and returned to Montreal in 1876 to establish a medical practice. McGill offered him a position as an assistant demonstrator of anatomy in 1876 under Francis Shepherd who was revising and expanding the anatomy laboratory course. The Montreal General appointed him to the staff where he worked in pathology and collaborated in reporting a number of cases with William Osler. In 1879 he became co-editor of the *Canadian Medical and Surgical Journal* with George Ross until 1882 and then with T.G. Roddick.

He married Ester Edith Shepherd (1854–1912), daughter of Captain R.W. Shepherd and the sister of F.J. Shepherd. They had two children, Edith and Hobart. The family lived in a grey stone house (today marked with a commemorative plaque) on the corner of McGill College Avenue and Sherbrooke Street, across from McGill University. Molson developed a large medical practice and did much charitable work for the Montreal poor, waiving his fee for indigent families. After Stewart left the General to be chief of medicine at the Royal Victoria in 1893, Molson was senior attending physician at the hospital. In all, he was attending physician at the General for over a quarter of a century. He became noted for never letting medical students see his hospital patients and never taking them on his ward rounds. He worked with and befriended many of his more famous contemporaries in the medical faculty. He died of cardiac disease on 4 January 1920.

References: Obituary, CMAJ 10 (1920): 208; K. Molson, *The Molsons: Their Lives and Times, 1780–2000* (Willowdale, Ont.: Firefly Books, 2001), 279, 283.

HORST OERTEL (1873–1956)

Oertel was born in Germany and graduated M.D. from Yale Medical School in 1894. He studied pathology in Berlin, Würzburg, and Bavaria, and philosophy and logic in Leipzig under Wundt, who taught him the broad view of the world outside of medicine. He returned to Yale in 1897 and then went to New York City and to London. In 1914 J.G. Adami invited him to come to Montreal as associate professor of pathology at McGill and pathologist at the Royal Victoria. The

Montreal General insisted in having its own pathologist and clinical laboratory director, so Oertel was appointed consulting pathologist. In 1919 he succeeded Adami as Strathcona Professor of Pathology and director of the department when Adami indicated he would not return to McGill but instead accepted an appointment at the University of Liverpool. Oertel was a peculiar academic in that although his students respected him, he was not popular amongst staff internists and surgeons. He felt strongly that the pathologist was not the handmaiden of medicine and surgery.

In 1924 he became director of a funded Pathological Institute that had been built for teaching and research, but his main interest was in teaching, an activity in which he excelled. Well educated in pathology, philosophy and humanities, he could put all this together in his lectures.

He lived as a bachelor in the Ritz Carlton Hotel. McGill was his life and yet it appeared he did not feel obliged to help his fellow staff members if it didn't suit him, particularly when it involved cooperation with the research interests of the clinicians. He befriended Vincent Meredith, president of the Royal Vic, and in the early 1920s defended Meredith's arbitrary appointments that were in the interests of the hospital and not McGill. He was compliant in the Sir Henry Gray affair and later refused to help Penfield in 1928 when he was looking for laboratory space for his neuropathology interests. Neither of these events endeared Oertel to his associates. He retired in 1938 at the age of sixty-five.

References: Obituary: CMAJ 74 (1956): 485; W.G. Barnard, "Horst Oertel: 1873–1956," Journal of Pathology and Bacteriology 72 (1956): 331–3.

WILDER GRAVES PENFIELD (1891–1976)

Born in Spokane, Washington, in 1891, Penfield graduated B.A. in 1913 from Princeton University. In 1914 he went to Oxford as a Rhodes Scholar where he was influenced by Sir Charles Sherrington and Sir William Osler. He lived at the Osler home in Oxford while recovering from a broken leg sustained on board a ship torpedoed in the English Channel. He returned to America to get his medical degree at Johns Hopkins Medical School in 1918. After graduation he continued his studies with Sherrington at Oxford and Sir Gordon Holmes, a famous clinical neurologist, at Queen Square, London. He was appointed to a position at the New York Neurological Institute in 1921 where he became assistant director and remained until 1928. During this time he studied histology in Spain with Ramón y Cajal, an anatomist who won a Nobel Prize for physiology and medicine in 1906, and neurosurgical techniques in Germany with Otfrid Foerster, the self-taught neurologist-neurosurgeon.

In 1928 Penfield came to McGill with William Cone to establish the neurosurgical unit at the Royal Victoria. Within a few years he wanted to establish an institute for neurosurgical training and the treatment of epilepsy. With the help of J.C. Meakins, E.W. Archibald, C.F. Martin, Principal Sir Arthur Currie, and the Rockefeller Foundation (which gave a $1,250,000 grant), he established the Montreal Neurological Institute (MNI) in 1934.

At the MNI Penfield developed a worldwide reputation for focal epilepsy surgery. His greatest contribution to neurosurgery was his capacity to keep a team working on the same subject – epilepsy – and generally speaking, to keep everyone happy. He won numerous awards, published books and papers, and received the Order of Merit from the queen (which essentially is knighthood outside of Great Britain), the Order of Canada, the Legion of Honour, and the U.S. Medal of Freedom. He was a candidate for appointment as governor general of Canada.

After retirement in 1960, Penfield travelled to China and later headed the Vanier Institute of the Family. He wrote his autobiography, completing it shortly before he died in 1976.

References: W.G. Penfield, *No Man Alone: A Neurosurgeon's Life* (Boston: Little Brown, 1977); J. Lewis, *Something Hidden: A Biography of Wilder Penfield* (Toronto: Doubleday, 1981).

SIR WILLIAM PETERSON (1856–1921)

A brilliant classicist, Peterson came to McGill from Scotland and never forsook his roots in the U.K., yet truly became a McGill man. In secondary school he graduated as a distinguished pupil and was first in his class on graduation from Edinburgh University in 1875. He won prestigious scholarships including the Ferguson Scholarship for the best candidate in Scotland and graduated with high honours in classics from Oxford University. So gifted was he that in 1882 he was appointed principal of Dundee University and chairman of classics. His reputation spread so that in 1895 when Sir William Dawson retired, Sir Donald Smith, then Chancellor of McGill and Canadian high commissioner in the United Kingdom, offered him the principalship of McGill. This started a twenty-four-year period of extraordinary growth in faculties, excellence, and endowment. He received honorary LL.D. degrees from St Andrew's, Princeton, Harvard, Yale, Queen's, and the University of Toronto, was awarded CMG in 1901, and was knighted in 1915.

During his principalship, McGill built a students' union, a music school, a dental school, a graduate school, the Strathcona Medical Building, and Macdonald College and acquired the property for Molson Stadium. Peterson helped to establish the first university military hospital unit in the British Empire in 1914 – the No. 3 Canadian General Hospital (McGill) – and the Officers' Training Corps (COTC), the first in Canada. The university endowment increased from $1,595,938 in 1895 to $12,033,020 by 1919, and disbursements in that period increased from $184,154 to $994,724.

Retiring as principal in 1919 after suffering a stroke, Peterson died in England in 1921. He left McGill a far better place than when he came but still in need of additional funds for development – a problem he left for his successor, Sir Arthur Currie, to solve. McGill owes a great deal to Peterson's leadership.

Reference: S.B. Frost, *McGill University,* vol. 2, *1895–1971* (Kingston and Montreal: McGill-Queen's University Press, 5–7, 109.

ROBERT FULFORD RUTTAN (1856–1930)

For more than forty years Ruttan taught chemistry at McGill and was one of Canada's most prominent chemists. Born in Newburg, Ontario, in 1856, after preliminary education he enrolled at the University of Toronto and graduated B.A. with a gold medal from the department of natural sciences. As an undergraduate he developed an interest in chemistry, and continued this interest after entering the McGill Faculty of Medicine in 1880, graduating M.D., C.M. in 1884 with the Sutherland Medal. Although he passed the examinations for membership in the Ontario College of Physicians and Surgeons, he decided not to enter the practice of medicine but to continue his interests in chemistry. For the next two years he studied in Berlin with A.W. von Hoffman, returning to Montreal in 1886 with an appointment as lecturer in the medical faculty, to assist G.P. Girdwood, professor of chemistry.

Ruttan rose to be assistant professor of chemistry in 1888, professor of practical chemistry and associate professor of medicine in 1891, and, after Girdwood retired, professor of organic and biological chemistry and chairman of the chemistry department in 1902. In addition he was registrar of the medical faculty from 1891 to 1901.

Prior to 1912, Ruttan's appointments were in the medical faculty. In that year there was a major reorganization at McGill, and Ruttan became director of the new university department of chemistry, while retaining his appointment in the medical faculty. In 1924 he became dean of the Faculty of Graduate Studies and Research. He retired from McGill in 1928 and died two years later.

As well as his work at McGill, Ruttan was an active member of several professional organizations including the National Research Council and the Society of Chemical Industries of England. A member of the Royal Society of Canada from 1896, he served as its president in 1919–20.

Reference: Obituary and appreciation, *CMAJ*, 22 (1930): 596–7; *Transactions of the Royal Society of Canada* 24 (1930): vii–xi.

FRANCIS ALEXANDER CARRON SCRIMGER (1880–1937)

Scrimger was born in Montreal in 1880, the son of the principal of the Presbyterian College at McGill. He graduated B.A. from McGill with honours in biology in 1901 and M.D., C.M. in 1905. He interned under James Bell at the Royal Victoria Hospital from 1905 to 1909. The program for surgery at the Royal Vic was for four years – a year of surgical pathology, two years as an intern on the surgical service, and the final year as resident surgeon on Professor Bell's service. The training was rigid and required great energy, effort, and discipline. In 1909, Scrimger went to Europe for further study in pathology. On returning to Montreal in 1910, he was appointed clinical assistant in surgery at the Royal Vic and demonstrator of surgery at McGill.

On the outbreak of World War I, he was appointed medical officer of the 14th Battalion of the Royal Montreal Regiment, training at Camp Valcartier in Quebec and on the Salisbury Plain in England. By April 1915 he was in Belgium and was involved in the 2nd Battle of Ypres. The events leading to his being awarded the Victoria Cross are described in chapter 3. Later in the war he directed surgery at the No. 1 Canadian General Hospital in France, the No. 3 Canadian General Hospital (McGill), and the Granville Hospital in England. He was advanced in rank to lieutenant colonel.

Scrimger married Ellen Carpenter, a nurse who had worked with him during the war. In 1919 he returned to Montreal and to the Royal Vic where he became surgeon-in-chief in January 1936 and professor and chairman of the McGill surgery department in 1936–37. A heavy smoker and a very intense person, he died suddenly of a heart attack at home on 13 February 1937 at the age of fifty-seven.

References: W.B. Howell, "Colonel F.A.C. Scrimger, VC," CMAJ 38 (1938): 279–81; S. Kingsmill, *Francis Scrimger: Beyond the Call of Duty* (Toronto: Hannah Institute, 1991); E.W. Archibald, "F.A.C. Scrimger," *Annals Surg* 107 (1938): 159.

JAMES O. STEWART (1846–1906)

One of the enigmas of the McGill Faculty of Medicine was the inscrutable James Stewart. Of the many physicians at McGill, some were giants in Canadian medicine and built the reputation of the faculty; others came and went in a year or two leaving little trace. Doers and thinkers like Stewart left the legacy that we enjoy today. A man of few words, he was known to have never spoken a word in excess and at times none at all. He did not fit into any mould.

Born on 19 November 1864 in Osgood, Ontario (a small town east of Ottawa), his secondary education was in Ottawa. In 1863 at the age of twenty-one he entered McGill and graduated M.D., C.M. in 1869. For the next fourteen years he established medical practices in four different towns. In 1883 he went to Edinburgh for postgraduate study and passed the examination of the Royal College of Physicians. On his return to Montreal he was appointed to the chair of materia medica and therapeutics to replace Reverend William Wright, who was forced to resign because of student protest. Despite his quiet nature, Stewart was appointed registrar of the medical faculty from 1884 to 1891, secretary to the CMA from 1884 to 1897, attending physician to the Montreal General in 1887, chairman of clinical medicine in 1891, physician to the Royal Victoria and professor of medicine in 1893; the latter two made him the most important consultant in medicine in Montreal. He had a major interest in neurology as a sub-specialty in medicine and became the first neurological consultant at McGill.

Despite his reticence, Stewart was an outstanding and brilliant diagnostician. He exemplified the conservative, reserved Victorian image that people wanted in a chief. He became the last word in medical consultation because of what he represented and not necessarily for what he did. Though he wrote little, he reached the highest academic position at McGill as professor of medicine because of his remarkable clinical expertise. He died in 1906 from complications of hypertension.

Reference: H.W. Kelly and W.L. Burrage, *Dictionary of American Biography* (New York: Appleton, 1928), 1166–7.

GEORGE WILKINS (1842–1916)

Wilkins had the distinction of being a ship's surgeon, a professor in the medical faculties at Bishop's University and McGill, and the first medical director of the Sun Life Assurance Company of Canada. Born in Ireland in 1842, he moved to Toronto with his parents early in his life. He attended the Toronto Grammar School before his medical education at the Toronto Medical School where he obtained M.D. at age twenty-four in 1866. After graduation he was a ship's surgeon for the Allan Steam Ship Line (owned by Sir Hugh Allan, whose home, Ravenscrag, is now the Allan Memorial Institute of McGill). In 1870 he passed the membership examination for the Royal College of Surgeons of England. In 1871 he came to Montreal and accepted the position of professor of pathology at Bishop's medical faculty. After a few years he was appointed professor of practical physiology. He resigned from Bishop's in 1882 when McGill offered him a position in medical jurisprudence and histology. He continued to teach histology for years after Osler's resignation in 1884, and for several decades he was an attending physician at the Montreal General Hospital.

Wilkins was the first physician in Montreal to become interested in the insurance industry. In 1880 he became the first medical examiner for the Sun Life Assurance Company and later its medical director. He was active in the Med-Chi and its president in 1897. In 1911 he became the president of the Association of Medical Directors of Life Insurance in Canada. He died on 7 August 1916.

Reference: Obituary and appreciation, CMAJ 6 (1916): 823–4.

Appendix Two

Officers of the McGill Faculty of
Medicine, McGill University, Montreal
General Hospital, and Royal Victoria
Hospital, 1829–1936

McGill Faculty of Medicine, 1829–1936

Dean	Dates
Andrew F. Holmes	1854–60
George W. Campbell	1860–82
R. Palmer Howard	1882–89
Robert Craik	1889–1901
George Ross, vice-dean	1889–92
Thomas G. Roddick	1901–08
Francis J. Shepherd	1908–14
Herbert S. Birkett	1914–21 (leave of absence 1915–18)
Alexander D. Blackader, acting dean	1915–18
Frederick G. Finley	1921–22
George E. Armstrong	1922–23
Charles F. Martin	1923–36
Grant Fleming	1936–40

Assistant Dean	Dates
J.W. Scane	1920–22

Associate Dean	Dates
J.C. Simpson	1936–40

Registrars	Dates
John Stephenson	1829
Archibald Hall	1842
William Wright	1864
Robert Craik	1869
William Osler	1877–83
Francis J. Shepherd, Acting Registrar	1883
James Stewart	1884–91
Robert F. Ruttan	1891–1902
E.M. Eberts	1902–03
J.W. Scane	1903–19
(Post abolished 1919)	

Secretary	Dates
J.C. Simpson	1923–36

Professors: Pre-Clinical Subjects (Chapter 5)

Anatomy	Dates
John Stephenson	1829
Oliver T. Bruneau	1842
William E. Scott	1856
Francis J. Shepherd	1883–1913
Endowed 1912; Robert Reford professors	
Auckland C. Geddes	1913–19
Samuel E. Whitnall	1919–34
Cecil P. Martin	1936–54

Histology	Dates
G. Wilkins	1886–1907
J.C. Simpson	1910–38

Physiology	Dates
J. Stephenson	1829

Physiology	*Dates*
S.C. Sewell	1842
R.L. MacDonnell	1845
W. Fraser	1849
J.M. Drake	1868
W. Osler	1874
Endowed 1897; Morley Drake Professors	
T.W. Mills	1888–1910
N.H. Alcock	1911–13
G.R. Mines	1914–15
John Tait	1919–40
Boris P. Babkin, Research Professor	1928–47

Pharmacology and Therapeutics	*Dates*
A.F. Holmes	1829
A. Hall	1835
S.C. Sewell	1842
A. Hall	1849
W. Wright	1854
J. Stewart	1883
A.D. Blackader	1891–1920

Pharmacology	*Dates*
H.G. Barbour	1921–23
R.L. Stehle	1924–40

Chemistry	*Dates*
Andrew F. Holmes	1829
Archibald Hall	1842
William Sutherland	1849
Robert Craik	1867
Gilbert. P. Girdwood	1879–1902
Robert F. Ruttan	1902–28
	(1924, Macdonald Professor and director of the department)

Practical Chemistry (founded 1872)	Dates
Gilbert P. Girdwood	1872–94
Robert F. Ruttan	1894–1902
(Post abolished 1902)	

Biochemistry and Pathological Chemistry	Dates
A.B. Macallum	1920–28
J.B. Collip	1928–36
D.L. Thomson	1937

Botany	Dates
A.F. Holmes	1829
Dr Papineau	1845
James Barnston	1857
J. W. Dawson	1855–56, 1858–83
P. Penhallow	1883–1911
(Post abolished in medical faculty, 1912)	
F. E. Lloyd (Faculty of Arts)	1912–34 (Macdonald Professor of Botany)

Zoology (Founded 1902 in Faculty of Medicine)	Dates
William Dawson	1886–93
W.E. Deeks	1893–1902
W. McBride	1902–09
A. Willey	1910 (Strathcona Professor of Zoology 1919)
(Post abolished in the Faculty of Medicine, 1912; continued in the Faculty of Arts)	

Pathology Endowed 1893; Strathcona Professors	Dates
J. George Adami	1892–1919
Horst Oertel	1919–1938

Bacteriology and Immunity	Dates
F.C. Harrison	1928–30
E.D.G. Murray	1930–55

Professors of Medicine and Medical Specialties (Chapter 6)

Medicine	Dates
William Caldwell	1829–33
William Robertson	1833–42
Andrew F. Holmes	1842–60
R. Palmer Howard	1860–89
George Ross	1889–92
James Stewart	1893–1906
Fred G. Finley	1907–24
	(McGill chairman, 1920)
Henri A. Lafleur	1907–24
Charles F. Martin	1907–36
W.F. Hamilton	1924–33
Jonathan C. Meakins	1924–47
	(McGill chairman, 1924–47)
Campbell P. Howard	1924–36
Alva H. Gordon	1937–39

Clinical Medicine	Dates
James Crawford	1845 and 1852
Robert L. MacDonnell	1849
Stephen C. Sewell	1850
R. Palmer Howard	1856–60
Duncan C. MacCallum	1860
Joseph M. Drake	1872
George Ross	1872–89
Richard L. MacDonnell	1889–91
James Stewart	1891–93
(Post abolished 1893)	

Pedriactics	Dates
A.D. Blackader	1919–21
H.B. Cushing	1937–38 McGill chairman of pediatrics (clinical professor, 1924–37)

Neurology and Clinical Neurology	Dates
Colin Russel	Clinical professor, 1922
Wilder G. Penfield	Clinical professor, 1928–32 Professor neurology and neurosurgery, 1932–60
F.H. Mackay	Clinical professor, 1928

Dermatology	Dates
G.G. Campbell	Clinical professor, 1923–28
J.F. Burgess	Clinical professor, 1928–50

Psychiatry	Dates
T.J.W. Burgess	Professor of mental diseases, 1899–1920 Professor of psychiatry, 1920–23
C.A. Porteus	Clinical professor, 1923

Professors Surgery and Surgical Specialties (Chapter 7)

Surgery	Dates
John Stephenson MGH	1829
G.W. Campbell MGH	1835
George E. Fenwick MGH	1875–90
Thomas G. Roddick MGH & RVH	1890–1907
James Bell MGH & RVH	1907–11
George E. Armstrong MGH & RVH	1907–23
J.A. Hutchison MGH	1913–23
E.W. Archibald RVH	1923–35; McGill chairman, 1923–35

Surgery	Dates
F.A.C. Scrimger RVH	1936–37; McGill chairman, 1936–37
A.T. Bazin MGH	1923–39; McGill chairman, 1937–38
E.M. Eberts MGH	1929

Clinical Surgery	Dates
James Crawford	1845
William E. Scott	1852
Duncan C. MacCallum	1856
Robert Craik	1860
George E. Fenwick	1867
Thomas G. Roddick	1876–90
James Bell	1894–1907
(Post abolished 1907)	

Obstetrics and Gynecology	Dates
William W. Robertson	1829
John Racey	1833
George W. Campbell	1835
Michael McCulloch	1842–54
Archibald Hall	1854–68
Duncan C. MacCallum	1868–83
Arthur A. Browne	1883–86
James C. Cameron	1886–1912
Walter W. Chipman	1912–29
J.R. Fraser, professor and director	1929–
H.M. Little	1929

Gynecology	Dates
William Gardner	1883–1910
Walter W. Chipman	1910–12
(Post abolished 1912)	

Ophthalmology and Otology	Dates
F. Buller	1883–1905
(Post abolished 1906)	

Ophthalmology	Dates
J.W. Stirling	1906–23
W.G. Byers	1923–34
G.H. Mathewson	Clinical professor, 1923–31
F.T. Tooke	1934–
S.H. McKee	Clinical professor, 1931–41

Laryngology	Dates
G.W. Major	1893–95
S. Birkett	1895–1906
(Post abolished 1906)	

Oto-Laryngology	Dates
Herbert S. Birkett	1906–32
E. Hamilton White	1932–33

Urology	Dates
F.S. Patch	Clinical professor, 1923
D.W. MacKenzie	Clinical professor, 1923

Orthopedic Surgery	Dates
A.M.T. Forbes MGH	Clinical professor, 1920–29
W.G. Turner RVH	Clinical professor, 1925–
J.A. Nutter MGH	Clinical professor, 1929–35

Neurological Surgery	Dates
W.G. Penfield	Clinical professor, 1928–31, professor of neurology and neurosurgery, 1932–60
W.V. Cone	Lecturer, 1928, professor, 1932–59

Professors of Other Subjects (Chapter 8)

Hygiene and Public Health	Dates
George Ross	1871–73
Thomas G. Roddick	1873–75
Robert T. Godfrey	1875–79
William Gardner	1879–83
R.L. MacDonnell	1886–89

Endowed 1893; Strathcona professors

R. Craik	1889–1901
Wyatt Johnston	1902
T.A. Starkey	1902–35
A.G. Fleming	Professor and acting director of the Department of Public Health and Preventive Medicine, 1926

Medical Jurispridence	Dates
William Fraser	1845–49
Francis Badgley	1849
Francis C.T. Arnoldi	1850
William E. Scott	1851
William Wright	1852–54
R. Palmer Howard	1854–60
Duncan C. MacCallum	1860–67
George E. Fenwick	1867–75
William Gardner	1875–83
George Wilkins	1884–1907
D.D. MacTaggart	1911–29

(Course absorbed into Public Health, 1929)

History of Medicine	Dates
A. Macphail	1907–1937

McGill University, 1885–1936

Chancellors	Dates
James Ferrier	1884–88
Sir Donald Smith (Lord Strathcona)	1889–1913
Sir William Macdonald	1914–17
Robert Laird Borden	1918–20
Edward Wentworth Beatty	1920–43

Principals and Vice-Chancellors	Dates
Sir John William Dawson	1855–93
Sir William Peterson	1895–1918
Sir Aukland Campbell Geddes	1919–20
General Sir Arthur William Currie	1920–33
Arthur Eustace Morgan	1935–37

Registrars, Secretaries, Bursars	Dates
William Craig Baynes	?–1887
Walter Vaughan	1897–1918
John Scone	1920–
Thomas H. Matthews	1925–

Montreal General Hospital, 1885–1936

Chairman of Board of Management (Presidents)	Dates
Andrew Robertson	1881–87
John Sterling	1888–92
Thomas Davidson	1893
H. Wolferstan Thomas	1894–99
James Crathern	1900–09
H. Stikeman	1910–12
David Morrice	1912–13

Chairman of Board of Management (Presidents)	Dates
Sir H. Montagu Allan	1913–16
Farquhar Robertson	1917–21
Herbert Molson	1922–38

Chairman of the Medical Board	Dates
R.P. Howard	1883–89
D.C. MacCallum	1889–1904
F.J. Shepherd	1904–14
F.G. Finley	1914–16
H.A. Lafleur	1916–19
J.M. Elder	1919
G.G. Campbell	1919–23
A.T. Bazin	1923–30
C.A. Peters	1930–32
F.S. Patch	1932–38

Royal Victoria Hospital, 1885–1936

Chairman of Board of Governors (Presidents)	Dates
Sir J.C. Abbott	1887–93
R.B. Angus	1893–1910
Sir Edward Clouston	1910–12
James Ross	1912 (Jan.–Sept.)
Sir H. Vincent Meredith	1912–29
Sir Herbert Holt	1929–41

Chairman of the Medical Board	Dates
Robert Craik	1894–1900
Sir Thomas. G. Roddick	1901–17
George E. Armstrong	1918–23
W.F. Hamilton	1923–36

Appendix Three

Medical Faculty
Examination Papers, Session 1900–1901

EXAMINATION PAPERS, SESSION 1900-1901

MEDICAL FACULTY.

ELEMENTARY BIOLOGY.

Part I. Zoology.

First Year.

TUESDAY, DEC. 18TH:—2 TO 5 P.M.

Examiner..........................PROF. E. W. MACBRIDE.

N.B.—Students belonging to the Medical Faculty must attempt only *six* questions to be selected from questions 1 to 7 and their answer-books must be returned at 4 p.m.

Students belonging to the Faculty of Arts may attempt *nine* questions of which *six* are to be selected from questions 1 to 7 and *three* from questions 8 to 11.

1. Describe carefully the means by which Amœba, Paramœcium and Hydra obtain their food.

Point out so far as you can why a different method is pursued in each case.

2. Describe carefully the reproductive organs of the Worm. Point out any *general resemblances* between the reproductive system of this animal and that of the Dog-fish.

[N.B.—A detailed description of the reproductive system of the Dog-fish is *not* to be given.]

3. Describe the heart, main arteries and principal veins of the Dog-fish. Point out what parts if any, of the blood system of the Worm have representatives in the vessels of the Dog-fish which you have described.

4. What exactly is meant by a ferment ?

Enumerate the principal ferments found in the Dog-fish pointing out where they are formed and what results follow from their action. Can you suggest any reason why this result occurs ?

29

5. Define carefully the terms *neuron* and *sense cell* describing carefully an example of each and indicating their functions.

Describe the various kinds of sense cells found in the animals you have studied.

6. Define exactly what function is carried out by an excretory cell. Describe the exact situation of the excretory cells in the worm and the *adult* Dog-fish pointing in each case how they are related to the coelom.

7. Carefully describe the spinal and sympathetic ganglia of the Dog-fish; pointing out how they are formed; in what relation they stand to the spinal cord and what are their functions.

Can you explain the phenomenon known as " referred pain " ?

8. Describe carefully and completely the means by which the oxygen of the air is brought in contact with the blood of the Frog—the whole process of aerial respiration.

Compare the means by which the Frog breathes when submerged in water with that adopted by the Dog-fish.

9. Compare together carefully the male reproductive organs of the Frog and Dog-fish.

10. Describe carefully the origin and development of all the structures in the Dog-fish which correspond to the back-bone in the Frog.

What is the great difference between the back-bone in the Frog and the correseponding parts in the Dog-fish ?

11. Describe and compare the skeleton of the limbs in the Dog-fish and the Frog.

Elementary Biology.

Part II. Botany.

DEC. 21ST, 1900:—ONE HOUR.

The candidate will answer three questions only.

1. Give an account of the cell structure in plants as exhibited in Saccharomyces and describe fully the nature of the reproductive processes in that plant.

2. Compare the processes of nutrition in Myxomycetes and in Pleurococcus: show what conditions are essential in each case and what distinctive terms are employed to indicate these differences.

3. Compare the reproductive processes in Spirogyra, Oedogonium and Fucus, with special reference to differentiation of the gametes, the special conditions under which conjugation takes place, and the value of such data as evidence of succession in development.

4. Give an account of the process of destructive metabolism in plants. Through what special function is this chiefly expressed ? What are the characteristic products ? Under what conditions does it occur ? Compare with the corresponding function in animals.

30

Physics and Chemistry.

First Year.

APRIL 30TH, 1901.

Examiner...................*Prof.* G. P. Girdwood, M.D.

1. Describe the different methods of taking specific gravity (*a*) of solids heavier than water, (*b*) of liquids, (*c*) of solids lighter than water.

2. What is sound ? How is it propagated and carried to the ear? At what rate is it carried in air and in water ?

3. What do you understand by radiant energy ? What are the laws which govern the transmission of heat and light ?

4. What do you understand by atmospheric pressure ? How is it measured, what effect is produced by reduction of atmospheric pressure (*a*) on boiling point of liquids, (*b*) on solubility of gasses, (*c*) on respiration ?

5. What are the different kinds of electricity, from what sources are they obtained ? How is electrical equilibrium restored ? What are the units of measurement ?

6. Describe the occurrence in nature of Hydrogen. What are its properties ? How can it be prepared ? Give its atomic and molecular weight and volume.

7. What the the laws of chemical combination the atomic theory," what do you understand by atomic weight, molecular weight, and equivalent weight ?

8. Describe experiments proving the composition of Hydrochloric acid by weight and by volume. Give its molecular weight and its specific gravity (air=1).

Physiology.

First Year.

MAY 2ND, 1901.

Examiners...................... { Prof. Wesley Mills, M.D.
Dr. W. S. Morrow.
Dr. J. W. Scane.
Dr. A. A. Robertson.

1. Explain the meaning of the following :—Blastoderm, germ layers, cleavage of the mesoblast, spanchnopleure, chorion, amnion (true and false), optic vesicle, gut, medullory folds.

31

2. *Muscle and Nerve*: Explain the meaning of the following terms: Latent period, fatigue of muscle, kathode, opening tetanus, ascending current, conduction, galvanotanus and demarcation current.

3. Write fully on blood-cells.

4. *Circulation of the Blood* : (*a*) Factors. (*b*) Blood pressure in arteries, veins and capillaries compared. (*c*) Ways in which general and local blood pressure may be made to vary, with an account of the mechanism involved. (*d*) Circumstances that favor the return of the blood from the capillaries.

5. Describe the experiments by which it has been demonstrated that there are two kinds of vaso-motor fibres in the Sciatic Nerve.

6. *Respiration*: Discuss in outline the process in its various relations so as to indicate all the various factors and their significance.

7. *Digestion and Absorption*: Trace in outline the physiological history of a meal of bread and meat (fat and lean) from the time it enters the mouth till it is represented in the blood.

8. Write, as time permits, on one only of the following themes: (*a*) The importance of general biology and embryology for physiology. (*b*) The relations of facts, technique and general principles in a course of Physiology. (*c*) The general bearing of one process on another in the animal economy. (*d*) Co-ordination in the widest sense in physiology. (*e*) Or any other broad theme you choose to select.

Note.—Throughout this paper, wherever possible, use diagrams, etc., to illustrate your meaning.

Bacteriology.

First Year.

FRIDAY, MAY 3RD, 1901.

Examiners............................ { PROF. J. G. ADAMI, M.D.
H. B. YATES, M.D.

1. What are the precautions to be taken to prevent contamination of (*a*) the culture vessels and (*b*) the culture media in the process of gaining pure cultures of bacteria.

2. What are the main features distinguishing (1) the Hyphomycetes, (2) the Blastomycetes, (3) the Schizomycetes ?

3. What do you understand by the terms:—facultative anaerobe: Pasteurisation, discontinuous sterilisation; Endspore; Extracellular fermentation; metachromatic granule; aerial hypha.

32

Pharmacology and Therapeutic

Second Year.

MAY 3RD, 1901.

Examiners............................. PROF. A. D. BLACKADER.
DR. HALSEY.
DR. R. A. KERRY.

1. Explain the difference between a Liquor, a water, an Infusion, a liquid extract, and a tincture.

2. What do you understand by the terms:—Suppositoria, Chartae Emplastra, Unguenta ?

3. Name the specimens which will be shewn to you and state the more important official preparations of them.

4. Compare the action on the circulation of Aconite and Digitalis.

5. How may the various Mercurial preparations be grouped ? Give an example of each class and state how they differ from each other in action.

6. Name the official preparations of Arsenic. How would you know that a patient was getting too much Arsenic ?

7. State what you know about the origin, physical properties and physiological action of the following drugs:—Strychnine and Atropine. Name official preparations of each with their doses.

8. Name two drugs which lower blood pressure in different ways, state briefly the difference in their mode of action and give the dose of one preparation of each drug.

Examination in Chemistry

Second Year.

MAY 1ST, 1901.

Examiners............................. { PROF. R. F. RUTTAN, M.D.
PROF. G. P. GIRDWOOD, M.D.

1. Describe the solar spectrum. How may it be produced ? Describe Frauenhoffer's lines. Where are the principal ones situated ? For what purposes in chemistry is the spectroscope used ?

2. Write an account of the chemistry of Phosphorus, giving its occurrence, manufacture, properties and chief compounds. Describe fully the chemistry of the compounds of Phosphorus with Hydrogen.

33

3. How much manganese dioxide will be required with sulphuric acide to oxidize 9.2 grammes of anhydrous oxalic acid ? What will be the nature and volume of the resulting gas, normal temperature and pressure ? mm=55.

4. Write a short account of the chemistry of (a) the alkali metals and (b) the Halogen elements.

5. Shew by equations how Ethyl Amine may be prepared from marsh gas and acetic acid from Ethyl Amine.

6. Describe the preparation and give characteristic reactions for (a) Urea and (b) Chloral.

7. Describe a practical method of making (a) Acetylene, (b. Salicylic acid, (c) Glycocoll (glycine), (d) oxalic acid.

8. Shew by a table the classification of simple sugars (mono saccharides). Give a concise account of the properties of (a) Glucose and (b) Cellulose.

9. Give the chemical relations and formulae of Tartaric Acid, Picric Acid, Gallic Acid, Stearine and Pyridine.

10. Define and give an example of (a) an etherial salt, (b) a glucoside, (c) an alkaloid, (d) a secondary alcohol. Give one reaction characteristic of each.

Physiology.

Second Year.

APRIL 30TH, 1901.

Examiners.......................
{
PROF. WESLEY MILLS, M.D.
DR. W. S. MORROW.
DR. J. W. SCANE.
DR. A. A. ROBERTSON.
}

1. Explain briefly the meaning of the following:—Allantois, placental villi, decidua reflexa, corpus luteum, electrotonus, electrotonic currents, polarizing current, law of contraction, reaction or degeneration, idio-muscular contraction, rheochord.

2. *Blood and Circulation* : (a) Reasons for considering them together. (b) Discuss the cardiac cycle and (c) the innervation of the heart.

3. *Respiration*: Discuss briefly, diffusion, vital action of epithelium, respiratory coefficient, intra thoracic pressure, effects of respiration on circulation and blood pressure in asphyxia.

4. *Digestion and Absorption*: Trace in outline the principal changes in a meal of bread and beeksteak (fat and lean) from the time it enters the intestine till it is returned to the outer world.

5. State and criticise the various theories of renal activity (urinary secretion).

2

34

6. Make the complete anatomico-physiological connections in the following cases:—(*a*) Tacile perception referred to the right index finger. (*b*) Voluntary motor impulses leading to conjugate deviation of the eyes to the right. (*c*) Crossed reflex of the left arm.

7. State with reasons, where the site of the operative lesion has probably been in the following cases:—(*a*) Left Hemianopsia in a monkey (left referring to the eye affected). (*b*) Staggering (reeling) gait in a dog. (*c*) Temporary loss of control of the rectal and vesical sphincters in a dog. (*d*) Ataxy of the legs in a monkey.

8. State and discuss (*a*) Theories of ocular accommodation. (*b*) Theories of color vision.

Note.—Wherever possible throughout this paper to use diagrams, etc., do so.

Histology.

Second Year.

DEC. 20TH, 1900.

Examiners............................ { PROF. G. WILKINS, M.D.
DR. N. D. GUNN, M.D.

1. Describe a serous gland. Mention where some typical examples are found.

2. Describe a section of Pancreas.

3. Describe a section through Cervix Uteri of adult at junction of Vagina.

4. Describe a section through eye-ball made from before directly backwards.

5. Name the various nerve endings and give drawing and description of each.

6. Draw a cross section of upper end of Medulla Oblongata and give short description. Compare spinal and sympathetic ganglion.

Anatomy.

Second Year.

MARCH 9TH, 1901.

Examiners.................. { PROF. F. J. SHEPHERD, M.D.
DR. J. A. SPRINGLE, M.D.
DR. J. G. McCARTHY, M.D.
DR. J. A. HENDERSON, M.D.

1. Dissection necessary to expose the Stylo-pharyngeus muscle.

2. Describe the solid viscera in relation with the left kidney.

3. Insertion, nerve supply and actions of the muscles attached to the fibula.

35

4. Trace the various constituents of the spermatic cord from their origins to termination.

5. Describe the Optic tract and Chiasm.   How does the optic nerve terminate ?

6. Name in order the parts it is necessary to remove to expose the right pulmonary artery.

Note.—Candidates are required to answer four question only, including the first two.

Pharmacology and Therapeutics.

Third Year.

MAY 10TH, 1901.

Examiners...................... { PROF. A. D. BLACKADER, M.D.
DR. R. A. KERRY.
DR. J. HALSEY.

1. State the various methods in which the following drugs may be directed to be dispensed, and give illustrative prescriptions:— Quinniae Sulphas. Copaiba. Extractum Colocynthidis Compositum. Extractum Filicis Liquidum.

2. Discuss the exact action of the following drugs on:—(*a*) the respiratory organs, (*b*) the circulatory organs, viz. :—Belladonna. Scilla. Aconitum. Ammonia.

3. Discuss the action on the secretions and excretions of the following drugs:—

> Pilocarpinae Nitras.
> Potassi Citras.
> Cubeba.
> Sodii Salicylas.

4. Name the more important conditions in which the therapeutic employment of the following drugs is indicated. Write illustrative prescriptions with appropriate dosage:—

> Potassii Iodidum.
> Liquor Trinitrini.
> Opium.
> Bismuthi Carbonas.

36

Hygiene.

Third Year.

MAY 4TH, 1901.

Examiners...................... { PROF. R. CRAIK, M.D., LL.D.
                                    PROF. WYATT JOHNSTON.
                                    PROF. R. F. RUTTAN.

1. Explain what is meant by ground water, self purification of soil, siphonage, damp-proof construction, DuChaumont's formula.

2. What special preventive measures should be adopted in dealing with (a) Consumption, (b) Diphtheria, (c) Glanders, (d) Trichinosis.

3. Mention the chief advantages and drawbacks of heating by hot air. Describe briefly some common methods of combining heating with ventilation.

4. Describe briefly the essential points connected with the drainage of a town house by the water carriage system.

5. What precautions should be taken to properly isolate a case of contagious disease ? How should disinfection be done at the close of the case ?

6. What are the main sanitary rules regarding schools?

7. Describe a method for determining the carbon dioxide and moisture in the atmosphere of a room. Within what limits should both be kept ?

8. Classify climates. Give instructions for systematic observations regarding the climate of a locality.

Obstetrics.

Third Year.

MAY 8TH, 1901.

Examiners...................... { PROF. J. C. CAMERON, M.D.
                                    DR. D. J. EVANS.

1. Define:—Inlet, Excavation, Axis, Plane, External Conjugate, Diagonal Conjugate, Vertex, Vertex presentation, Second position.

2. Describe the phenomena of Menstruation.

37

3. How is the menstrual process affected by (*a*) Conception and (*b*) Lactation ?

4. What bearing have flexion and extension upon the way in which the foetus presents ?

5. Liquor Amnii: what are its sources and uses ?

6. How would you manage:—

        (*a*) The second stage of labour.

        (*b*) The third stage of labour.

Mental Diseases.

Third Year.

APRIL 29TH, 1901.

Examiner.................PROF. T. J. W. BURGESS, M.D.

1. What conditions are prerequisite for the proper treatment of an insane patient outside of an institution for the insane ?

2. Mention the leading points in the history of an alleged lunatic with what a physician should familiarize himself prior to examining the patient.

3. When is the use of Opium indicated in insanity, and when that of hyoscine ?

4. In what mental disorders is efeeblemet of memory likely to be found a prominent symptom ?

5. State the leading symptoms usually found in the second stage of general paresis.

Bacteriology.

Third Year.

JAN. 19TH, 1901:—9.30 TO 12.

Examiners.....................{ PROF. J. G. ADAMI, M.D.
PROF. WYATT JOHNSTON, M.D.
DR. H. B. YATES.

1. Construct tables showing the morphological, cultural and other distinctions between:—

    (1) The Streptococcus pyogenes and the Pyococcus aureus.

    (2) The Diplococcus pneumoniae and the diplobacillus of Friedlaender.

    (3) The Bacillus Typhosus and the Bacillus coli.

    (4) The Spirillum Cholerae and either the Vibrio Metchnikovi or the Spirillum of Finkler Prior.

38

2. (a) What, in order of frequency, are the modes of infection of the human being by the tubercle bacillus ? (b) What the means to be taken to lessen the spread of tuberculosis ? (c) What is Tuberculin and (d) What are its uses ?

3. (a) Classify the different methods whereby acquired immunity can be developed, and (b) discuss the relative value of the immunity acquired by the different methods. (c) State briefly the nature of the methods now practiced to induce immunity against:—(1) Smallpox. (2) Anthrax. (3) Cholera. (4) The Plague and (5) Diphtheria.

4. What is the evidence that (1) the B. typhosus is the cause of Typhoid fever; (2) the B. Tetani of Tetanus; (3) the Amoeba coli of dystentery; and (4) the Sp. Cholerae of Cholera ?

Pathology.

Third Year.

MARCH 23RD, 1901:—9.30 TO 12.30.

Examiners..................... {
PROF. J. G. ADAMI,
DR. A. G. NICHOLS.
DR. D. MACTAGGART.
DR. D. P. ANDERSON.
}

1. What conditions would you expect to find in the gross and microscopical examination of the tissues and organs of one who had died from peritonitis in the third week of Typhoid Fever ?

2. Explain the following terms, giving examples :—Atavism. Spontaneous variation.   The non-inheritance of acquired defects. The inheritance of acquired constitutional states.   Heteromorphous inheritance. Parasitic double monster. Congenital anomaly. Parasyphilitic lesion. Teratoma. Hermaphrodite.

3. From your knowledge of the degrees and stages of acute inflammation of the cornea deduce the changes which may occur locally in acute inflammation of the outer portion of the Cusps of a cardiac valve and from your knowledge of the properties of the blood deduce the added changes, both local and general, which are likely to occur in such a case as the result of the inflamed regions being bathed in the circulating blood.

4. Under what conditions do we encounter " shock " and " collapse " respectively ? Mention any observations and experiments indicating a difference between these two states .

5. Give briefly the arguments for and against: (1) the microbic theories of causation of malignant tumours and (2) the " cell rest " theory of origin of tumours in general; in either case give the conclusion to which you are led upon weighing the arguments.

39

6. What do you understand by the terms:—Ulcer.   Metaplasia.
Vicarious hypertrophy.   Pseudochylous ascites.   Amyloid bodies.
Mulberry calculus.   Caseation.   Vitreous degeneration.   Serous
cyst. Haemosiderin.

Medical Jurisprudence.

Third Year.

MARCH 9TH, 1901.

Examiners.............. .... { PROF. G. WILKINS.
PROF. WYATT JOHNSTON.

1. What are the three modes of dying? Give examples of each,
also the characteristic post-mortem appearances.

2. What appearances would indicate that incised wounds, bruises
and burns were inflicted a few hours before death ? What are the
appearances of similar injuries inflicted after death ?

3. In examining for Life Insurance, you find an applicant to all
appearances perfectly healthy with a history of never having had
any serious illness. Nothwithstanding this, what points in family
and personal history would cause aplicant not to be considered a
first class life ?   What do you understand by " reserve " on the
policy ?

4. How would you treat the apparently drowned—only two or
three minutes submerged ?   What are the characteristic post-
mortem appearances of an individual recently drowned and just
removed from the water ?

5. How would you treat poisoning by alkalies and acids ? What
characteristic lesions are found in each ?

Ophthalmology and Otology.

Fourth Year.

MAY 30TH, 1901.

Examiners.........................{ PROF. F. BULLER, M.D.
DR. J. J. GARDNER.
DR. J. W. STIRLING.

1. Write a brief account of Asthenopia, including causes, symptoms, and treatment.

2. State what you know of the Bacteriology of the Conjunctiva.

3. Describe Phlyctoenular Keratitis, giving its etiology, pathology,
symptoms and treatment.

40

4. Mention the different varieties of cataract and state how you would determine whether a cataract was mature and the eye otherwise in such a condition as to justify removal of the cataract by operation.

5. Describe Opthalmia Neonatorum and its treatment.

6. Give indications and contra-indications for the use of Atropine, Eserine and Nitrate of Silver in Ophthalmic practice.

7. Give the signs and symptoms of Mostoiditis following acute suppuration of middle ear and state what you would do to prevent its occurrence when threatened.

8. Give a brief outline of the functional examination of the ears.

Surgery.

Fourth Year.

MAY 29TH, 1901.

Examiners.......................... { PROF. T. G. RODDICK.
DR. J. M. ELDER.
DR. A. E. GARROW.

1. What forms of Heart and Kidney Disease contra-indicate operations ? What precautions should be taken in this connection before operation ?

2. Describe the symptoms and treatment of Diabetic Gangrene.

3. Discuss Anel's and Hunter's operations for the cure of Aneurism.

4. Describe the symptoms and treatment of Angular Curviture of the Spine. With what complications may a surgeon have to deal in this disease ?

5. A child seven years old has a right-sided Empyaema following Pneumonia: what would be your plan of treatment, giving details of any operative measures employed ?

6. Bronchocele: Give (a) Differential diagnosis from other tumours of the neck. (b) Classification. (c) Surgical treatment of Cystic form.

7. Name the conditions which simulate Stone in the Kidney and state the essential points of difference in each instance cited.

8. Give the symptoms and signs of fracture through the middle fossa of the base of the skull. How would you treat such an accident ?

41

Gynæcology.

Fourth Year.

MAY 2ND, 1901.

Examiners.............................{ PROF. WM. GARDNER.
DR. LOCKHART.
DR. CHIPMAN.

1. Gonorrhœa in woman, the structures it involves, symptoms and physical signs.
2. The causes and symptoms of Cystitis.
3. The accidents and complications of Ovarian Tumours.
4. The classification, minute structure, course and terminations of uterine fibro-myoma.

Medicine.

Fourth Year.

MAY 27TH, 1901.

Examiners.........................{ PROF. JAS. STEWART.
PROF. A. D. BLACKADER.
PROF. H. A. LAFLEUR.
PROF. F. G. FINLEY.
PROF. C. F. MARTIN.

1. (25) What conditions give rise to paroxysmal dyspnœa ? Describe fully the physical signs of one of them.
2. (25) What features would lead you to give a favorable prognosis in a case of pulmonary tuberculosis ? Describe the main points in the treatment of such a case.
3. (25) What are the important etiological factors in infantile entero-colitis ? State what treatment might be employed in the case of a child one year old suffering from a acute attack.
. 4. (20) Give the causes and symptoms of (1) Peripheral Facial Paralysis. (2) Paralysis of the musculo-spiral nerve.
5. (25) Discuss the etiology and the diagnosis of two forms of meningitis.
6. (30) Outline the early symptoms and treatment in a case of Chronic Interstitial Nephritis.
7. (20) What various forms of motor insufficiency of the stomach are described, and what are the individual features of the differential diagnosis ?

3

42

8. (30) A farmer, aged 34, gives a history of illness lasting about 3 months, beginning with severe pain over the lower ribs on the right side and in the epigastrium. Associated with the pain there was a cough with fever of an irregular character, some chilliness, but no sweating. The expectoration was at first whitish, then frankly purulent, and once or twice tinged with blood, and during the first part of the illness very foul. The quantity varied from day to day, but was never very large at any time. The cough has been all along of a paroxysmal character and very distressing; worse when the man was lying down. During the first two months there was a loss in weight of twenty pounds, part of which was regained in the third month. The patient has no shortness of breath, is not anæmic, has a fair appetite and sleeps well when not disturbed by coughing. He has had no other illness. Physical examination shows only a half-moon shaped area, 4 by 2 inches, of impaired resonance (not absolute dullness) in the extreme right lower axilla between the anterior and posterior axillary lines, over which the breath sounds are very slightly diminished in intesity without any qualitative change and without adventitious sounds. There is a mark of a blister in the epigastrium. The temperature at 5 p.m. was 98 and 2-5°, but there had been fever on the previous day. The patient shewed half an ounce of rather thin reddish brown homogeneous, not offensive pus, which he had coughed up on that day. Staphylococci but no tubercle bacilli were found in the specimen. Discuss the probable diagnosis and what additional examination might be necessary to come to a definite conclusion ?

Obstretics.

Fourth Year.

APRIL 29TH, 1901.

Examiners...................... { PROF. J. C. CAMERON, M.D.
DR. D. J. EVANS.

1. (40) A case of threatened abortion at the beginning of the 4th month.
    (a) Give the symptoms.
    (b) Prognosis.
    (c) Describe fully the treatment you would prefer, giving your reasons for the choice which you make.
2. (35) A case of R.O.P., describe fully the mechanism of delivery.
3. (35) Face presentations: give causes, symptoms and treatment.

43

4. (55) A III para, æt. 40, who menstruated last on 31st May, 1900, comes under your care on January 2nd, 1901. In two previous pregnancies she was delivered at full term with great difficulty, on the first occasion, craniotomy was performed. The children weighed 6½ and 6 lbs. The patients measures 5 ft. 2 in., weighs 105 lbs., and is of highly nervous temperament. At both confinements she lost a great deal of blood. She is anxious to have a living child if possible. Her pelvic measurements are as follows:—

Spines..	24	cm.
Crests	25	cm.
Ext. Conj..	17	cm.
Diag. Conj.	10.5	cm.
Interischial..	10	cm.

How would you manage the case ? Give your reasons for the line of treatment you decide to pursue.

5. (35) Give the varieties and treatment of:—

(a) Harelip in infants.

(b) Asphyxia Neonatorum.

(c) Ophthalmia Neonatorum.

Appendix Four

Holmes Gold Medallists
(established 1865)[1]

1885	Edwin C. Wood	1909	E.H. Funk
1886	Herbert S. Birkett	1910	T.A. Robinson
1887	Edward Evans	1911	W.O. Glidden
1888	Neil D. Gunn	1912	Fred Mackay
1889	Alexander E. Garrow	1913	R.H. Malone
1890	Robert E. McKechnie	1914	Cecil R. Joyce
1891	W.A. Brown	1915	W.A.S. Browne
1892	Thomas Jameson	1916	Louis Gross
1893	William E. Deeks	1917	Harold A. Desbrisay
1894	Andrew A. Robertson	1918	Robert H. MacLauchlan
1895	William A. Feader	1919	P.M.H. Savory
1896	George D. Robins	1920	C.M. Eaton
1897	John G. McDougall	1921	Peter Heinbecker
1898	W.O. Rose	1922	Atholl M. McNabb
1899	Alva H. Gordon	1923	Archibald L. Wilkie
1900	E.R. Secord	1924	John S. Henry
1901	R.H. Ker	1925	Donald E. Tinkess
1902	R.M. van Wart	1926	Kenneth I. Melville
1903	Edmund M. McLaughlin	1927	Neil Feeney
1904	J.A. Nutter	1928	Robert J. Caldwell
1905	H.C. Mersereau	1929	John S.L. Browne
1906	R.S. MacArthur	1930	J. Wendell MacLeod
1907	R.M. Benvie	1931	Katherine H. Dawson
1908	V.J.P. MacMillan	1932	Frank L. Horsfall

1933	Ruth P. Dow	1935	W.D.A. Maycock
1934	William R. Foote	1936	Ebert E. Judd

Wood Gold Medallists

(established 1905)[2]

1906	T.A. Lomer	1922	Jessie Boyd Scriver
1907	R.M. Benvie	1923	H.M. Elder
1908	F.C. Clarke	1924	Clarence A. McIntosh
1909	R.G. Bugbee	1925	Nicholas P. Hill
1910	Sidney B. Peele	1926	Arthur A. Haig
1911	Harold J.G. Geggie	1927	Victor E. Donawa
1912	D. Sclater Lewis	1928	Maurice Brodie
1913	No award	1929	Howard L. Elliot
1914	A.L. Jones	1930	Jacob Land
1915	No award	1931	Homer C. Oatman
1916	H.B. McEwen	1932	Frederick D. Mott
1917	T.M. Rischardson	1933	William M. Couper
1918	Harold E. Skeete	1934	John V. Nicholls
1919	Walter W. Read	1935	Charles L. Yuile
1920	Lorne C. Montgomery	1936	David D. MacKenzie
1921	E.A. Bell		

Notes

Full book and journal citations relating specifically to McGill and the medical faculty are given in the bibliography.

INTRODUCTION

1 S.B. Frost, *McGill University*, vol. 1, chapters 1–3 and 6; H.E. MacDermot, *A History of the Montreal General Hospital*, chapters 1–3; J. Hanaway and R. Cruess, *McGill Medicine*, vol. 1, *1829–1885*, chapter 1; B.R. Tunis and E.H. Bensley, "William Leslie Logie: McGill University's First Graduate and Canada's First Medical Graduate," *Canadian Medical Association Journal* 105 (1971): 1259–63.
2 Hanaway and Cruess, *McGill Medicine*, vol. 1, 179–83; M. Bliss, *William Osler*, 86.
3 See chapter 2, "The Flexner Report."
4 Bliss, *Osler*, 382–90.

CHAPTER ONE

1 W. Osler, *Aphorisms*, 48.
2 M Fac Med, 6 January 1885: addition to the Medical Building proposed; 5 May 1885: cost estimate for a new wing; 1 January 1886: cost overrun of completed wing discussed; 18 December 1886: discussion of plans for the new addition costing $32,000 to $33,000; numerous dates in 1887, discussion of plans and finances. The official opening celebration was on 1 August 1888.

3 S.B. Frost, *McGill University,* vol. 2, 243; Dawson Papers, MUA, box 37: "The greatest gift ever made to the cause of natural science and the noblest building dedicated in the Dominion."

4 Biographical sketch of Sir John William Dawson in Hanaway and Cruess, *McGill Medicine,* vol. 1, 159.

5 "Benefactors of McGill," *Faculty of Medicine Series* no. 1, 1932: William Christopher Macdonald, 17–20; Lord Strathcona, 3–16, W.B. Howell; see also S.E. Woods, Jr, *The Molson Saga 1763 to 1983* (Toronto: Doubleday, 1983), 166.

6 Lainchoil: personal communication from Sinclair Ross of Morayshire, Scotland, to Roy MacGregor of St Andrews, Fyfe, Scotland, 10 December 1993. Alexander Smith, after trying the army and farming, set up as a merchant in Grantown in 1810 when he was twenty-nine. Soon afterwards he met Barbara, daughter of Donald Stuart, of the Manor of Lethna-coyle (Lainchoil) in the neighbouring parish of Abernathy. The young lady's mother was Janet, daughter of Robert Grant of Cromdale. The courtship of Alexander Smith and Barbara Stuart proved a long one. They were married in 1813. After the birth of a daughter, Margaret, the Smiths moved to Forres where two sons were born, the eldest christened John Stuart after a famous uncle, and the younger Donald Alexander. Thus the Lainchoil bequest to McGill by Sir Donald Smith was in memory of his mother's birthplace in Scotland.

7 "The New Building of the Medical Faculty of McGill University," *Annual Announcement of the Medical Faculty* (1885): 6; also *Canada Medical and Surgical Journal* (June 1885): 1–3.

8 All of the teaching in the pre-clinical subjects was by lectures, except for the work in the anatomy dissection room.

9 Biographical sketch for Wyatt Galt Johnston in Hanaway and Cruess, *McGill Medicine,* vol. 1, 186.

10 Biographical sketch for T. Wesley Mills in Hanaway and Cruess, *McGill Medicine,* vol. 1, 171.

11 W. Osler, "Professor Wesley Mills," CMAJ: 338–41.

12 Girdwood, unlike most of the other professors, did not have a medical practice.

13 Biographical sketch for George Ross in Hanaway and Cruess, *McGill Medicine,* vol. 1, 171.

14 M Fac Med, 8 January 1876: The summer course for medical students was instituted in 1876.

15 P. Robb, *Development of Neurology at McGill,* 11–12.

16 The Verdun Asylum was renamed the Verdun Protestant Hospital for the Insane, then the Verdun Protestant Hospital, and finally the Douglas Hospital.

17 Biographical sketch for William Gardner in Hanaway and Cruess, *McGill Medicine,* vol. 1, 169.

18 Blackader was professor of pharmacology and therapeutics. Cameron was
   professor of obstetrics. Biographical sketch for Alexander Blackader in
   Hanaway and Cruess, *McGill Medicine*, vol. 1, 177.
19 J.B. Scriver, *The Montreal Children's Hospital*, 15. In 1937 Harold Cushing was appointed chairman of the department of pediatrics for one year
   because he was one year from retirement. In 1938 Rolf R. Struthers succeeded him (he had been a staff pediatrician at the Children's Memorial
   Hospital). Struthers served as chairman until 1944 when Alton Goldbloom was appointed physician-in-chief at the Children's Memorial
   Hospital and professor of pediatrics at McGill from 1944 to 1953.
20 See Hanaway and Cruess, *McGill Medicine*, vol. 1, 43, for the Latin text
   and note 24 for the English text of the *sponsio academica*.
21 M Fac Med, 22 March 1902, 219, the Faculty of Medicine adopted the
   six-year B.A./B.S.C., M.D., C.M. "double course"; see 22 October 1904,
   261, for details of the double course, including the fees.
22 M Fac Med, February 1896: Faculty approved the first postgraduate
   courses at the MGH and the RVH to be held in the summer of 1897.
   Shepherd (MGH) and Bell (RVH) were in charge of organizing the courses.
23 The diploma course in public health was initiated in the 1899–1900
   session. The details of the course are recorded in M Fac Med, 12 May
   1900, 168.
24 M Fac Med, 21 April 1893.
25 J.G. Adami, *The Principles of Pathology*, vols. 1 and 2.
26 The first medical textbook from McGill was W. Mills's *Textbook of
   Comparative Physiology* (1890).
27 Further discussion in chapter 5, "Pathology and Bacteriology."
28 Francis Bagdley, M.D. (1807–1863). According to Harold Segall in *Pioneers of Cardiology in Canada*, 24–5, Bagdley, who had apprenticed with
   William Robertson until 1826 and obtained a degree from the Royal College of Physicians of Edinburgh in 1827, learned the techniques of auscultation in Scotland. When he returned to Montreal in 1842, he became
   involved in the formation of a francophone medical school, L'école de
   Médecine et Chirurgie de Montréal (1843). Bagdley practised and taught
   auscultation after 1842. He was appointed to the McGill staff in 1849,
   so he probably was one of the first to promote the use of a stethoscope
   in Montreal.
29 A.F. Holmes performed auscultation. He referred to the use of the stethoscope in a valedictory address to McGill students in 1850. *British American Medical and Physical Journal* 5 (1850): 263–4.
30 J. Duffin, *To See with a Better Eye: A Life of R.T.H. Laënnec* (Princeton,
   N.J.: Princeton University Press, 1998).
31 The Montreal Veterinary College (1866–89) became the McGill Faculty
   of Comparative Medicine and Veterinary Science in 1889–90. That faculty
   closed in 1903.

32 Maude Abbott was the first female employed by McGill's medical faculty. See D. Waugh, *Maudie of McGill*, 50–1; H.E. MacDermot, *Maude Abbott: A Memoir*, 59–64.

33 A.H. Gordon, "Medicine in Montreal in the Nineties," CMAJ 53 (1945): 495–9.

34 Members of the Montreal General board of management (a committee of the life governors) were required to make annual inspections of the hospital and record their findings in a large ledger. Most of the annual comments were perfunctory and short. However, on Tuesday, 13 December, and Thursday, 15 December 1898, G. Summers and F. Carsley inspected the hospital in detail. In five pages they wrote a major condemnation of the hospital, room by room.

35 C.F. Martin's "The Montreal General Hospital in Osler's Time" is a well-written condemnation of the MGH with details.

36 Hanaway and Cruess, *McGill Medicine*, vol. 1, 207–8n19.

37 Thomas J.W. Burgess, M.D., was the first superintendent of the Verdun Protestant Hospital for the Insane in 1896 and the first psychiatrist at McGill in 1895. See Robb, *Neurology at McGill*, 5–6.

38 For further information about the use of surgical gloves, see S.B. Day, "Postscript to the Surgical Legend of William Stewart Halsted and the Introduction of Rubber Gloves to Surgery," *Surgery, Gynecology & Obstetrics* (July 1963); 121–2.; J. Randers-Pehrson, *The Surgeon's Glove* (Springfield, Ill.: Charles C. Thomas, 1962).

39 George Stephen, first Lord Mount Stephen (1829–1921), GCVD. H. Gilbert, *The Life of Lord Mount Stephen*; vol. 1, *Awakening Continent*, vol. 2, *The End of the Road* (Aberdeen: University Press, 1965 and 1977).

40 F.J. Shepherd, *History of the Montreal General*; H.E. MacDermot, *History of the Montreal General Hospital*; F.N. Gurd, *The Gurds*.

41 M Fac Med, 8 November 1889, 103; the negotiations between the Montreal General and the Royal Vic are reported in D.S. Lewis's *Royal Victoria Hospital*, 10–17. In 1996 the Montreal General, Royal Victoria, Montreal Children's, and Montreal Neurological Institute amalgamated to form the McGill University Health Centre.

42 H. Saxon Snell, a British architect with a reputation for hospital design, was given the contract for the design of the RVH in 1887. See Lewis, *Royal Victoria Hospital*, 18.

43 Iodoform was a popular antiseptic agent used in the operating room and as a disinfectant throughout hospitals. Obtained by the action of iodine and alcohol in the presence of alkalis and their carbonates, the result was a compound of very high vapour pressure which when used could be smelled throughout the hospital. Most hospitals in the first third of the twentieth century smelled strongly of iodine. See J.S. Billings, *The National Medical Dictionary*, vol. 2 (Philadelphia: Lea & Brothers), 189.

44 The Holmes Medal honours the memory of the first dean of the McGill

medical faculty, Andrew Ferdinando Holmes. Established in 1865, the terms for awarding the Holmes Medal have changed over the years. At first the medal was awarded on the basis of excellence for a thesis and a special written examination. For many years the Holmes Medal has been awarded to the student graduating with the highest total marks in the different branches of the medical curriculum. It is the senior award for scholastic achievement in medicine. See E.H. Bensley, "The Holmes Medal," *McGill Medical Journal* 34, no. 1, February 1965: 3–7.

45 Holmes Medallists: Gunn 1888, Brown 1891, and Deeks 1893.

46 There were more than one hundred life governors at the Montreal General.

47 The casebooks for medical and surgical patients at the Montreal General were large, folio-size ledgers into which the history, physical examination, and the hospital course of patients were written, including temperature charts. The casebooks were kept in the departmental offices. Introduced in 1863, they were used until the early 1950s. Follow-up notes were written approximately once a week for patients with prolonged hospital stays, usually dictated by the attending staff doctors to the house officers on ward rounds. McGill University Archives, MGH Case Books, 1863–1951 (C62–64, C130, C146, C226–247, C253–256).

48 See Lewis, *RVH*, on the ambulance service, 112–15.

49 The first motor ambulance was donated to the RVH in 1909 by Sir Vincent Meredith, president of the RVH from 1912 to 1929. It was underpowered, and as it was of no use in the winter, it was usually stored then until better equipment was provided (Lewis, 114).

50 K. Ludmerer, *Learning to Heal* (New York: Basic Books, 1985).

51 Full union of the McGill medical faculty and its teaching hospitals was not accomplished until 1975. See D.A.E. Shephard, *Royal College of Physicians and Surgeons of Canada, 1960–80* (Ottawa: RCPSC, 1985), 199–205.

52 The Johns Hopkins Medical School was founded in 1893. From the beginning the medical school also administered its own university hospital. This unique arrangement helped make the Hopkins the best clinical training centre on the continent. See M. Kaufman, *American Medical Education, 1765–1910* (London: Greenwood, 1976), 149–52.

53 This refers to the Sir Henry Gray affair of 1923–25. Details in chapter 4. See Lewis, *RVH*, 76–7.

54 Francis Buller introduced the ophthalmoscope to McGill. He was the first ophthalmologist appointed to the Montreal General in 1877. He subsequently opened a department of ophthalmology at the Royal Vic. He learned ophthalmoscopy in Berlin and London during his training and brought the technique to Montreal. See biographical sketch for Francis Buller in Hanaway and Cruess, *McGill Medicine*, vol. 1, 170.

55 J. Babinski, a Russian physician in Paris, described his famous physical sign in 1896. He discovered that patients with lesions or pressure involving the

central nervous system would manifest this by the toes going upwards, particularly the large toe, when the sole of the foot was scratched. The original description describes the great toe going up and the other toes fanning. See J. Babinski, "Sur le 'reflex cuetane' plantaire dans certains affections organiques du system nerveau central," *C R Soc Biol (Paris)* 48: 207–8, 1896.

56 H. Nelson, "Experiments with Sulfuric Ether," *British American Journal of Medical and Physical Science* 3 (1847): 34–6.

57 D. Bain, "On the Use of Carbolic Acid in Surgery," *Canadian Medical Journal* 4 (1868): 388. This is the first article in Canada on the use of antiseptic techniques learned from Lister. See R. Craik, "Two Cases of Ovariotomy, One Unsuccessful and One Successful," *Can Med J* 6 (1869): 1–10. Craik was probably the first to use antisepsis at McGill, but since he didn't follow the technique perfectly, he didn't have good results. Roddick, starting in 1877, followed the Listerian techniques in detail with excellent results and really introduced antisepsis in a practical way to McGill.

58 MGH *Operation Book, 1881–1890*, MUA.

59 First mention of an operation for appendicitis was recorded in the Montreal General annual report in 1890. The *Operation Book* records that the first operation for appendicitis at the MGH was done by James Bell and the second by Francis Shepherd in 1889. MUA, MGH *Operation Book, 1881–1890*; C.W. Harris, "Abraham Graves of Fergus, Ontario: The First Elective Appendectomy," *Canad J Surg* 4 (1961): 405–10.

60 E.A. Graham and W.H. Cole, "Roentgenological Examination of the Gallbladder," *Journal of the American Medical Association* 82 (1924): 613–14. This is the first description of contrast radiology of the gallbladder, known as the Graham–Cole Test.

61 N.B. Friedman, "Medical Practice in Montreal in 1840s," *L'Action Médicale* 23 (1947): 45–7.

62 A.H. Gordon, "Medicine in Montreal in the Nineties," *CMAJ* 53 (1945): 495–9.

63 William Withering (1741–99), *An Account of the Foxglove and Some of Its Medical Uses* (Birmingham: Swinney, 1785).

64 N.A. Howard-Jones, "Critical Study of the Origins and Early Development of Hypodermic Medication," *J Hist Med* 2 (1947): 201–49.

65 C.G. Roland, "Sunk under the Taxation of Nature: Malaria in Upper Canada," in *Health, Disease and Medicine*, C.G. Roland, ed. (Toronto: Hannah Institute for the History of Medicine, 1984), 154–70.

66 E.H. Behring and S. Kitasato, "Uber des Zustendekommen der Diphtherie-Immunitat und der Tetanus-Immunitat bei Thieren." *Disch Med W Schr;* 16 (1890): 1113–14; 1145–8.

67 E. Jenner, *An Inquiry into the Causes and Effects of Variolae Vaccinae* (London: S. Low, 1798).

68 Osler, *Principles and Practice of Medicine*.

69 Louis Riel (1844–1885) was an articulate and educated spokesman for the Métis population in Manitoba and Saskatchewan. After leading an unsuccessful rebellion against Canada from March to July 1885 (the Riel Rebellion), he was apprehended and hung for treason on 16 November 1885 in Regina.

70 Darby Bergin, 1826–1896. See C.G. Roland, "The Life and Times of Canada's First Surgeon-General," *Ontario Medicine 6,* no. 8 (1987): 29; *Dictionary of Canadian Biography,* vol. 12, 94–7.

71 There was no regular army medical corps. Volunteer regimental surgeons were usually untrained and unreliable. Darby Bergin, surgeon general at the time of the Riel Rebellion, began to establish a corps of doctors trained in military medicine, a sort of medical militia that would be trained annually and ready to be called for active duty. For instance, James Bell of McGill taught first aid and stretcher drill. Volunteers for the medical corps came from Montreal and Toronto. Nursing sisters volunteered from the U.S. and Canada. The performance of the medical corps during the Riel Rebellion proved the feasibility and practicality of a permanent Canadian Army Medical Corps.

72 M Fac Med, 13 April 1889, 108.

73 Dean Robert Craik (1829–1906) reviewed the history of McGill medical school at the opening of the addition to the Medical Building 8 June 1895 (recorded in the official program, 4–17). This is the first fairly accurate review of the history of the faculty. See R. Craik, *Papers and Addresses,* 103–17.

74 Principal Sir William Dawson resigned in May 1893. In May 1895 William Peterson was appointed as his successor.

75 Biographical sketch for Craik in Hanaway and Cruess, *McGill Medicine,* vol. 1, 166.

76 Craik's *Papers and Addresses* contains speeches at opening days of the faculty, graduations and other occasions. F.J. Shepherd wrote the introduction.

77 Ibid., 36.

78 Ibid., 55.

79 See biographical sketch for Robert Jarred Bliss Howard, this volume.

80 Medical student enrolment in 1900 was 457. The 1901 addition to the Medical Building was to accommodate an even larger enrolment.

81 D. McDonald, *Lord Strathcona: A Biography of Donald Smith,* 447–9.

82 Medical students had to purchase a hospital card in order to enter the MGH for clinical instruction. There were two types of hospital card, regular and perpetual; the latter was more expansive. A regular hospital card was valid for a specific period and there was a space on the obverse to record attendance at hospital clinics, etc. A perpetual card was valid for an indefinite period. Octavia Ritchie advised Maude Abbott to purchase a perpetual card.

83 Women were admitted to McGill College in 1884 with the aid of a five-year

$50,000 grant from Sir Donald Smith. Because of his generosity, the women were known as "Donaldas." Women were admitted to Bishop's University Medical School in 1890, to the McGill Medical School in 1918, and to the McGill Dental Faculty in 1922. See M. Gillett, *We Walked Very Warily*, 70–112, 274–302; M.A. Rogers, *A History of the McGill Dental School*, 33–4.

84 Craik, *Papers and Addresses*, 47.

85 There are several biographies of Florence Nightingale and descriptions of the St Thomas's School for Nurses: Sir Edward Cook, *Florence Nightingale*, vols. 1 and 2 (London: Macmillan, 1913); Cecil Woodham-Smith, *Florence Nightingale* (Harmondsworth, Middlesex, U.K.: Penguin Books, 1955); Maude E. Seymour Abbott, "Florence Nightingale, As Seen in Her Portraits," *Boston Medical and Surgical Journal*, 14 September 1916, 14, 21, 28. One of the most concise is Lytton Strachey's *The Eminent Victorians* (London: Chatto & Windus, 1918), 115–76.

86 J.M. Gibbon and M.S. Mathewson, *Three Centuries of Canadian Nursing* (Toronto: MacMillan, 1947).

87 H.E. MacDermot, *History of the School of Nursing of the Montreal General Hospital*. First published in 1940 to commemorate the fiftieth anniversary of the school, the 1961 edition contains the names of all graduates from the MGH from 1891 to 1961 and graduates of the Western Hospital from 1889 to 1926. See also MacDermot, *History of the Montreal General Hospital*.

88 MGH annual reports, 1890–1919.

89 M.D. Munroe, *The Training School for Nurses, Royal Victoria Hospital, 1894–1942*; Lewis, *RVH*, 79.

90 S.B. Frost, *McGill*, vol. 2, 116–7, 222–3, and 393; B.L. Tunis, *In Caps and Gowns: The Story of the School for Graduate Nurses, 1920–1964*.

CHAPTER 2

1 Osler, "Specialization in the General Hospital," *Johns Hopkins Hospital Bulletin* 24 (1913): 167–71.

2 M Fac Med, 18 January 1902, 213. Roddick was the fifth dean of the medical faculty.

3 In 1889 McGill accepted the Montreal Veterinary College as its Faculty of Comparative Medicine and Veterinary Science, which qualified students for the Degree of Doctor of Veterinary Medicine (D.V.M.) on graduation. Duncan McEachran was the leader in the new faculty. When he retired in 1903, there was no one to reorganize the school to make it competitive with other institutions. The operation of the faculty was terminated. The last graduate received the McGill D.V.M. at the summer convocation in 1903. See S.B. Frost, *McGill*, vol. 2, 46.

4 The Bishop's Dental School Building was located on Phillips Square, Montreal. The dental school had little to do with Bishop's University.

5 M.A. Rogers, *A History of the McGill Dental School*, 1–8; Frost, *McGill*, vol. 2, 45–7, 169, 396.

6 M Fac Med, 14 November 1903. A committee was established to investigate the arrangements for the establishment of a department of dental medicine in the McGill medical faculty. Follow-up discussion occurred at subsequent faculty meetings.

7 The McGill Corporation regulated the academic affairs of the university. Governors, deans, and elected representatives from each faculty were the members of corporation. In 1935 the corporation was renamed the McGill Senate. Frost, *McGill*, vol. 2, 55, 207. See chapter 9, "Governance."

8 The Bishop's Dental Faculty that came to McGill in 1904 included Peter Brown, D.D.S., professor of operative dentistry; Fred Henry, D.D.S., professor of dental pathology and dental materia medica; James Berwick, D.D.S., professor of prosthetic dentistry; E.R. Barton, D.D.S., lecturer in dental anatomy; James Morrison, D.D.S., lecturer in orthodontics; A.D. Angus, D.D.S., demonstrator in operative techniques; and W.D. Smith, D.D.S., demonstrator in prosthetic dentistry. Regarding the Bishop's dental students, McGill did not allow them to transfer to the McGill dental department. Bishop's dental students continued dental studies at McGill but graduated with a Bishop's degree. One student did apply to McGill and had to start in the first year of the McGill dental program. See Rogers, *History*, 22.

9 M Fac Med, 8 October 1909, 354; MacDermot, *History of the Montreal General Hospital*, 103.

10 Rogers, *History*, 21.

11 Faculties of Arts, Applied Science, and Law.

12 M Fac Med, November 1904 to May 1905; McGill Board of Governors, 26 May 1905; Frost, *McGill*, vol. 2, 50. Shepherd and Adami disagreed on the terms "union" and "amalgamation." In the minutes and resolutions the two terms are used interchangeably.

13 Biographical sketch for Robert Tait McKenzie, this volume.

14 Major James Farquarson, "The Life of a Remarkable Man," *Canadian Army Journal* (1955): 96–106; J. McGill, *The Joy of Effort*; F. Cosentino, *Almonte's Brothers of the Wind: R. Tait McKenzie and James Naismith*.

15 R.T. McKenzie, *Exercise in Education and Medicine* (Philadelphia: W.B. Saunders, 1909); R.T. McKenzie, *Reclaiming the Maimed: Handbook of Physical Therapy* (New York: Macmillan Co., 1918).

16 Four small bronze masks measuring about four inches by eight inches stand on the top of bookshelves at the MGH Medical Library. They are probably little noticed by those who enter. They are copies of the four famous masks done by R. Tait McKenzie. The original masks are in

Philadelphia (University of Pennsylvania) and Cambridge University. See A.J. Kozar, *The Sport Sculpture of R.T. McKenzie*, 38–40.

17 Letters from D.G. Keddie, curator of the R. Tait McKenzie Museum, the Mill of Kintail, RR1, Almonte, Ont., MUA, 27 January and 2 July 1977.

18 F.W. Campbell was born in Montreal 1837. He graduated M.D., C.M. from McGill in 1860. He practised medicine in Montreal and had activities in several fields, including being president of the Montreal Med-Chi in 1877 and vice-president of the CMA in 1879 (*Canadian Dictionary of Biography*, vol. 13, 153).

19 Maude Abbott was admitted to Bishop's medical faculty in 1890 and graduated M.D., C.M. with honours in 1894. See C. Nicholl, *Bishop's University, 1843–1970* (Montreal and Kingston: MQUP, 1994), appendix 3, the Faculty of Medicine, 317–47; D.C. Masters, *Bishop's University: The First 100 Years* (Toronto: Clarke, Irwin, 1950); E.H. Bensley, "Bishop's Medical School," *CMAJ* 72 (1955): 463–5.

20 F.W. Campbell's elder son, Rollo Campbell, died from typhoid in May 1904. His second son, F.W. Campbell, Jr, died of typhoid in April 1905.

21 The Western General Hospital was incorporated in 1874 and opened in 1880. It shared the facilities with the Women's Hospital of Montreal until 1894 when the Women's Hospital moved further west on St Catherine Street In 1907 suggestions were made on several occasions to merge the Western General Hospital with the MGH. The merger finally succeeded in 1924; the Western General Hospital became the Western Division (private pavilion) of the MGH. Although the staff of the Western General Hospital was mostly from McGill, Bishop's students were taught there from 1880 until 1904 when Bishop's medical faculty closed and amalgamated with McGill's medical faculty.

22 M Fac Med, 4 November 1905, 422: terms of amalgamation of Bishop's Faculty of Medicine with McGill.

23 M Fac Med, 19 September 1908, 288; 4 December 1909, 371.

24 In 1912 the McGill faculty considered establishing a date after which no more McGill *ad eundem* degrees would be granted to Bishop's medical graduates.

25 M Fac Med, 30 April 1914, 102.

26 "McGill Again Victim from Fire," *Montreal Gazette*, 16 April 1907.

27 Ibid.

28 Ibid.

29 M Fac Med, 16 April 1907.

30 "McGill Fire Believed to Be Work of Incendiary," *Montreal Gazette*, 17 April 1907.

31 Percy Erskine Nobbs was born in Scotland in 1875. After living in St Petersburg, Russia, he came to Canada in 1903. He was the second Macdonald Professor of Architecture at McGill and directed the department from 1910 to 1945. For many years he had a private architectural firm, Nobbs

& Hyde. He designed several buildings at McGill including the Student Union and the Pathological Institute. He also designed the Osler Memorial Library in the SMB. In 1909 he married Cecelia Shepherd, F.J. Shepherd's elder daughter. See S. Wagg, *Percy Erskine Nobbs, Architect, Artist, Craftsman.*

32 M Fac Med, 11 April 1894: discussion as to whether the academic year should be extended from four sessions of six months to four sessions of nine months, or else adding a fifth year to the medical curriculum.

33 The perpetual card from the MGH allowed students to enter the hospital and the wards. There was also an annual card. Students had to purchase these cards.

34 By 1907 approximately 10 per cent of the graduating class (those with high academic standing) obtained positions as house officers at the MGH or the RVH. Over the years the terminology for medical graduates who had recognized appointments at a teaching hospital for further training prior to starting practice changed. At first they were "house surgeons"; then the title "house officer" was more frequently used. Starting in the 1920s, the title intern(e) – junior, rotating, or senior – was used for the first or second postgraduate year. For further postgraduate hospital training, medical graduates were "residents" or "fellows." It is difficult to give a definite date when these changes occurred because they varied from hospital to hospital.

35 F. Buller, "Introductory Lecture, McGill University, Faculty of Medicine, 1881–82," *Canada Medical and Surgical Journal* 10 (1881): 193–204; also in Buller's Valedictory Address to the graduating class in 1903 in the *Montreal Medical Journal* 32 (1903): 500: "Let me tell you first of all that the student who leaves college and immediately goes abroad to study some specialty for six months or a year, during which time he merely attends the clinics, and then returns home and starts as a specialist, is nothing short of an impostor, a superficial, narrow-minded, ill-trained egoist, too ignorant to understand his own incapacity." Quoted in MacDermot, *MGH*, 93.

36 M Fac Med, 6 May 1911, 474.

37 M Fac Med, 5 December 1908, 302.

38 A. Macphail, *History of the Canadian Forces in the Great War, 1914–19.*

39 Actually W.W. Francis was Osler's second cousin, "with nephew status," as Osler liked to say. He was the son of Osler's cousin Marian Francis. See Bliss, *William Osler, A Life in Medicine,* 494.

40 Starting in 1877, Roddick promoted antisepsis at the MGH through talks and papers about his results with Lister's techniques. Although Roddick did not introduce antisepsis, he was its main promoter in Quebec. By 1880 he had convinced the General's operating room staff to adopt his procedures to standardize antisepsis.

41 Sir Wilfred Laurier, Liberal prime minister of Canada, 1896–1911.

42 The final vote on the Roddick Bill on 19 May 1911 established the Medical

Council of Canada under the Canadian Medical Act. The effective date of the formation of the Medical Council of Canada was 7 November 1912. Roddick had spent eighteen years working on this worthy project.

43 The Dominion Medical Council would become the Medical Council of Canada. See R.B. Kerr, *History of the Medical Council of Canada.*

44 Ibid., 25.

45 M Fac Med, 13 June 1907, 217. Although he was senior attending surgeon at the MGH, Shepherd was not a candidate for the posts of professor of surgery or professor of clinical surgery since he was already heavily committed as professor of anatomy. Shepherd was "lecturer in operative surgery," a title relating to his participation in summer postgraduate courses.

46 M Fac Med, 8 June 1908, 286.

47 Biographical sketch for F.J. Shepherd in Hanaway and Cruess, *McGill Medicine*, vol. 1, 183.

48 At the MGH there were four attending surgeons. Two were on duty for the winter term October to March, and the other two for the summer term, April to September. Shepherd always took the summer term since he taught anatomy during the winter term. See Howell, *Shepherd.*

49 Ibid., 207–11.

50 Shepherd's residence at 152 Mansfield was one block south of the McGill grounds.

51 Como is a small town on the southern shore of the Lake of Two Mountains, west of Montreal.

52 MUA, Shepherd Album. In 1913 Dean Shepherd and his daughter, Dorothy Shepherd, sent written invitations to an At Home in the recently completed Strathcona Medical Building.

53 The 1913 trip was Shepherd's thirteenth and last trip to Europe. The main purpose of the trip was to receive an honorary fellowship in the Royal College of Surgeons of England.

54 The Pabos River is on the south shore of Quebec's Gaspé Peninsula and flows into the Baie de Chaleur (Howell, *Shepherd*, 187).

55 M Fac Med, 31 May 1911, 483.

56 M Fac Med, 10 July 1912, 548. In 1912 the estate of the late James Cooper bequeathed $60,000 to McGill for the support of the medical faculty. Amongst others, the Department of Experimental Medicine and J.C. Meakins and J. Kaufmann received support from the Cooper Fund.

57 M Fac Med, 17 October 1912, 553.

58 M Fac Med, 10 October 1913, 58.

59 M Fac Med, 4 October 1919, 391.

60 A. Flexner, *Medical Education in the United States and Canada*

61 Flexner, *The American College: A Criticism* (New York: Century Corporation, 1908). This little-known book by Flexner (his first) was a criticism of the American college system written while he was in Germany.

62 Flexner, *I Remember, An Autobiography of Abraham Flexner* (New York: Simon & Schuster, 1940), 109–11.
63 M Fac Med, 28 September 1914, 117.
64 Howell, *Shepherd*, 207–25.
65 M Fac Med, 15 June 1914, 110.

CHAPTER THREE

1 Osler, "The Fixed Period," *Aequanimitas*, 377.
2 R. Kipling, "The White Man's Burden," stanza 1.
3 Montreal merchant Jesse Joseph built his house at the corner of Sherbrooke and McTavish Streets in 1860 and called it "Dilcoosha," a Hindu word meaning "the heart's desire." After Joseph died in 1904, the house was vacant for several years. See E.A. Collard, *Oldest McGill*, 95–6.
4 Some of the military units were the Black Watch, Royal Montreal Regiment, Victoria Rifles, and 17th Hussars.
5 The Canadian Army Medical Corps (CAMC) was established in 1904.
6 By the end of World War I, Birkett had been promoted to brigadier general. King George V decorated him with Companion of the Order of the Bath.
7 Other Canadian universities followed McGill's example and recruited medical units – Toronto, Queen's, Laval, and University of Western Ontario. See A. Macphail, *History of the Canadian Forces in the Great War, 1914–19*; R.C. Fetherstonhaugh, *No. 3 Canadian General Hospital (McGill), 1914–1919*.
8 Macphail, *History*, 214–33 and 644–73.
9 Camp Valcartier is west of Quebec City.
10 The Battle of the Somme (1915–16) was the first battle in which Canadians were involved. The Canadians experienced German gas attacks and had enormous casualties. Approximately one thousand soldiers were killed during those battles.
11 In October 1915, 650 wounded were admitted; 450 operations were performed; there were 21 deaths (Fetherstonhaugh, *McGill*, 32).
12 Fetherstonhaugh listed different numbers for medical treatment in August and September 1917: 117, 5,109 admitted; 129, 4,192 admitted (Fetherstonhaugh, *McGill*, 129).
13 See biographical sketch for John McCrae, this volume.
14 McCrae, *In Flanders Fields and Other Poems*, 5–7 (introduction by A. Macphail); J.F. Prescott, *In Flanders Fields: The Story of John McCrae*.
15 Fetherstonhaugh, *No. 3 Canadian General Hospital (McGill)*, 249.
16 Biographical sketch for F.A.C. Scrimger, this volume.
17 The Victoria Cross was created during the Crimean War, 29 January 1856, to recognize outstanding deeds of gallantry. It is a bronze Maltese Cross made from captured Russian cannons. There is a Royal Crest in the

centre and a scroll with the words "for valour." The ribbon is dark red. On the back of the bar is the recruit's identification; the date of the deed is inscribed on the back of the cross. During World War I, 579 Victoria Crosses were conferred, twelve to personnel of the medical services, of which two were to Canadians. Scrimger received the Victoria Cross for his actions on 25 April 1915 and B.S. Hutchison for valour on 2 September 1918.

18 About 400 metres west of the main road between Ypres and St Julien is a large farmhouse on a hill called "Mouse Trap Farm," where Scrimger performed his heroic deeds in 1915. See N. Christie, *For King and Empire.*

19 Captain Harold McDonald, 16th Canadian Scottish and 3rd Brigade, received severe wounds that were cared for by Francis Scrimger who carried the helpless officer on his back to an advanced dressing station. McDonald miraculously survived his wounds and the war.

20 Biographical sketch for C.F. Martin, this volume.

21 H. Segall, "Goldbloom, Goldblatt, Greenspoon and Gross," *Canadian Jewish Historical Society Journal* 6 (1982): 17–32

22 Ibid.

23 M Fac Med, 4 November 1916.

24 M Fac Med, December 1917, 295.

25 M Fac Med, 5 January 1918, 286.

26 M Fac Med, 18 June 1918, 324.

27 In 1910 Abraham Flexner encouraged his friend Richard Burdon Haldane (later Viscount Haldane) to have a Royal Commission on Medical Education in the London-area, hospital-based medical schools. Flexner and Osler testified that there needed to be a serious restructuring of London medical education along university lines as at Johns Hopkins "to break the existing level of mediocrity" (*Royal Commission on University Education in London, Final Report, Chairman, Viscount Haldane, London, 1913);* A. Flexner, *Medical Education in Europe* (New York: Carnegie Foundation Bulletin no. 6, 1912).

28 See Bliss, *William Osler: A Life In Medicine,* 463–6, for a discussion of Osler and the full-time system.

29 Fred Finley returned to McGill after overseas service with the CAMC and replaced Martin as chairman of the Education Committee.

30 Lewis, *RVH,* 71.

31 Ibid., 69–71.

32 Letters sent by Osler to dean of medicine General Herbert Birkett, 29 July 1919, 31 July 1919, 19 August 1919, 28 August 1919, 12 September 1919, 1 November 1919; to George Armstrong, 11 January 1919; to William Welch, August 1919; to John D. Rockefeller, Jr, 28 August 1919 (OL).

33 M Fac Med, 28 February 1921.

34 Letters: George Vincent, Rockefeller Foundation, to H. John Scone, registrar, McGill University, 24 December 1919; George Vincent, Rockefeller

Foundation, to Acting Principal Frank Adams, McGill University, 28 January 1920 (OL and RF Archives).

35 Letters, Charles Cason, Rockefeller Foundation, to Acting Principal Frank Adams, 13 February 1920, regarding visit to Montreal by Dr Richard Pearce and George Vincent (OL and RF Archives).

36 Frank Dawson Adams, a geologist, was dean of the Faculty of Applied Science. He became acting principal when Sir William Peterson suffered a stroke in 1919. Later Adams was vice-principal of the Khaki University and then returned to McGill in the 1920s as the first dean of the Faculty of Graduate Studies. See Frost, *McGill*, vol. 2, 106.

37 The latter new building was the Biology Building. In the 1960s it was remodelled and became the F. Cyril James Building for the Office of the Principal and administrative offices.

38 Pathological Institute was the official name of the building, although most people referred to it as the Pathology Institute.

39 Many letters between the Rockefeller Foundation and McGill exist. Dr Richard Pearce visited McGill on 13 March, 11 May, and 4–9 June 1921 (OL and RF Archives).

40 Frost, *McGill* vol. 2, 114.

41 Salary of $17,500, a house, and assurance that he would be appointed as a director of the Bank of Montreal for which he would receive an honorarium of $3,000 to $4,000 a year. See Frost, *McGill*, vol. 2, 109–10, 113–15, 116–18; H.M. Urquhart, *Arthur Currie*, 61–2; M. Denison, *Canada's First Bank*, vol. 2 (Toronto: McClelland & Stewart, 1967), 422.

42 Currie did not have a university degree.

43 Dr George Vincent wrote to Chancellor Sir Edward Beatty on 11 June 1920 for assurance of McGill's willingness and ability to raise $900,000 (OL and RF Archives). A letter from Chancellor Beatty, 28 June 1920, assured the Rockefeller Foundation of McGill's intentions. The $900,000 was raised as part of a $6,321,511 fund-raising completed on November 25, 1920. With the money in hand for McGill, on 1 December 1920 the Rockefeller Foundation pledged $1,000,000 (OL and RF Archives).

44 Octavia Grace Ritchie, a remarkable woman and educational activist, was admitted to McGill in 1884 as one of the first woman students at the university. Supported by a gift from Sir Donald Smith (later Lord Strathcona), she graduated B.A. in 1888 (a "Donalda," in honour of Donald Smith). She gave the valedictorian address for the women and complained of the failure of the university to open the doors of the medical faculty to women. Denied admission to McGill, she went to Women's Medical College in Kingston, Ontario, in the autumn of 1888. In 1890 Bishop's medical faculty decided to accept women. In 1890 Ritchie transferred to Bishop's and graduated M.D., C.M. in 1891, the first Donalda to become a medical doctor.

Ritchie studied in Europe and then returned to Montreal. She married

Dr F.R. England and practised medicine in Montreal. A medical activist, she was one of the pioneer women medical graduates in Canada. She worked tirelessly to get women admitted to the medical faculty. This was accomplished in 1918 with the admission of four women, all of whom graduated in 1922. See M. Gillett, *We Walked Very Warily.*

45 M Fac Med, 10 May 1889, 117; the medical faculty recommended no co-education to the McGill Corporation.

46 M Fac Med, 1 Feb. 1889, 100.

47 The Women's Medical College in Kingston, Ontario, was founded in 1883 as a spin-off from the Royal College of Physicians and Surgeons of Kingston. The latter college was associated with Queen's University, which did not have a medical faculty until 1892. Lectures actually began at the Women's College in 1890. Some of the lectures were given in conjunction with the Royal College students. There was separate anatomy instruction and some lectures for the women.

Jennie Gowanlock Trout, one of the pioneers of women's medical education in Ontario and Canada, was a strong supporter of this school, which graduated twenty-six students. After 1893 the Women's Medical College in Kingston closed, and thereafter women in Ontario received medical education in Toronto. Queen's medical faculty did not admit women students until 1943. Cf. C. Godfrey, *Medicine in Ontario* (Belleville, Ontario: Mika Publishing, 1979), 188–90.

48 M Fac Med, 19 October 1901, 206.

49 M Fac Med, 12 May 1905, 68.

50 M Fac Med, April 1910.

51 M Fac Med, 3 June 1913, 605.

52 M Fac Med, 7 February 1914, 92.

53 The Ritz-Carlton Hotel is on the south side of Sherbrooke Street, west of McGill University. For many years it has been a fashionable site for entertainment for the McGill community.

54 Gillett, *We Walked Very Warily*; J.B. Scriver, "McGill's First Women Doctors," 131–5, in *The McGill You Knew*, E.A. Collard, ed.; Frost, *McGill,* vol. 2, 176.

CHAPTER FOUR

1 Osler, "The Hospital As a College," in *Aequanimitas*, 316.

2 S.B. Frost, *McGill University*, vol. 2, 169: "In 1923 Currie announced the appointment of Charles F. Martin as dean of the faculty, without limitation on the term of appointment."

3 R.P. Howard, *The Chief: Dr. William Osler*, 115–78.

4 Biographical sketch for George E Armstrong, this volume.

5 Biographical sketch for Henry Gray, this volume.

6 Lewis, *RVH*, 77.

7 Sir Arthur Currie's diary, 28 February 1923 (OL).

8 Sir Arthur Currie's diary, Monday, 14 May 1923; letter: R.M. Pearce to Currie, 11 June 1923 (OL).

9 W.G. Penfield, "Edward Archibald, 1872–1945." *Canad J Surg;* 1:167–74, 1954; D.S. Lewis, "A Pioneer of Modern Surgery: Dr. Edward Archibald," in E.A. Collard, ed., *The McGill You Knew.*

10 W.B. Spaulding, "Charles F. Martin, 1868–1953: A Notable Dean of McGill University": 29–31.

11 Martin was president of the CMA in 1923–24.

12 Letters, Sir Henry Gray to Principal Sir Arthur Currie, 28 September 1925; Sir Henry Gray to editor of *CMAJ*, 9 October 1925 (a handwritten note at the bottom of Gray's letter from the *CMAJ* editor stating that Gray's long, rambling letter should not be published) (OL); M.A. Entin, *Edward Archibald*, chapter 6.

13 Lewis, *RVH*, 169–82.

14 Ibid., 188–9.

15 Ibid., 186–9.

16 W.G. Penfield, *No Man Alone*, 151–2.

17 After Sir Vincent Meredith's resignation late in 1928, the RVH board of governors appointed Sir Herbert Holt, a Montreal financier, as acting president of the RVH and president in 1929. See Lewis, *RVH*, 249.

18 Letters, Martin to Pearce, 15 November 1928; Pearce memo to Rockefeller Foundation, 20 December 1928.

19 Sir Edward Beatty was an active chancellor of McGill from 1920 to 1943. In 1928 Beatty appointed Dean Martin as acting principal of McGill during Principal's Currie's absence in India. See Frost, *McGill*, vol. 2, 189.

20 M Fac Med, 17 April 1924, 11: entrance requirements defined; pre-med course established.

21 M Fac Med, 26 May 1931, 109.

22 M Fac Med, 25 April 1934, 132.

23 At the RVH in 1932 a new four-storey fireproof building was erected for the intern staff with a lounge and a billiard room. The building could accommodate forty interns. In 1939 this building was enlarged by the addition of a further twenty rooms (Lewis, *RVH*, 249).

24 M Fac Med, 14 October 1935, 154.

25 T.G. Roddick was the first chief surgeon at the RVH.

26 Lewis, *RVH*, 297.

27 E.W. Archibald, "Surgical Affections and Wounds of the Head," in *American Practice of Surgery*, J.D. Bryant and R.H. Buck, eds. (New York: Wood, 1908).

28 D.A. Murphy, "James Bell's Appendicitis," *Canad J Surg* 15 (1972): 335–8.

29 Penfield, *No Man Alone*, 141.

30 Ibid., 141, 144–6, 299–307, 330–8; Lewis, *RVH*, 229, 302, 398; Penfield,

"Dr. Penfield Describes How His Work at McGill Began," in *The McGill You Knew*, E.A. Collard, ed., 146–50.

31 Gratton D. Thompson was the architect for the Roddick Memorial Gates. See *McGill News* 6, no. 3 (June 1925); S.B. Frost, "Roddick Gates Honour Canada's Foremost Physician," *McGill News*, fall 2001, 40.

32 Bliss, *William Osler*, 421. Prima: works that made up a biographical-bibliographical account of the evolution of science, including medicine; secunda: secondary works on the same theme; litteraria: literary works written by or about physicians; historica: books on medical history; biographica: lives; bibliographica: books about books; incunabula: books from the dawn of printing; manuscripts.

33 M Fac Med, 8 April 1920, 433.

34 E.H. Bensley, "Samuel Ernest Whitnall (1876–1950)," *McGill Medical Luminaries*, 107–9.

35 M Fac Med, 26 November 1921.

36 M Fac Med, 27 January 1923, 538.

37 M Fac Med, 23 May 1927, 71.

38 H. Cushing, *The Life of William Osler* (Oxford: Clarendon Press, 1925), 717; Bliss, *Osler*, 483–93, 496–7; Osler Library newsletters, numerous references, June 1969 to present.

39 On 12 June 1935 Professor Stephen Leacock received the following form letter from A.P.S. Glassco, treasurer of the university: "Resolved: that all teachers and officers of the University shall automatically retire on reaching the age of 65 years, the Board [of governors], however, reserves the right to retain the services of any officer or teacher beyond that age if it be considered in the interests of the University to do so. Pursuant to the above resolution, the Governors have instructed me to notify you that you will be retired from the University on 31 May 1936." See A. and T. Moritz, *Leacock, a Biography* (Toronto: Stoddart, 1985), 272. Presumably Professor Martin received a similar letter.

40 Spaulding, "Notable Dean": 29–31; D.S. Lewis, "McGill's First Full-Time Dean of Medicine," in *McGill*, E.A. Collard, ed., 136–8.

CHAPTER FIVE

1 Osler, "The Leaven of Science," *Aequanimitas*, 92.

2 For anatomy prior to 1885, see Hanaway and Cruess, *McGill Medicine*, vol. 1, 73–5.

3 W.B. Howell, *Francis John Shepherd*, 170–5.

4 Gurd, *The Gurds*, 171.

5 F.J. Shepherd, "On the Teaching of Anatomy to Medical Students," *Montreal Medical Journal* (November 1900): 807–12.

6 M Fac Med, 1 May 1907.

7 M Fac Med, February 1912, 485.

8 M Fac Med, 9 April 1908, 270. Lecturers: J.A. Springle and J.A Henderson; five demonstrators and five assistant demonstrators.

9 When the medical faculty moved from the SMB to the MacIntyre Medical Building on Pine Avenue in 1966, the anatomy department remained in the SMB, which was renamed the Strathcona Anatomy and Dental Building.

10 Shepherd's colleagues and students organized a dinner on 28 March 1913 to mark the occasion of his twenty-five years as professor of anatomy and presented him with some silver plate (Howell, *Shepherd,* 203).

11 C.L.N. Robinson, *J.C. Boileau Grant: Anatomist Extraordinary* (Toronto: Association of Medical Services, 1993).

12 M Fac Med, 13 June 1913, 605–6.

13 M Fac Med, January 1912, 416; 3 February 1912, 515.

14 M Fac Med, June 1913, 592: Geddes was appointed Reford Professor of Anatomy.

15 Howell, *Shepherd,* 209.

16 M Fac Med, October 1914, 130. Geddes had been a combatant officer in the Boer War (ibid.).

17 Frost, *McGill University*, vol. 2, 109–10.

18 Samuel Ernest Whitnall (1876–1950) received his medical degree from Oxford University in 1909. He taught anatomy at Oxford from 1909 to 1914 and 1918–19; see E.H. Bensley, *McGill Medical Luminaries*, 107.

19 Gurd, *The Gurds,* 171.

20 M Fac Med, 24 September 1934, 136.

21 A revised and enlarged second edition was published in 1933 (London: Arnold).

22 S.E. Whitnall, *Anatomy of the Human Orbit and Accessory Organs of Vision* (London: Oxford University Press, 1st ed., 1921; 2nd ed., 1932).

23 Osler Society of McGill University, a medical student group devoted to "reflecting Osler's ideas of a liberal medical education."

24 M Fac Med, 13 October 1936: C.P. Martin, professor of anatomy, introduced to the faculty.

25 Histology prior to 1885 described in Hanaway and Cruess, *McGill Medicine*, vol. 1, 95.

26 Biographical sketch for G. Wilkins, this volume.

27 M Fac Med, January 1908: shared responsibility for teaching of histology.

28 J.C. Simpson was secretary of the McGill medical faculty from 1921 to 1936, associate dean from 1936 to 1940, and dean 1940–41.

29 For physiology prior to 1885, see Hanaway and Cruess, *McGill Medicine*, vol. 1, 95.

30 Biographical sketch for T.W. Mills in ibid., 176–7.

31 Ibid., 68.

32 In 1912 W.B. Howell's salary as a lecturer in the department of physiology

was $600 per year. In the same year he resigned to start a department of anesthesia at the MGH. After serving in the CAMC, he became head of anesthesia at the RVH.

33 He died on 15 February 1915 of myocardial infarction.

34 M Fac Med, 31 May 1911: Alcock appointed professor of physiology.

35 M Fac Med, 3 June 1914: G.R. Mines, M.A., appointed professor of physiology.

36 M Fac Med, 1 April 1916, 225, report of the search committee for the chair of physiology. Mottran was running the department as acting chairman.

37 E.H. Bensley, "Boris Petrovitch Babkin (1877–1950)," *Medical Luminaries,* 111–14.

38 J. Tait and W.J. McNally, *Collected Papers, 1925–1935, The Physiology of the Internal Ear* (Ottawa: RCPSC Library); W.J. McNally, "Five Lectures on the Physiology of the Ear," *Annals of Otology, Rhinology and Laryngology* 38 (December 1929): 1163; 39 (March 1930): 248.

39 Biographical sketch for Reverend W. Wright in Hanaway and Cruess, *McGill Medicine,* vol. 1, 165.

40 Biographical sketch for J. Stewart, present volume.

41 Biographical sketch for Blackader in Hanaway and Cruess, *McGill Medicine,* vol. 1, 177.

42 R.C. Stehle was professor of pharmacology from 1921 to 1940.

43 For chemistry prior to 1885, see Hanaway and Cruess, *McGill Medicine,* vol.1, 95.

44 Ibid., 5.

45 Biographical sketch for G.P. Girdwood in ibid., 167.

46 M Fac Med, 13 May 1886: R.F. Ruttan appointed assistant to the professor of chemistry (Girdwood) with the title of lecturer ($250 per annum) to assist with the practical chemistry class. See biographical sketch for Ruttan, this volume.

47 M Fac Med, April 1888: Ruttan in charge of organic chemistry; guaranteed $1,000 per year with some student fees paid to him.

48 M Fac Med, 20 June 1894, 245: Ruttan appointed professor of practical chemistry.

49 M Fac Med, September 1909, 360: physiological and pathological chemistry to be taught in the medical faculty; M Fac Med, 6 April 1912, 534: course in biological chemistry, and laboratory course in clinical chemistry.

50 M Fac Med, March 1912, 543: teaching of general chemistry transferred from the medical faculty to the Chemistry Building under the aegis of the Faculty of Arts and Science. See Frost, *McGill,* vol. 2, 145. In 1913 Ruttan was professor of chemistry in the Faculty of Arts and Science.

51 M Fac Med, 17 April 1924, 11.

52 Transactions of the Royal Society of Canada, 34: xix–xxi, 1934.

53 Biographical sketch for J.B. Collip, this volume.

54 This section is based on a monograph written by Professor Rose John-
   stone, whose independent research is responsible for the material included.
   She served as chair of the biochemistry department from 1981 to 1991.

55 Hanaway and Cruess, *McGill Medicine*, vol. 1, 57.

56 M Fac Med, 3 May 1902: botany and zoology to be taught in the medical
   faculty; M Fac Med, January 1903, 284: the faculty debated whether
   botany would continue to be taught in the medical faculty or the arts faculty; M Fac Med, 16 May 1907: biology would not be taught in the Medical Building because of the fire, but in the arts faculty; M Fac Med, 6
   April 1912, 524: botany eliminated from the medical curriculum; 553:
   course in zoology for medical students.

57 Biographical sketch for W.G. Johnston in Hanaway and Cruess, *McGill
   Medicine*, vol.1, 186.

58 M Fac Med, 23 July 1892, 179: faculty discussed ten candidates for the
   chair of pathology. Adami of Jesus College, Cambridge, was one of the
   ten candidates. M Fac Med, 8 September 1892, 181: several of the ten
   candidates did not want to be considered. (The faculty recommended
   Adami to the university board of governors at an annual salary of £600
   per annum.) M Fac Med, 6 May 1899: Adami given McGill M.D., C.M.,
   M.A., *ad eundem*.

59 Biographical sketch for J.G. Adami, this volume.

60 Relationship of McGill professor of pathology to pathologists at the MGH
   and the RVH. This subject was debated at numerous medical faculty executive meetings, and there were several lengthy reports. Adami was offered
   the title of "advisory pathologist" at the MGH and the RVH. In his opinion, outside of Montreal the title would be regarded as purely honorary
   and this would be detrimental to his reputation. Subsequently Adami was
   appointed pathologist to the RVH and continued as advisory pathologist to
   the MGH. M Fac Med, Oct. 1908: relationship of McGill professor of
   pathology to RVH and MGH. M Fac Med, 31 May 1911, 484: McGill professor of pathology to be pathologist-in-chief at RVH. The MGH wanted to
   appoint its own pathologist. M Fac Med, 10 October 1913, 56: L.J. Rhea
   was appointed pathologist to MGH and McGill assistant professor and
   later associate professor of pathology.

61 In the 1911 textbook Adami was listed as "Advisory Pathologist to the
   MGH and the RVH; Fellow Jesus College, Cambridge"; McCrae was lecturer in pathology and clinical medicine at McGill and a senior assistant
   physician at the RVH.

62 Biographical sketch for H. Oertel, this volume.

63 The official name of the new building was the Pathological Institute but
   it was generally known as the Pathology Institute.

64 M Fac Med, 14 October 1899, 149.

65 Bensley, *Medical Luminaries*, 131.

CHAPTER SIX

1 Osler, "The Hospital As a College," in *Aequanimitas*, 327–42.

2 See chapter 1, n81, for a description of regular and perpetual hospital cards.

3 H.E. MacDermot, *History of the Montreal General Hospital*, 74.

4 The official opening ceremony for the RVH was in December 1893. The first patients were admitted in 1894.

5 Biographical sketch for William Alexander Molson, this volume. Molson (1852–1920), McGill M.D., C.M., 1874, married. F.J. Shepherd's sister. See Bliss, *William Osler: A Life in Medicine*, 102, 115–16.

6 Biographical sketches for F. Finley and H. Lafleur, this volume. In 1894 Finley was thirty-three and Lafleur thirty-two. They were promoted assistant professors in 1895, associate professors in 1899, and professors of medicine in 1907.

7 M Fac Med, 1904, 352: For the 1903–04 session there were five assistant demonstrators for clinical medicine.

8 M Fac Med, 5 November 1898, 119. For clinical training one-half the class was assigned to the RVH and the other half to the MGH. A student could elect to have all clinical training at one hospital.

9 M Fac Med, 1 February 1902, 217.

10 In 1900 clinical demonstrators received an honorarium of $100 per annum; assistant demonstrators received $50.

11 The first four salaried members of McGill's Faculty of Medicine were Wesley Mills, physiology (1886); J. George Adami, pathology (1892); Robert F. Ruttan, practical chemistry (1894); and Auckland Geddes, anatomy (1913).

12 Gurd, *The Gurds*, 131 and 162.

13 R.P. Howard, *The Chief: Dr. William Osler*, 185.

14 Between 1936 and 1956 there were six editions of Meakins's *The Practice of Medicine*. Each edition had more contributing editors. The sixth edition in 1956 was a multi-authored textbook with Meakins as editor-in-chief.

15 Proprietors of a large department store in Montreal.

16 Chloroform anesthesia was associated with a high incidence of hepatic damage and undesirable circulatory effects (hypotension, cardiac arrest, and arrhythmias). See L.S. Goodman and A. Gilman, *The Pharmacological Basis of Therapeutics*, 4th ed. (Toronto: Macmillan, 1970), 84.

17 R. Bodman and D. Gillies, *Harold Griffith: The Evolution of Modern Anesthesia*, 39–40.

18 MacDermot, MGH, 94.

19 Gurd, *The Gurds*, 99.

20 *Montreal Medical Journal* 38: 518, 1909.

21 Lewis, RVH, 144–8.

22 W. Bourne, *Mysterious Waters to Guard* (Oxford: Blackwell, 1955);

J.C. Bevan and M.A. Pacelli, *Wesley Bourne* (Montreal: McGill University Library, 1996).

23 Bodman and Gillies, *Harold Griffith*, 30.

24 Renamed the Queen Elizabeth Hospital in 1951.

25 Osler, ed., *Montreal General Hospital: Reports Clinical and Pathological*, vol. 1.

26 In the first edition of *Principles and Practice of Medicine* in 1892, Osler included twenty-five pages on diseases of the nervous system and muscles.

27 P. Robb, *Development of Neurology at McGill*.

28 The major centre for neurological diseases at Queen Square, London, was named the National Hospital for the Paralytic and Epileptic. In the mid-1920s the name was changed to the National Hospital for Neurology and Neurosurgery, and more recently to the Institute of Neurology. It is generally referred to as Queen Square.

29 Robb, *Neurology*.

30 R.A. Cleghorn, "The Emergence of Psychiatry at McGill": 552–6.

31 T.G. Roddick, "A Remarkable Case of Favus," in Osler, ed., *Montreal General Hospital Reports: Clinical and Pathological*, vol. 1, 227–32; also in *Canadian Dermatological Association Journal* 1, no. 2 (1987), 4–5, with an introduction by R.R. Forsey.

32 W.B. Howell, *Francis John Shepherd, Surgeon*, 37, 38, 47.

33 M Fac Med, 19 October 1901, 207.

34 Shepherd was professor and chairman of anatomy. There is no record of his holding a specific faculty appointment in dermatology.

35 M Fac Med, September 1909, 360.

36 Dr James E. Graham was the first Canadian member of the American Dermatological Association.

37 Howell, *Shepherd*, 150.

38 G.G. Campbell, *Common Diseases of the Skin, with Notes on Diagnosis and Treatment* (New York: Macmillan Co., 1920). M Fac Med, 28 April 1923, 556: G.G. Campbell appointed clinical professor of dermatology.

39 Lewis, *RVH*, 53, 62, 143, 180, and 184–6.

40 R.R. Forsey, "Did You Know?", *Canadian Dermatological Association Journal* 1, no.1, 8–10.

41 Verdun is a suburb of Montreal on the south shore of the Island of Montreal.

42 W.C. Röntgen, "Uber Eine Neue Art von Straklen." *S B Phys-Med Ges* (25 December 1895): 132–41.

43 *Montreal Medical Journal* 24 (1896): 661.

44 C.G. Roland, "Priority of Clinical X-Ray Reports: A Classic Dethroned," *Canad J Surg*, 5 (1962): 247–51.

45 Lewis, *RVH*, 155–9, 210–16.

46 MacDermot, *History of the MGH*, 36, 96, 103–4, 110.

47 Charles Hayter, paper delivered at the Congress for Social Sciences and

Humanities, Quebec City, May 2001, "Tarnished Adornment: The Troubled History of Quebec's Institut du Radium, 1923–1967."

48 Lewis, *RVH*, 214.

49 MacDermot, *History of the MGH*, 110.

CHAPTER SEVEN

1 Osler, "Teacher and Student," *Aequanimitas*, 30.

2 There were two surgical services at the MGH with two attending surgeons on each service. On each service, one surgeon was on duty for the winter session and the other surgeon for the summer session.

3 Dr Abraham Groves performed the first elective appendectomy in North America in 1883 on a kitchen table in a farmhouse near Fergus, Ontario, north of Guelph.

4 Howell, *Shepherd*, 176–84.

5 Biographical sketch for George Armstrong, this volume.

6 Gurd, *The Gurds*, 99.

7 The MGH Operations Book covers the period of 1880 to 1890. The name of the patient, age, the home address, the dates of admission and operation, the surgeon, the pre-operative diagnosis, and the operative procedure are listed (MUA).

8 Biographical sketch for James Bell, this volume.

9 In 1894 Shepherd, Armstrong, Sutherland, and Kirkpatrick were the MGH attending surgeons.

10 Lewis, *RVH*, 59.

11 Biographical sketch for Edward Archibald, this volume.

12 D.A. Murphy, "James Bell's Appendicitis," *Canad J Surg* 15 (1972): 335–8.

13 Lewis, *RVH*, 137–8.

14 Entin, *Edward Archibald*, chapter 6.

15 The Ross Memorial Pavilion (J.K.L. Ross) at the RVH for private patients was opened in 1916 by HRH Duke of Connaught. Located to the north of the hospital it was connected to the main building by a tunnel. The front door was reached by a circuitous road from Pine Avenue.

16 Lewis, *RVH*, 76; biographical sketch for Sir Henry Gray, this volume.

17 Details in chapter 4.

18 Howell, *Shepherd*, 201.

19 The attending surgeons at the MGH were Hutchison, Elder, Bazin, and Eberts.

20 Hanaway and Creuss, *McGill Medicine, 1829–1885*, vol. 1, 34.

21 Biographical sketch for Michael McCulloch in ibid., 147.

22 Biographical sketch for Archibald Hall in ibid., 154.

23 Biographical sketch for Duncan MacCallum in ibid., 163

24 Biographical sketch for William Gardner in ibid., 169.

25 Biographical sketch for Arthur Browne, this volume.
26 Biographical sketch for James Cameron, this volume.
27 Howell, *Shepherd*, 134–5.
28 Biographical sketch for Walter Chipman, this volume.
29 Biographical sketch for Frank Buller in Hanaway and Cruess, *McGill Medicine*, vol.1, 170.
30 Biographical sketch for George Wilson Major in ibid., 186.
31 The Western General Hospital was incorporated in 1874 on Essex Street, Montreal. It became the Western Division of the MGH on 1 January 1924. Following this merger, a private pavilion was built on the site facing Tupper Street and opened in October 1934.
32 J.D. Baxter, *The History of Otolaryngology in Canada*; MacDermot, MGH, 92; Lewis, RVH, 206–9.
33 Lewis, RVH, 152–4.
34 Ibid., 53, 151–4. MacDermot, MGH, 87, 97, and 113 .
35 Biographical sketch for MacKenzie Forbes, this volume.
36 MacDermot, MGH, 97; Lewis, RVH, 63, 142–3.

CHAPTER EIGHT

1 At that time students paid a fee for each course directly to the professor.
2 Biographical sketch for Robert Craik in Hanaway and Cruess, *McGill Medicine*, vol. 1, 166.
3 M Fac Med, 15 September 1895: hygiene course changed to public health and preventive medicine.
4 Biographical sketch for Wyatt Galt Johnston in Hanaway and Cruess, *McGill Medicine*, vol. 1., 186.
5 M Fac Med, 12 May 1900, 168.
6 M Fac Med, spring 1902, 258: T.A. Starkey appointed professor of hygiene and bacteriology.
7 Population of Montreal in 1891 was 219,616; in 1921 it was 618,506.
8 See "Medical Jurisprudence" in appendix 3.
9 Biographical sketch for George Wilkins, this volume.
10 M Fac Med, 24 February 1900: faculty approved the details of a course in forensic medicine.
11 H.E. MacDermot, *One Hundred Years of Medicine in Canada*, 163.
12 A.D. Blackader was acting editor of CMAJ during the war years and editor 1919 to 1929.

CHAPTER NINE

1 M Fac Med, 16 April 1885, 1.
2 M Fac Med, May 1893, 204.
3 Three of the four professorships were endowed: pathology, hygiene, and

physiology; see appendix 3. In 2002 there were thirty-seven endowed chairs and appointments in the medical faculty. See *McGill Focus: Medicine*, winter 2001–02.

4 M Fac Med, 7 January 1893, 191.

5 M Fac Med, 11 April 1896, 40.

6 Medicine, surgery, midwifery, anatomy, chemistry, physiology, pharmacology and therapeutics, biology (botany), medical jurisprudence, ophthalmology and otology, gynecology, hygiene, and pathology.

7 The university board of governors decreed that associate professors had the same status as professors, so Finley and Lafleur were members of the faculty executive when they were promoted to associate professors in 1897, as was C.F. Martin after 1900.

8 The principal could do this because at the turn of the century there were five faculties at McGill: Arts, Medicine, Law, Applied Science, and Veterinary Medicine. Principal Peterson travelled to Scotland each year after the Spring Convocation and returned to Montreal in September. See S.B. Frost, *McGill University*, vol. 2, 7.

9 M Fac Med, 14 January 1899, 124.

10 For instance, the Education Committee made recommendations regarding the curriculum, the duration of the course, reciprocity with other Canadian medical schools, and relations with the medical licensing authorities.

11 M Fac Med, 5 March 1910, 402.

12 M Fac Med, 2 April 1910, 409; 20 April 1910, 415.

13 M Fac Med, 12 October 1910, 437.

14 M Fac Med, 6 April 1912, 524.

15 Ibid., 527 and 534.

16 M Fac Med, 19 December 1914, 143. The dean was *ex officio* member of the associate faculty and was required to be informed of all meetings of the associate faculty and its business.

17 M Fac Med, 5 January 1918, 286; 1 February 1919, 356.

18 See Frost, *McGill University*, 169–70, on the reorganization of the medical faculty.

19 M Fac Med, April 1921, 490.

20 The three members of the standing committee were: 1923, Chipman, Bazin, and Whitnall; 1924, Meakins, Bazin, and Tate; 1925, Meakins, Oertel, and Eberts; 1928, Stehle, Patch, and Chipman.

21 M Fac Med, 24 November 1923: there were four special committees – museum policy, degree course in pharmacology, entrance requirements, and B.SC. (Med).

EPILOGUE

1 K. Ludmerer, *Learning to Heal: The Development of American Medical Education* (New York: Basic Books, 1995).

2 T.N. Bonner, *Becoming a Physician: Medical Education in Great Britain, France, Germany and the United States, 1750–1945* (New York: Oxford University Press, 1995).
3 The 1910 Flexner Report is discussed in chapter 2.
4 Ludmerer, *Time to Heal: American Medical Education from the Turn of the Century to the Era of Managed Care* (New York: Oxford University Press, 1999).

APPENDIX 4

1 For information about the Holmes Gold Medal, see chapter 1, n44.
2 The Wood Gold Medal was endowed in 1905 by Dr Casey A. Wood, the noted ophthalmologist, ornithologist, and historian. It is awarded annually by the McGill medical faculty to the student graduating in medicine with the highest aggregate marks in the clinical examinations of the final year. It is the lineal descendant of a Bishop's Medical Faculty Wood Gold Medal. The Wood family was originally connected with Bishop's University at Lennoxville, Quebec. The Bishop's Medal was established in 1878 by Dr. Orrin C. Wood of Ottawa, Dr Casey Wood's father. Dr O.C. Wood's interest in Bishop's arose from the fact that his son Casey Wood had received his medical degree from Bishop's, and after Dr O.C. Wood's death in 1884, Dr Casey Wood continued the award on behalf of the Wood family. The medal was awarded annually by Bishop's Medical Faculty from 1878 to 1905. In the latter year the Bishop's faculty was absorbed by McGill University and, at Dr Casey Wood's request, the Wood Gold Medal, suitably redesigned, became a McGill award.

Selected Bibliography of Books and Articles on McGill University and Medical Faculty

Additional references are included in the notes for each chapter.

Abbott, M.E.S. "An Historical Sketch of the Medical Faculty of McGill University." *Montreal Medical Journal* 31 (1902): 561–672.
– *History of Medicine in the Province of Quebec.* Montreal: McGill University Publications 1931.
– *McGill's Historic Past, 1821–1921.* Montreal: McGill University Publications 1921.
Adami, J.G. *The Principles of Pathology.* Vol. 1, *General Pathology;* vol. 2, *Systemic Pathology.* Philadelphia: Lea & Febiger 1908 and 1909.
Adami, J.G., and J. McCrae. *A Textbook of Pathology for Students of Medicine.* Philadelphia: Lea & Febiger 1912.
Adami, M. *J. George Adami: A Memoir.* London: Constable 1930.
Barrett, C.V., and J.R. Fraser. *The Royal Victoria Montreal Maternity Hospital, 1843–1943.* Montreal: Printed privately 1943.
Baxter, J.D. *The History of Otolaryngology in Canada.* Hamilton, Ont.: Decker 1998.
Bensley, E.H. *McGill Medical Luminaries.* Montreal: Osler Library 1990.
Bliss, M. *William Osler: A Life in Medicine.* Toronto: University of Toronto Press 1999.
Bodman, R., and D. Gillies. *Harold Griffith: The Evolution of Modern Anesthesia.* Toronto: Hannah 1992.
Christie, N. *For King and Country.* Winnipeg: Bunker 1996.
Cleghorn, R.A. "The Emergence of Psychiatry at McGill." *Canadian Journal of Psychiatry* 29 (1984): 52–6.

Collard, E.A. *Oldest McGill*. Toronto: Macmillan Co. 1946.

Collard, E.A., ed. *The McGill You Knew: An Anthology of Memories, 1920–1960*. Don Mills, Ont.: Longman 1975.

Cosentino, F. *Brothers of the Wind: R. Tait McKenzie and James Naismith*. Burnstown, Ont.: General Store Publishing 1996.

Craik, R. *Papers and Addresses*. Montreal: Gazette Printing Co. 1907.

Davenport, H.T., ed. *Anaesthesia at McGill*. Montreal: Printed privately 1996.

Entin, M. *Edward Archibald, Surgeon of the Royal Vic*. McGill University Libraries 2004.

– "History of Surgery: The Dynasties of Research at the Royal Victoria Hospital, Montreal." *Canadian Journal of Surgery* 30 (1987): 449–50.

Fetherstonhaugh, R.C. *McGill University at War, 1914–1918, 1939–1945*. Montreal: McGill University 1947.

– *No. 3 Canadian General Hospital (McGill), 1914–1919*. Montreal: Gazette Printing Co. 1928.

Flexner, A. *Medical Education in the United States and Canada*. Bulletin no. 4. New York: Carnegie Foundation for the Advancement of Teaching 1910. Facsimile edition, 1960.

Frost, S.B. *McGill University: For the Advancement of Learning*. Vol. 1: *1801–1895*; vol. 2: *1895–1971*. Kingston and Montreal: McGill-Queen's University Press 1980 and 1984.

Gilbert, H. *The Life of Lord Mount Stephen*. Vol. 1: *Awakening Continent*; vol. 2: *The End of the Road*. Aberdeen: University Press 1965 and 1977.

Gillett, M. *We Walked Very Warily: A History of Women at McGill*. Montreal: Eden Press 1981.

Gillett, M., and K. Sibbald. *A Fair Shake: Autobiographical Essays by McGill Women*. Montreal: Eden Press 1984.

Goldbloom, A. *Small Patients*. Toronto: Longmans, Green & Co. 1959.

Graves, D. *A Crown of Life: The World of John McCrae*. St Catherines, Ont.: Vanwell 1977.

Gurd, F.N. *The Gurds: The Montreal General and McGill: A Family Saga*. Edited by D. Waugh. Burnstown, Ont.: General Store Publishing 1996.

Hanaway, J., and R. Cruess. *McGill Medicine: The First Half Century*. Vol. 1, *1829–1885*. Kingston and Montreal: McGill-Queen's University Press 1996.

Howard, R.P. *The Chief: Dr. William Osler*. Canton, Mass.: Science History Publications 1983.

Howell, W.B. *Francis John Shepherd, Surgeon: His Life and Times, 1851–1929*. Toronto: J.M. Dent 1934.

Kerr, R.B. *History of the Medical Council of Canada*. Ottawa: Medical Council of Canada 1979.

Kingsmill, S. *Francis Scrimger: Beyond the Call of Duty*. Toronto: Hannah 1991.

Kozar, A.J. *The Sport Sculpture of R. Tait McKenzie*. 2nd ed. Ontario: Human Kinetic Publishers 1992.

Lewis, D.S. *Royal Victoria Hospital, 1887–1947*. Montreal: McGill University Press 1969.

MacCallum, D.C. *Addresses*. Montreal: Desbarats & Co. 1901.

McCrae, J. *In Flanders Fields and Other Poems*. Toronto: Briggs 1919.

MacDermot, H.E. *History of the Montreal General Hospital*. Montreal: Montreal General Hospital 1950.

– *History of the School of Nursing of the Montreal General Hospital*. Montreal: The Alumnae Association 1940.

– *Maude Abbott: A Memoir*. Toronto: Macmillan 1941

– *One Hundred Years of Medicine in Canada*. Toronto: McClelland & Stewart, 1967.

– *Sir Thomas Roddick: His Work in Medicine and Public Life*. Toronto: Macmillan 1938.

McDonald, D. *Lord Strathcona: A Biography of Donald Smith*. Toronto: Dundurn 1996.

McGill, J. *The Joy of Effort: A Biography of R.T. McKenzie*. Ontario: Clay Publishing 1980.

MacIntosh, F.C. "Boris Petrovich Babkin, 1877–1950." *Revue canadienne de biologie* 10, no.1 (1951): 3–7.

MacLennan, H., ed. *McGill: The Story of a University*. London: George Allan & Unwin 1960.

MacMillan, C. *McGill and Its Story, 1821–1921*. Toronto: Oxford University Press 1921.

Macphail, A. *History of the Canadian Forces in the Great War, 1914–19: The Medical Services*. Ottawa: King's Printer 1925.

MacPhedran, T. *Two Centuries of Medical History, 1822–1922*. Montreal: Harvest House 1993.

Martin, C.F. "The Montreal General Hospital in Osler's Time." *Montreal General Hospital Bulletin* 2, no. 7 (1955): 11–15.

Molson, K. *The Molsons: Their Lives and Times, 1780–2000*. Willowdale, Ont.: Firefly 2001.

Mills, T.W. *Textbook of Comparative Physiology*. N.p.: n.p. 1890.

Munroe, M.D. *The Training School for Nurses, Royal Victoria Hospital, 1894–1942*. Montreal: Alumnae Association 1943.

Murphy, D.A. "James Bell's Appendicitis." *Canadian Journal of Surgery* 15 (1972): 335–8.

Osler, W. *Aequanimitas; with Other Addresses to Medical Students, Nurses and Practitioners of Medicine*. 3rd ed. New York: Blakiston 1947.

– *Aphorisms*. W.B. Bean, ed. Springfield, Ill.: Chas. C. Thomas 1961.

– *Principles and Practice of Medicine*. New York: D. Appleton & Co. 1892.

– "Professor Wesley Mills." *CMAJ* 5 (1915): 338–41.

Osler, W., ed. *Montreal General Hospital, Pathological Reports, No. 1*. Montreal: Dawson 1877.

– *Montreal General Hospital Reports: Clinical and Pathological by the Medical Staff.* Montreal: Dawson 1880.

Penfield, W.G. "Boris Petrovich Babkin, 1877–1950." *Proceedings/Transactions of the Royal Society of Canada* 44 (1950): 65–6.

– "Edward Archibald, 1872–1945." *Canadian Journal of Surgery* 1 (1954): 167–74.

– *No Man Alone: A Neurosurgeon's Life.* Boston: Little Brown 1977.

Prescott, J.F. *In Flanders Fields: The Story of John McCrae.* Erin, Ont.: Boston Mills 1985.

Robb, P. *Development of Neurology at McGill.* Montreal: Printed privately 1990.

Robertson, H.R. "Dedication of the Archibald Amphitheatre." *Canadian Journal of Surgery* 24 (1981): 447.

Rogers, M.A. *A History of the McGill Dental School.* Montreal: McGill University 1980.

Scriver, J.B. *The Montreal Children's Hospital: Years of Growth.* Montreal and Kingston: McGill-Queen's University Press 1979.

Segall, H. *Pioneers of Cardiology in Canada, 1820–1970.* Willowdale, Ont.: Hounslow Press 1988.

– "Stories of and about Goldbloom, Goldblatt, Greenspoon and Gross: The Four 'Gs' of the McGill Medical Class of 1916." *Canadian Jewish Historical Society Journal* 6 (1982): 17–32.

Shepherd, F.J. "The First Medical School in Canada." *CMAJ* 15 (1925): 418–25.

– *History of the Montreal General Hospital.* Montreal: Printed privately 1924.

–"On the Teaching of Anatomy to Medical Students." *Montreal Medical Journal* (November 1900): 13–25.

– *Reminiscences of Student Days and the Dissecting Room.* Montreal: Printed privately 1919.

Spaulding, W.B. "Charles F. Martin (1868–1953): A Notable Dean of McGill University." *Annals RCPSC* 24 (1991): 29–31.

Tunis, B.L. *In Caps and Gowns: The Story of the School for Graduate Nurses, 1920–1964.* Montreal: McGill University Press 1966.

Urquhurt, H.M. *Arthur Currie: The Biography of a Great Canadian.* Toronto: Dent 1950.

Wagg, S. *Percy Erskine Nobbs, Architect, Artist, Craftsman.* Kingston and Montreal: McGill-Queen's University Press 1982.

Waugh, D. *Maudie of McGill: Dr. Maude Abbott and the Foundations of Heart Surgery.* Toronto: Hannah 1992.

Index

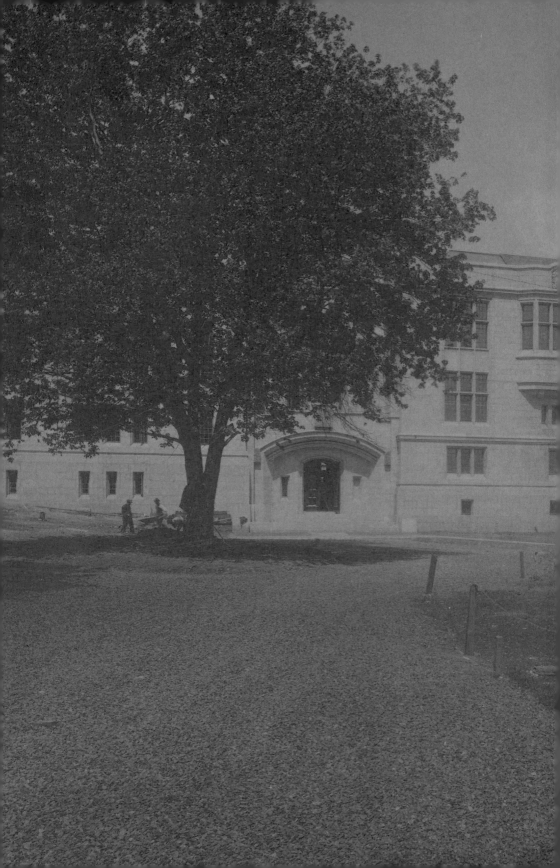